EPIDEMIOLOGY OF CANCER OF THE DIGESTIVE TRACT

DEVELOPMENTS IN ONCOLOGY 6

Previously published in this series:

1. F.J. Cleton and J.W.I.M. Simons, eds., Genetic Origins of Tumor Cells
   ISBN 90-247-2272-1
2. J. Aisner and P. Chang, eds., Cancer Treatment Research
   ISBN 90-247-2358-2
3. B.W. Ongerboer de Visser, D.A. Bosch and W.M.H. van Woerkom-Eykenboom, eds.,
   Neuro-Oncology: Clinical and Experimental Aspects
   ISBN 90-247-2421-X
4. K. Hellmann, P. Hilgard and S. Eccles, eds., Metastasis: Clinical and Experimental Aspects
   ISBN 90-247-2424-4
5. H.F. Seigler, ed., Clinical Management of Melanoma
   ISBN 90-247-2584-4

Series ISBN: 90-247-2338-8

EPIDEMIOLOGY OF CANCER OF THE DIGESTIVE TRACT

edited by

PELAYO CORREA
Professor of Pathology,
Louisiana State University Medical Center,
New Orleans, Louisiana, USA

and

WILLIAM HAENSZEL
Professor of Epidemiology,
University of Illinois and Senior Epidemiologist,
Illinois Cancer Council,
Chicago, Illinois, USA

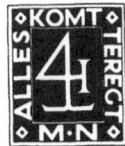

1982

MARTINUS NIJHOFF PUBLISHERS

THE HAGUE/BOSTON/LONDON

Distributors:

for the United States and Canada
Kluwer Boston, Inc.
190 Old Derby Street
Hingham, MA 02043
USA

for all other countries
Kluwer Academic Publishers Group
Distribution Center
P.O.Box 322
3300 AH Dordrecht
The Netherlands

Library of Congress   Cataloging in Publication Data   **CIP**

Main entry under title:
Epidemiology of cancer of the digestive tract.

   (Developments in oncology ; v. 6)
   Includes index.
   1. Gastrointestinal system–Cancer.
2. Epidemiology.   3. Digestive organs–Cancer.
I. Correa, Pelayo.   II. Haenszel, William.
III. Series.   [DNLM: 1. Digestive system neoplasms–Occurence.
W1 DE998N v. 6 / WI 149 E64]
RC280.D5E64   616.99'43071   81-18986
                                AACR2

ISBN-13:978-94-009-7504-0   e-ISBN-13:978-94-009-7502-6
DOI: 10.1007/978-94-009-7502-6

Table of Contents

Preface

The digestive organs are the most frequent site of cancer in the world, accounting for approximately 30% of all malignant tumors. This prominent position has been present for many decades in spite of marked shifts in the frequency of cancer of specific organs. The most remarkable shift has been the decrease in gastric cancer rates occurring concomitantly with an increase in colon cancer rates in most 'western' industrialized societies. Important exceptions to this rule, as well as other epidemiologic evidence, indicate that the opposite trends for gastric and colon cancers are not inevitable consequences of each other. Although genetically determined precancerous syndromes are well recognized, it is generally agreed that environmental factors play an overriding role in digestive cancer causation. The most obvious environmental factors seem to be the result of what we eat, drink, or smoke. Although the nutritional component of the diet is of unquestionable importance, the nonnutrient elements in our diet have also proven to be influential causative factors. Several studies have focused on the microenvironment at the level of the mucosa or the digestive organs as a microcosmos where forces promoting and inhibiting carcinogenesis are operating for a prolonged period of time. Their interaction eventually determines the presence or absence of a malignant tumor. Our understanding of such modulating forces, hopefully, will someday allow us to modify the microenvironment in a favorable way and attain the goal of cancer prevention. Epidemiologic studies have already indicated that the cancer-related microenvironment is different in each digestive organ. Ongoing epidemiologic studies throughout the world most probably will contribute new information in the near future and better clarify the role of the different components of the microenvironment.

This volume brings together updated epidemiologic information pointing out similarities and differences between the etiologic pathways observed in the several digestive organs. We hope that it will be helpful to all professionals concerned with digestive cancer causation by bringing them up to date, preparing them for better use of forthcoming information, and helping them design a rationale for preventive measures.

Pelayo Correa
William Haenszel

List of Contributors

CORREA, Pelayo, M.D., Department of Pathology, Louisiana State University Medical Center, 1901 Perdido St., New Orleans, LA 70112, USA

DAY, Nicholas E., Ph.D., Biostatistics Programme, Division of Epidemiology and Biostatistics, International Agency for Research on Cancer, 150 cours Albert Thomas, 69372 Lyon Cédex 2, France

DEVOR, Eric J., Ph.D., Dept. of Psychiatry, Washington University School of Medicine, 216 S. Kingshighway Blvd., St. Louis, MO 61378, USA

FONTHAM, Elizabeth T.H., M.P.H., Department of Pathology, Louisiana State University Medical Center, 1901 Perdido St., New Orleans, LA 70112, USA

GEORGE, Stephen L., Ph.D., Biostatistics Section St. Jude Children's Research Hospital, 332 North Lauderdale, P.O. Box 318, Memphis, TN 38101, USA

GHADIRIAN, Parviz, M.Sc., Institute of Public Health Research, University of Teheran, Teheran, Iran

HAENSZEL, William, D.P.H., Illinois Cancer Council, 36 South Wabash, Chicago, IL 60603, USA

HEATH, Clark W., Jr., M.D., Director, Chronic Diseases division, Center for Environmental Health, Centers for Disease Control, 1600 Clifton Road, N.E., Atlanta, GA 30333, USA

LINSELL, Allen, M.B.B.S., F.R.C.PATH., Director, Division of Epidemiology and Biostatistics, International Agency for Research on Cancer, 150 cours Albert Thomas, 69372 Lyon Cédex 2, France

MACK, Thomas M., M.D., M.P.H., Department of Family and Preventive Medicine, University of Southern California School of Medicine, and Cancer Surveillance Program, Los Angeles County/University of Southern California Cancer Center, Los Angeles, CA 90033, USA

MENCK, Herman R., C.Phil., Department of Family and Preventive Medicine, University of Southern California, Los Angeles, CA 90033, USA

MUÑOZ, Nubia, M.D., Analytical Epidemiology Programme, Division of Epidemiology and Biostatistics, International Agency for Research on Cancer, 150 cours Albert Thomas, 69372 Lyon Cédex 2, France

PRATT, Charles B., M.D., St. Jude Children's Research Hospital, 332 North Lauderdale, P.O. Box 318, Memphis, TN 38101, USA

SMITH, Elaine M., M.P.H., Ph.D., University of Iowa, School of Medicine, Department of Preventive Medicine, and Downstate SEER Program, Iowa City, IA 52242, USA

1. Epidemiology of Cancers of the Oral Cavity and Pharynx

ELAINE M. SMITH

Introduction

Despite the relative visibility of oral and pharyngeal cancers (ICD-A 140-149, 9th revision) which should make them easier to diagnose than other digestive cancers, most of these tumors are found in later stages and have poor survival. For some buccal cavity and pharyngeal sites lethality is even higher than that of the stomach, colon, or rectum.

Epidemiologic data of oral and pharyngeal cancers are limited. The most reliable information comes from areas with population-based cancer registries, but more information is needed to determine the accuracy of the international differences in incidence, mortality, and survival.

Detailed investigations on various sites are uneven. Those of the lip, mouth, and nasopharynx have drawn more attention than have other oral and pharyngeal tumors because of their relatively high frequency in certain parts of the world or because of their correlation with specific etiologic conditions. The sites referred to in this chapter include ICD 140-149, 7–9th revision. Despite some inadequacies, there are some extreme differences in international incidence patterns that are difficult to account for completely as artifacts due to differences in methodology.

Morbidity and mortality

Relative frequency often has been used to assess the morbidity risk for oral cavity and pharynx cancer when incidence data are unavailable. In North America and Western Europe (1–8) the frequency is between 2–5%, while in Asia, Southeast Asia, Middle East, and USSR (2) it accounts for as much as 50% of all cancers. The ranking of sites in order of frequency varies, but in general the order among North American and Western European countries is lip with highest, pharynx with lowest, and mouth, gum, floor of mouth, salivary glands, and tongue of similar frequency (1, 8, 9).

The major sources of international figures on age-specific and adjusted incidence are the three volumes of 'Cancer incidence in five continents' (2, 12–13). A

Correa, P. and Haenszel, W. (eds.), Epidemiology of Cancer of the Digestive Tract.
© *1982 Martinus Nijhoff Publishers. The Hague/Boston/London. ISBN-13:978-94-009-7504-0*

Table 1. Age-adjusted incidence per 100,000 of oral and pharyngeal cancers, in selected populations, by sex.

Area	Lip (140)		Tongue (141)		Salivary gland (142)		Mouth (143–5)		Oro (146)		Pharynx naso (147)		Hypo (148)	
	♂	♀	♂	♀	♂	♀	♂	♀	♂	♀	♂	♀	♂	♀
UK														
Birmingham	1.2	0.1	1.0	0.4	1.0	1.2	1.5	0.5	0.6	0.2	0.4	0.2	0.8	0.6
Liverpool	1.8	0.1	1.1	0.5	1.0	1.3	1.6	0.7	0.6	0.3	0.4	0.2	0.8	0.9
Oxford	1.9	0.2	0.7	0.4	1.5	2.0	1.0	0.4	0.4	0.2	0.4	0.2	0.6	0.4
Sheffield	1.3	0.1	0.7	0.4	0.9	0.8	1.2	0.4	0.6	0.2	0.4	0.1	0.5	0.5
Canada														
British Columbia	4.7	0.3	1.6	1.0	0.9	0.9	1.9	1.2	0.9	0.3	1.1	0.5	0.4	0.1
Maritime Province	10.6	0.4	0.9	0.4	1.0	0.6	2.5	0.9	1.0	0.3	0.4	0.1	0.3	0.3
Newfoundland	27.1	0.8	1.2	0.4	0.5	0.6	1.6	0.4	0.8	0.3	1.2	0.3	0.8	0.3
Quebec	5.0	0.2	2.4	0.7	1.1	1.2	3.5	0.8	2.5	0.6	0.6	0.2	0.8	0.2
Saskatchewan	16.4	0.8	1.3	0.4	1.0	1.3	1.3	0.5	0.1	0.2	0.3	0.2	0.3	0.2
US														
Alameda														
White	4.0	0.2	3.0	1.6	0.9	1.1	3.7	2.2	2.2	1.0	0.5	0.1	1.1	0.8
Black	0.6	0.0	2.2	0.8	0.2	0.8	4.1	1.6	2.2	0.3	1.1	0.2	1.5	0.0
San Francisco Bay														
White	3.7	0.4	3.2	1.6	0.9	1.0	4.2	2.3	2.6	1.1	0.7	0.3	1.5	0.5
Black	0.6	0.1	2.1	1.4	1.0	1.4–	4.8	1.5	3.3	0.7	1.1	0.3	1.5	0.1
Chinese	0.0	0.0	1.6	0.0	0.7	0.4	4.2	1.8	1.0	0.0	19.1	6.4	1.1	0.0
Hawaii														
Caucasian	5.6	0.7	3.4	1.7			5.3	2.3			1.0	0.9		
Chinese	0.0	0.0	0.0	1.8			0.0	0.9			10.3	5.1		
Hawaiian	0.0	0.0	3.5	2.4			5.1	1.4			4.4	1.6		
Japanese	0.4	0.0	2.0	0.8			1.5	0.4			1.0	0.2		
El Paso														
other White	7.9	0.0	4.6	1.2	0.7	0.4	3.3	2.7	4.8	1.1	0.0	0.7	0.0	0.4
Spanish	0.0	0.0	0.0	0.0	2.0	1.5	1.3	2.2	1.3	1.9	0.0	0.6	0.0	0.6
New Mexico														
other White	3.2	0.2	2.2	0.4	1.2	0.5	2.8	1.4	1.4	0.7	0.3	0.1	0.3	0.2
Am Indian	1.1	0.0	1.3	0.0	0.0	0.0	0.0	0.0	0.0	0.0	1.3	0.0	0.0	0.0
Spanish	0.8	0.0	0.4	0.3	0.8	0.3	0.7	0.7	0.4	0.2	0.8	0.1	0.2	0.0

	1	2	3	4	5	6	7	8	9	10	11	12	13	14
Utah White	12.3	1.0	2.1	0.7	1.1	0.4	2.5	1.1	0.9	0.2	0.6	0.3	0.4	0.1
Detroit White	1.3	0.1	2.7	0.8	0.8	0.9	3.3	1.3	2.0	0.5	0.7	0.4	1.2	0.2
Detroit Black	0.1	0.0	3.3	1.5	1.3	0.6	3.3	1.4	2.1	0.4	0.2	0.4	1.1	0.2
Puerto Rico	1.5	0.5	7.5	1.5	0.4	0.3	7.8	2.4	4.3	1.1	0.4	0.2	4.4	0.6
Brazil Sao Paulo	6.2	1.7	5.7	1.0	0.7	0.7	7.0	1.2	3.8	0.2	0.6	0.3	0.9	0.0
Denmark	4.8	0.4	0.3	0.3	0.9	0.9	0.7	0.6	0.7	0.3	0.9	0.6	0.5	0.2
Iceland	5.3	0.4	0.3	0.7	0.6	0.5	1.2	0.4	0.3	0.1	0.4	0.2	0.6	0.2
Finland	5.8	0.4	0.8	0.5	0.7	0.7	0.7	0.5	0.4	0.1	0.4	0.2	0.7	0.4
Norway	4.2	0.2	0.8	0.5			1.2	0.6			0.5	0.3		
Sweden	2.7	0.2	0.6	0.4			1.1	0.6						
FRG Hamburg	0.7	0.1	1.2	0.4	0.2	0.2	1.2	0.4	1.4	0.5	0.1	0.1	0.3	0.1
Poland Warsaw rural	7.9	0.7	0.1	0.0	0.2	0.2	0.4	0.1	0.6	0.3	0.1	0.3	0.1	0.0
Hungary Szabolcs	12.1	1.0	0.6	0.0	0.2	0.2	0.9	0.2	0.5	0.2	0.2	0.1	0.2	0.0
Switzerland Geneva	0.2	0.0	2.9	0.6	0.5	0.7	3.0	0.7	4.7	0.4	0.4	0.2	2.9	0.5
Israel Jews	4.2	1.4	0.5	0.5	1,0	0.7	1.0	0.5	0.3	0.1	1.1	0.5	0.4	0.2
Japan Miyagi	0.3	0.0	0.7	0.6	0.3	0.1	0.4	0.3	0.1	0.1	0.3	0.1	0.3	0.0
Okayama	0.0	0.1	1.6	0.5	0.3	0.4	0.6	0.1	0.4	0.0	0.1	0.0	0.2	0.0
Osaka	0.1	0.0	1.3	0.6	0.3	0.2	0.7	0.3	0.2	0.1	0.4	0.2	0.4	0.1
Singapore Malay	0.2	0.0	2.0	0.0	0.7	0.2	3.1	1.1	0.4	0.0	4.8	0.6	0.2	0.3
Indian	0.0	0.0	4.1	3.8	2.5	0.0	8.6	16.9	2.8	2.3	0.9	0.0	4.1	2.5
Chinese	0.0	0.1	1.9	0.6	0.5	0.5	2.1	0.5	1.5	0.2	18.7	7.1	0.9	0.0
India Bombay	0.3	0.4	12.6	3.1	0.3	0.2	6.7	5.4	5.6	1.2	0.4	0.3	7.7	1.8

4

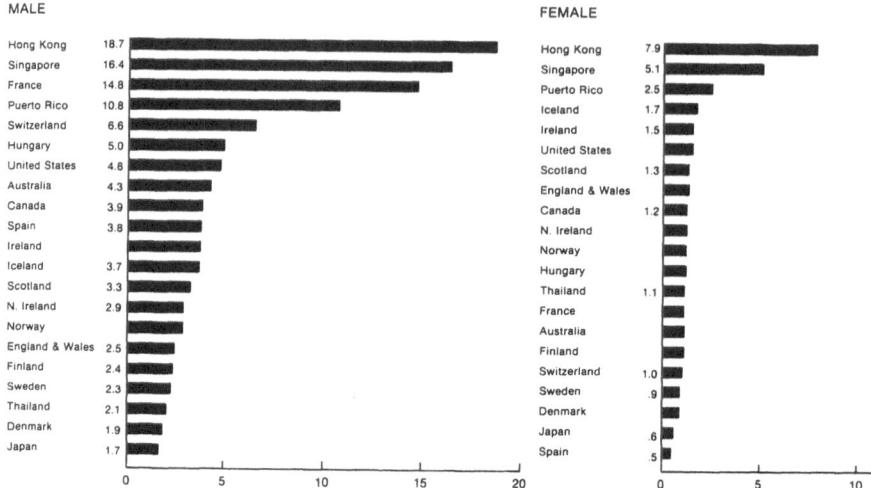

Figure 1. Age-adjusted (world population) mortality per 100,000 of oral and pharyngeal cancers by sex in selected areas, 1974.

number of countries publish similar data based on regional or national cancer registry statistics. In order ro facilitate comparisons between countries in morbidity (Table 1) and mortality (Fig. 1), data standardized to the world population are used (2).

Table 1 represents statistics published in Vol. III of 'Cancer incidence in five continents' of mean annual age-adjusted incidence in countries between the late 1960s and early 1970s (2). Earlier publications dating from the mid 1950s show few changes in these incidence patterns (12, 13). Notable exceptions occur among ethnic groups (Hawaiian, Japanese, Caucasian) in Hawaii, which may reflect real as well as artifactual changes due to improved reporting. There is a rise in neoplasms of the lip among Caucasian males (2), tongue among Japanese and Hawaiian males, and (3) mouth among all male and Hawaiian female ethnic groups.

Figure 1 represents Segi's work on age-adjusted (world) mortality in 1974 (14). As with incidence, males have higher mortality than do females (14–18). Comparisons in oral and pharyngeal mortality between 1950–51 (15), 1966–67 (15) and 1975 (19) show little change for high risk countries: France, Switzerland, US, Australia, or Canada. The British countries including Ireland, have slowly reduced their death rates since the early 1950s. Other high incidence areas, Hong Kong, Singapore, and Puerto Rico, were not included in the earlier mortality reports. Incidence and mortality patterns since the mid 50s suggest no major international changes have occurred among cancers of the buccal cavity and pharynx.

The site with highest survival is lip cancer, between 65 and 90% over a five-year period (1,3); lowest survival are observed for tumors of the pharyngeal sites, approximately 25%; survival for tumors of the tongue, salivary gland, and mouth, gum, and other sites in the buccal cavity are somewhat in between, 35-55% (CD 8, 143-145) (1,3).

The male/female ratio of incidence and mortality is usually greater than 1.0, and increases with age. The highest frequency for both sexes is between the sixth and eighth decades (1,8,9,11,20,21). Women generally have higher survival ratios than men.

Histopathology and precancerous lesions

There is scarcity of international epidemiologic investigations utilizing information on histology. Available pathology reports from cancer registries and population-based studies indicate that most neoplasms are squamous cell carcinoma (1,9,20,22–26). A small percentage of lip, salivary gland, and pharyngeal cancers are distributed in other types. Poorest survival, however, is found for squamous cell type (1,25).

The most common histopathologies for salivary gland tumors are mucoepidermoid tumors followed by adenocarcinomas or adenoid cystic tumors (27–32). Nasopharyngeal tumors have been characterized by poorly or undifferentiated squamous cell type (33,34), some with lymphoid stroma (28).

A number of studies have investigated various tissue changes in the oral cavity, proposing that they are precancerous (35–39). These changes include preleukoplakia, leukoplakia, hyperkeratosis, nicotine stomatitis, lichen planus, and dysplasia. Their results, however, do not support the preneoplastic hypothesis. Most individuals with leukoplakia revert to normal, remain unchanged, or develop cancer at other sites in the mouth or pharynx (37,40–45). In one major study (35,46) only 0.13% of leukoplakia cases developed oral cancer. Most of the leukoplakias had disappeared (32%) or remained unchanged (57%) in a two year follow-up. Several surveys (37,41,43–44) indicate that leukoplakia is more likely to regress among chewers than among smokers. Nicotine stomatitis is associated most often with reverse chutta use, but in the investigations this habit did not usually lead to oral cancer of the hard palate (47).

Site specific characteristics

Lip (140). This site is prone to misclassification because in diagnosis failure to specify skin of the lip and differentiate lip from the mucosa occurs frequently (48).

Incidence (Table 1) is not uniformly highest for both sexes in any one country or area. Newfoundland, Canada, with a rate of $27.1/10^5$, and Saskatchewan with $16.4/10^5$ report the highest proportions of lip cancer among males, more than found in any other nation. In contrast, the highest incidence among women in Canada is extremely low ($0.8/10^5$) compared to males. This low female rate holds true in all countries. Unlike men, women show little variability in incidence. Lowest proportions of lip cancer are reported among oriental, black and Hispanic populations regardless of sex (2). Intermediate incidence is found among other Caucasian groups: the USA (other than Hispanic), Northern Ireland, Australia, British Columbia, Scandinavia, and Western Europe.

The high incidence of lip cancer in Newfoundland has been observed among fisherman. Scottish fisherman also experienced a high frequency of lip tumors (10,49). In this regard actinic radiation has long been implicated in causing lip cancer, particularly among Caucasians, who are said to be at higher risk due to less melanin, and among those whose occupation is outdoors (48,50–54). Results form a questionnaire administered in Finland over four time periods between 1940–73, requesting information on occupation: indoor/outdoor, geographic residence, detailed smoking habits, noted that 73 percent of males with malignancies of the lip (male: female ratio, 6.8:1) had outdoor work such as farming and forestry as compared with skin cancer controls and were more likely to live in rural areas; there were no significant differences among women (51,52). Male cases were much more likely to smoke, with relative odds correlated to dose-response. Using data from the Finnish Cancer Registry between 1953–73, Lindquist found an inverse correlation between mean annual solar radiation and lip cancer incidence suggesting that other factors are involved (52). Higher incidence of lip cancer among rural vs urban dwellers has been reported in Norway between 1955–67 (55–58). Other research suggested that although there is no difference in amount of actinic radiation between Finland and Sweden, Finland had twice the age-adjusted incidence among males (56–61). According to the Swedish Cancer Registry between 1958–67, the oral site with highest frequency was the lip (26).

Mortality patterns in the USA showed higher rates among white males in several agricultural midwestern states, and similar trends occurred among white females in several southern states (17,18). Among non-whites, however, regardless of sex, there were significantly fewer deaths than expected in all states. Szpak et al., in another study in the USA, however, showed no correlation between incidence of lip cancer and latitude (62). Comparative trends of lip and skin neoplasms in four major cities in the Third National Cancer Survey (1969–71) showed an increased incidence for skin tumors varying directly with latitude, but no similar relationship for lip cancer. These findings suggest that whereas actinic radiation may play a major role in the development of skin cancers, the lip also may be subject to other major competitive factors such as exposure to alcohol or tobacco carcinogens. Nonetheless, countries with high incidence of neoplasms of the lip are composed primarily of Caucasians (63,64). Contrasts between races for incidence in the USA are most apparent: proportions for whites are higher as compared to Hispanic, Black, Oriental and American Indian (Table 1).

Salivary glands (142). Salivary glands have the lowest average incidence of any oral cancer site throughout the world. Unlike other sites, sex differences are minimal. Non-white populations are more likely to record lowest rates. International comparisons reveal no correlation between the incidence of salivary gland cancer and other buccal and pharyngeal cancers. Indians in Singapore have high rates of salivary gland tumors and low rates for other sites, while for those in Bombay the reverse relationship holds.

Parotid glands are more likely to be malignant followed by submandibular and palatal glands (26,65,66). The majority of salivary gland tumors are pleomorphic adenomas (mixed tumors) (26,65,66). Cases in Greenland and those admitted into Danish hospitals between 1955–74 showed greater age-adjusted incidence (European population (2)) than other countries (66).

Atomic Bomb Casualty Commission (ABCC) investigations have shown an increased prevalence of salivary gland tumors among survivors of atomic radiation in 1945 in Hiroshima and Nagasaki (27,67). Radiation exposure was based on 'air dose' in rads. A study of exposed and non-exposed persons (those who moved to these areas after the bomb) comparing age-standardized incidence showed a statistically significantly higher incidence of malignancy among cases vs controls $(1.0/10^5; 0.1/10^5)$ between 1953–71. The excess was slightly more pronounced among males (1.2 vs 0.8).

Nasopharynx (147). Squamous cell carcinoma of the nasopharynx (NPC) is rare in most countries (< 1/100,000), but its incidence is high in Chinese populations, particularly those living in the southern region of China (2,5,7,68). As shown in Table 2, age-adjusted rates are highest in Hong Kong (5), Singapore Cantonese, Teochews, Hokkien (7), and San Francisco (2). While these investigations suggest that a racially determined genetic susceptibility may exist, other evidence suggests an environmental component exists as well. Rates are somewhat lower among Chinese migrants (2,69–72) and among those with part-Chinese ancestry, but generally still higher than other ethnic or racial groups living in the same habitat. For example, Chinese living in California show a decreased risk to NPC in successive generations as compared to native Chinese (69,70,73,74). Japanese (68), Eskimos (75), and Hawaiians (2) of Chinese ancestry have rates somewhat lower than other Chinese. On the other hand, there is an increased risk among low-risk racial groups such as whites who migrate to Southeast Asia (74) or to Alaska (75,76). These circumstances support the hypothesis that NPC is more likely to be caused by shared environmental exposures found in some Chinese or Asian groups (68). Further support for environmental factors is evident in the

Table 2. Age-adjusted incidence per 100,000 per year of nasopharyngeal cancer in Chinese populations.

Country/area	♂	♀
Hong Kong (5)	24.3	10.2
San Francisco (2)	19.1	6.4
Singapore (2)	18.7	7.1
Cantonese (7)	29.4	10.3
Teochew (7)	17.4	5.9
Hokkien (7)	13.7	4.0
Taiwan (77)		
Mainland	11.4	11.7
Taiwanese	5.9	2.8
Hawaii (2)	10.3	5.1
Eskimos (75)	9.6	3.8
Japan (33)	6.8	3.0

repeated sex differences among all ethnic and racial groups (Table 2); males maintain a higher, albeit variable, incidence compared to females.

Particularly intriguing is the serological association of this tumor with Epstein-Barr virus (EBV). It is not found for other tumor types of the nasopharynx or carcinomas of the buccal cavity and pharynx. Case-control studies suggest that both place of birth and high anti-EBV antibody titer significantly increase the risk of NPC (33,68,78,79). A number of genetic studies have linked EBV with NPC, but the data are not conclusive (5,34,80,81). Most researchers have not adequately investigated sociocultural factors which may influence the higher correlation between EBV and NPC seen among groups of Chinese, but not among descendants whose rates decline in low incidence areas. Whether NPC is virally induced or simply associated with higher viral infections is unknown (34,82,83). Titers of healthy Chinese and Japanese of similar age who live in Japan and have low incidence of NPC show only minimal differences in an antiviral capsid antigen (VCA) antibody (33). Yet, healthy Japanese living in Taiwan have anti-VCA titers similar to Taiwanese living in high incidence areas (33). Sawaki et al. reported no significant differences in titer values between disease-free Chinese born in China, or in those of Chinese-Japanese mixture. They concluded that titers are influenced by cultural and environmental factors, but not by hereditary ones. Nonetheless, the relative frequency of NPC (and presumably the absolute risk) is much higher among Chinese than among Japanese residing in Japan.

A few environmental factors have been investigated in relation to NPC (84). Exposure to smoke (cooking, work, tobacco) has been studied with mixed results (Table 3). Poor ventilation and occupational fumes have been hypothesized as producing increased risks, 20–30 fold for Chinese, and for Eskimos and whites moving to Alaska who heat and cook indoors with inadequate ventilation (75).

Table 3. Relative risk of environmental factors for nasopharyngeal cancer.

Risk factor	Reference	RO
Tobacco		
(> 40 cig/day)	Henderson et al. (6)	1.0
(> 10 years)	Shamugaratnam (85)	0.9
(> 1 pkg cig/day)	Hu (86)	1.8
Air pollution		
cooking fumes - wood	Hu (86)	1.5
	Shamugaratnam (85)	0.9
industrial fumes	Henderson (6)	2.0
	Lin et al. (76)	2.6
	Lin et al. (76)	2.2

Yet women, who are more likely to be at risk from this exposure, have lower incidence to NPC. In contrast, 'boat' people, Chinese who live on boats all their lives, cook their food in open air, have high incidence. Some studies have pointed out certain dietary items such as salted fish (which may contain nitrosamines) might explain why 'boat' people suffer from high NPC incidence despite adequate ventilation (6,68,75,87).

Heavy cigarette smoking is not thought to be a risk factor. Differences in usage and carcinogenicity between Western and Asian substances are unknown, however. It is conceivable that because routine smoking is relatively uncommon among Chinese, particularly in rural regions, that amount and duration of this exposure is insufficient to produce an apparent increased risk (88,89). The need for additional analytic epidemiologic research of environmental (chemical carcinogens such as nitrosamines, EBV) as well as genetic factors remain.

Tongue (141). Indians in Bombay and in Singapore (females) have the highest incidence of tongue cancer. Puerto Rico and Brazil are a distant second among males with most other nations reporting low risk for either sex. Areas in the USA, regardless of population composition have similar risks – only Spanish origin and Chinese in Hawaii have incidence which may vary from this pattern, with rates less than $1/10^5$. Research has suggested that Plummer-Vinson's syndrome increases the frequency of tongue cancers among women in Sweden (26); nonetheless, the female incidence does not exceed that for males in that country and is lower than that for females in other countries.

Mouth (143–5). Indian women in Singapore have the highest incidence of mouth cancer ($16.9/10^5$, ICD-A 143-145, 8th rev.), even higher than seen among Indian males ($8.6/10^5$). Indians in Bombay have a higher incidence of these tumors than other populations, but still significantly lower than Indians in Singapore (2). As with tongue cancer, males, and to a lesser degree females, in Brazil and Puerto

Rico are at high risk to developing neoplasms of the mouth. A number of Westernized countries that have low incidence for tongue cancer also have low incidence for this site, particularly among oriental populations: indigenous Japanese, and Japanese and Chinese living in Hawaii. Other racial groups in Hawaii have rates similar to whites in the continental USA, however, Caucasians in Europe and Scandinavia have even lower incidence than US whites.

Oro, hypo- and other parts of the pharynx (146,148,149). Age-adjusted rates of oro- and hypopharyngeal tumors among males (Table 1) are high in Indians, Swiss, and Puerto Ricans; their rates of nasopharyngeal cancers, however, are very low. These findings suggest different etiologic components, most likely attributable to environment exposures.

Etiologic factors

Alcohol and tobacco

Alcoholic beverages and tobacco are the major etiologic factors implicated in oral and pharyngeal tumors throughout the world (21,90–33). Additional factors such as actinic rays, ionizing radiation and viruses have been identified for tumors of the lip, salivary gland, and nasopharynx.

Although people in most countries use cigarettes, cigars, pipe, or chewing tobacco, a few of the Southeast Asian countries report an increased risk from specific regional tobacco-like substances to which they are exposed; betel nut or pan chewing, chutta cigars, and bidi cigarettes (35,40,41,46,47,97–109). Dried betel leaves, which come from a climbing pepper bush, are chewed with the nut and may be coated with slaked lime, tobacco, and occasionally other substances. Chutta, which is made from dried tobacco leaves tied at one end, is easier to smoke with the lighted end in the mouth. Bidi cigarettes are uncured tobacco that has been wrapped in banana or other dried leaf.

Two major studies in India suggest that use of pan is correlated with the development of oral and pharyngeal tumors. In a follow-up study of over 57,500 male workers, pan was the most commonly used tobacco product, by 85% of the group (35,97). Most cancers were of the tongue and oropharynx. The authors felt that, although a low correlation existed and data were not examined for confounders, the tobacco agents used, particularly pan, increased the risk to oral cancer. This conclusion is supported by Jussawalla et al. (99). In a matched case-control study of over 2000 individuals from Bombay, smokers or pan chewers had a significantly increased risk to all the oral and pharyngeal sites compared to controls who were non-tobacco(like) users.

Studies of age and sex-matched controls and cases of oral cancer in Ceylon and in Travancore)India) indicated that frequency and duration (chain chewers: < 4 min; > 1 hr/chew) of chewing tobacco quid was associated with an increasing relative risk in the development of oral cancer regardless of sex (108). The risks were similar in the two samples and were as high as 63 times that of non-chewers. In Ceylon and southern India the majority of neoplasms occur in the oral cavity because of their habit of chewing, primarily tobacco mixed with shell lime. In northern India, Mainpuri, where oral cancers also are high, a mixture of tobacco, lime, and betel nut is chewed. The quid is kept in different parts of the mouth in these geographic locations but tumors predominate at the site of the quid. Major sites affected are buccal mucosa, the anterior tongue, and the oropharynx, although the lower lip is involved among those who hold the tobacco on its inner side in the gingivolabial fold.

Among white rural females who work in the southeastern United States, oral and pharyngeal cancer mortality is elevated (110). Several studies of southern female populations have reported that oral cancer cases are more likely to use snuff than controls (111,112). In another study, Smith et al. (112), studying 15,000 snuff users in Tennessee by duration of use, found no association.

Reverse chutta smoking, with the combustible end in the mouth, is a habit in greater use among Indian women while conventional chutta smoking is greater among men. Whether the habit of reverse smoking or the use of chutta produces a greater risk, however, is unclear. Women showed more tissues changes of the hard palate from reverse chutta use in one investigation, but there was no correlation between other tobacco habits and malignancies among either sex (105). Other research comparing cases and controls of Indian populations in Sri Kahulua and Visakhapatnam produced an increased risk among reverse chutta smokers for palatal cancer in males (102). The Parsi population who have a different religion, higher SES, and are more Westernized that the rest of Bombay, smoke little an have lower incidence rates of oral and pharyngeal cancers than the rest of India and Western countries (100). The relative risk among those who used both chutta and pan was greater, particularly in the oro- and hypopharynx, and larynx (31.7, 16.9, 20.1, respectively). Smoking bidi alone accounted for the highest risk: soft palate (12.6), pharynx (1.8), base of tongue (9.7), tonsils (8.1) and larynx (7.7); chewing pan produced the highest risk for hypopharynx (6.2). The authors suggest that it is not genetic but rather environmental habits that play a role in the lower incidence among the Parsi (100).

Alcohol also is correlated with oral and pharyngeal cancers, particularly in such countries as France, Switzerland, Puerto Rico and Ireland where per capita alcohol consumption is among the highest in the world (35,40,97,98,101,102, 114–117). Alcohol has been correlated with cancers of the tongue, hypopharynx, larynx, and esophagus (42–45,118). Age-specific cohorts among Western populations in the United States, England and Wales, Australia, and France show evidence of changing incidence and mortality patterns of chronic alcoholism, liver cirrhosis, and upper alimentary tract cancers (tongue, oropharynx, esophagus) that correlate with time trends since 1900 in per capita alcohol consumption (42,44,113,115,119–122). These cancer patterns are consistent with each other and in contrast to the sharp rise in tobacco use and lung cancer rates in these countries (44,113,119–123). The carcinogenic effect is far less among females because of lower dose and less use and is reflected in lower incidence (Table 1) and relative risk. After adjusting for confounding effects of tobacco, dental conditions, and sociodemographic factors, the relative risk of alcohol consumption is between 2.0–17.7 for both men and women (95,96). Difference in sites examined and in amount, type, and duration of each product by site may explain why there are such large variations in relative risk for both alcohol and tobacco, inasmuch as the areas of the mouth and upper digestive tissues are exposed differently to these two substances.

In Japan, a low risk country, age-adjusted death rates over a twenty-year period, 1950–71, showed no change (123). There is speculation that with increasing Westernization, the ensuing increased alcohol and tobacco consumption will produce higher mortality. Although this has not yet been reflected in mortality statistics, incidence is rising (2,12,13,123,124). There is evidence (123,125) that alcohol associated cancers (viz., tongue, hypopharynx, esophagus) have risen in age-specific incidence and cohort mortality among younger Japanese since World War II. The trend in alcohol consumption between 1951–1972 correlated with increased urbanization particularly in large Japanese cities, not just increased economic growth (21,126). Furthermore, foreign beer and liquor use rose at a higher rate than traditional Japanese products: sake and shochu (115,116,127,128). Age-standardized incidence and mortality have risen considerably for tobacco-related cancers, lung, bronchus, and trachea, among both sexes (ratio: ♂ 6.13; ♀ 5.06); and Kono et al. demonstrated an increasing standardized mortality ratio (SMR) for esophageal and lung tumors (116).

Hirayama, in a population-based study in 1965, interviewed and followed up individuals over an 8-year period on use of risk factors (alcohol and tobacco) and survival (death certificates) (129). A significant association between smoking and cancer ratio was reported among males. The elevated SMR were pronounced when the habit was initiated early: mouth (7.04), hypopharynx (2.81), as well as esophagus (2.57) and lung (2.03). Similar conclusions were drawn for alcohol users, although no alcohol units or sex-specific SMRs were reported: mouth (3.53), esophagus (1.82), and lung (1.28). Combinations of alcohol and tobacco reportedly enhanced the carcinogenic risk to the mouth as well as to the esophagus and the liver.

A few studies have proposed that alcohol and tobacco provide not only an independent but also a synergistic effect in producing oral and pharyngeal tumors (21,43,95). Rothman (21), and Tuyns et al. (43) reported greater relative excess risk among cases who smoke and drink. Other research, however, using both additive and multiplicative synergistic models, found no such effect, which leaves this conclusion in question (95,130). These conflicting results may be due to the differences in definitions of substances, sites and populations. Indeed several theories propose that alcohol may act only as a promoter or cocarcinogen with tobacco, by (1) enhancing the carcinogenic effect of tobacco, (2) irritating tissues thus increasing their susceptibility to carcinogenic agents, (3) replacing or compromising nutritional requirements of tissues allowing cell alteration to occur, (4) weakening the immune system, or (5) acting as solvent of tobacco carcinogens (131–133).

In sum, although there are much data describing the correlation of alcohol and tobacco in conjunction with oral and pharyngeal tumors, more research emphasis is needed to define their synergistic effects on these upper alimentary tract neoplasms.

Dental conditions

Dental conditions such as oral hygiene, trauma, dentures, and jagged teeth have been suggested as etiologic factors producing biochemical alterations. These changes are thought to lead to the development of cancers in the buccal cavity (95,130,134). Alternatively, it is possible that dental conditions are correlated with socioeconomic status, a confounder which also is related to exposure to etiologic factors, alcohol and tobacco. In a 40-year study at a Swedish medical institution, dental status among cases showed no association with oral cancer (135). Similar results were found by Mashberg and Meyers in a prospective study in the United States (136). Dental trauma generally was not located at the disease site.

Environmental/occupational exposures

A few studies have investigated occupational exposures in England and Wales and the US with mixed results (110,137–142). Moss and Lee reported significantly higher proportionate mortality ratios (PMR) for tongue, mouth, and pharynx cancers among fiber preparers, and lower ratios for other cotton and wool textile workers (138,139).

A later study of the two main textile regions in England and Wales showed no greater risk between textile workers (140). Although more refined definitions of risk factors (e.g. smoking, drinking) were made in this investigation, confounding and synergistic effects in cases and controls were not assessed. An interview study in one English burough, Stoke-on-Trent, was conducted on identified cancer registry cases between 1957–71 (141). Subjects were similarly matched as the Moss study (139). No significant differences were found for occupation, although alcohol, tobacco, and dental conditions showed some differences between cases and controls.

Studies in the US reported that between 1950–69 mortality was elevated for males in counties with leather, paper and chemical industries, and for females with apparel and textile manufacturing (110,142). The higher mortality remained after demographic factors, and alcohol and tobacco consumption were assessed.

Summary

The several sub-sites of oropharyngeal cancer do not show the same pattern of high or low risk in different populations. These conditions suggest that etiologic effects vary by site. Caucasians are at highest risk for lip cancer, Indians for mouth, and Chinese for nasopharynx. Suspected causes are both genetic and environmental in nature.

The major etiologic factors identified are smoking and drinking, which seem to be linked with the highest relative risk. Although these two substances are also thought to produce the highest attributable risks, studies have not systematically examined this important epidemiologic phenomenon. Increasingly, however, other environmental sources have been identified in the development of neoplastic diseases. Occupational agents that are inhaled or chemicals that are ingested may provide new or hitherto unknown carcinogens in the development of oral and pharyngeal tumors. Unfortunately, to date the major causes identified are behaviorally related. They require the individual to take action and thus, are the most difficult to prevent or control.

References

1. Axtell M, Asire AJ, Myers MH (eds): Cancer Patient Survival. Report No 5 SEER Program. DHEW Publ No 77-992. Washington, DC: US Govt Print Off, 1976, 315 pp.
2. Waterhouse J, Correa P, Muir C, et al. (eds): Cancer incidence in five continents. Vol III. IARC, Scientific Publ No 15. Lyon, France, 1976.
3. Binnie WH: Epidemiology and etiology of oral cancer in Britain. Proceed Roy Soc Med 69:737–740, 1976.
4. Garnjana-Goochorn S, Chantarakul N: Nasopharyngeal cancer at Siriraj Hospital, Dhouburi, Thailand. In: Muir CS, Shanmugaratnam K (eds): Cancer of the nasopharynx. UICC. Monogr No 1. Copenhagen: Munksgaard, 1967, pp. 33–37.
5. Ho HC: Current knowledge of the epidemiology of nasopharyngeal carcinoma-A review. In: Biggs PM, de-Thé G, Payne LN (eds): Oncogenesis and herpesviruses. IARC, Scientific Publ, No 2, Lyon, 1972, pp 357–366.
6. Henderson BE, Louie E, Jing JS, et al: Risk factors associated with nasopharyngeal carcinoma. New Engl J Med 295:1101–1106, 1976.

7. Shanmugaratnam K: Cancer in Singapore – Ethnic and dialect group variations in cancer incidence. Singapore Med J 14:69–81, 1973.
8. Fischel R: Diseases affecting the oral cavity observed in Costa Rica and Central America. Int Dent J 15:326–330, 1965.
9. Correa JN, Bosch A, Marcial VA: Carcinoma of the floor of the mouth. Review of clinical factors and results of treatment. Amer J Roentgen 99:302–312, 1967.
10. Spitzer WO, Hill GB, Chambers LW, et al.: The occupation of fishing as a risk factor in cancer of the lip. N Engl J Med 293:419–424, 1975.
11. Cutler SJ, Young JL (eds): Third National Cancer Survey: Incidence Data. Natl Cancer Inst Mongr 41:1–454, 1975.
12. Doll R, Payne P, Waterhouse J (eds): Cancer incidence in five continents. Vol I. IARC. Switzerland: Springer-Verlag, 1966.
13. Doll R, Payne P, Waterhouse J (eds): Cancer incidence in five continents. Vol. II. IARC. Switzerland: Springer-Verlag, 1966.
14. Segi M: Age-adjusted death rates for cancer for selected sites (A-classification) in 51 countries in 1974. Nagoya, Japan: Segi Institute of Cancer Epidemiology, 1979.
15. Segi M, Kurihara M: Cancer mortality for selected sites in 24 countries. No 6 (1966–1967). Japan Cancer Society, 1972.
16. WHO Statistics Quarterly Report. Vol 31:67, 1978. Geneva: WHO.
17. Mason TJ: Atlas of cancer mortality for US counties: 1950–1969. DHEW Publ No 75-78. Washington, DC: US Govt Print Off, 1975, 103 pp.
18. Burbank F: Patterns in cancer mortality in the US: 1950–67. Natl Cancer Inst Monogr 33:1–90, 1971.
19. Segi M: Age-adjusted death rates for cancer for selected sites (A-classification) in 46 countries in 1975. Nagoya, Japan: Segi Institute of Cancer Epidemiology, 1980.
20. Edington GM, Sheiham A: Salivary gland tumors and tumors of the oral cavity in Western Nigeria. Br J Cancer 20:425–433, 1966.
21. Rothman K, Keller A: The effect of joint exposure to alcohol and tobacco on risk of cancer of the mouth and pharynx. J Chronic Dis 25:711–716, 1972.
22. Shedd DP, von Essen CF, Ferraro RH, et al.: Cancer of the tongue in Connecticut, 1935–1959. Cancer 21:89–96, 1968.
23. Shedd DP, von Essen CF, Connelly RR, et al.: Cancer of the floor of the mouth in Connecticut, 1935–1959. Cancer 21:97–101, 1968.
24. Shedd DP, von Essen CF, Connelly RR, et al.: Cancer of the buccal mucosa, palate, and gingiva in Connecticut, 1935–1959. Cancer 21:440–446, 1968.
25. Keller AZ: Cellular types, survival, race, nativity, occupations, habits and associated diseases in the pathogenesis of lip cancer. Am J Epidemiol 91:486–499, 1970.
26. Söder Per-Östen: The incidence of malignant tumors in the mouth-pharynx region in Sweden 1958–1967. Swed Dent J 66:419–428, 1973.
27. Takiuhi N, Hirose F, Yamamoto H: Salivary gland tumors in atomic bomb survivors, Hiroshima, Japan. I. Epidemiologic observations. Cancer 38:2462–2468, 1976.
28. Robbins SL, Cotran RS (eds): Pathologic basis of disease. Second edition. Philadelphia: WB Saunders, 1979.
29. Loke YW: Salivary gland tumors in Malaya. Br J Cancer 21:665–674, 1967.
30. Frazell EL: Observations on the management of salivary gland tumors. CA 18:235–240, 1968.
31. Dunn EJ, Kent T, Hines J, et al.: Parotid neoplasms: A report of 250 cases and review of the literature. Ann Surg 184:500–506, 1976.
32. Sharkey FE: Systematic evaluation of the world Health Organization. Classification of salivary gland tumors. Amer J Clin Path 67:272–278, 1977.
33. Sawaki S, Hirayama T, Sugano H: Studies on nasopharyngeal carcinoma in Japan. In: Hirayama T (ed): Cancer in Asia. Baltimore: University Park Press, 1976, pp 63–74.
34. Ho HC: Epidemiology of nasopharyngeal carcinoma. In: Hirayama T (ed): Cancer in Asia. Baltimore: University Park Press, 1976.
35. Silverman S Jr, Bhargava K, Mani NJ, et al.: Malignant transformationa and natural history of oral leukoplakia in 57,518 industrial workers in Gujarat, India. Cancer 38:1790–1795, 1976.

16

36. Gangadharan P, Paymaster JC: Leukoplakia – An epidemiologic study of 1504 cases observed at the Tata Memorial Hospital, Bombay, India. Br J Cancer 25:657–668, 1971.
37. Mehta FS, Schroff BC, Gupta PC, et al.: Oral leukoplakia in relation to tobacco habits. A ten-year follow-up study of Bombay policemen. Oral surg 34:426–433, 1972.
38. Mehta FS, Pindborg JJ: Spontaneous regression of oral leukoplakias among Indian villagers in a 5-year follow-up study. Comm Dent Oral Epidemiol 2:80–84, 1974.
39. Pindborg JJ, Daftary DK, Mehta FS, et al.: A follow-up study of sixty-one oral dysplastic precancerous lesions in Indian villagers. Oral surg 43:383–390, 1977.
40. Mehta FS, Pindborg JJ, Gupta PC, et al.: Epidemiological and histologic study of oral cancer and leukoplakia among 50,915 villagers in India. Cancer 24:832–849, 1969.
41. Mehta FS, Gupta PC, Daftary DK, et al.: An epidemiologic study of oral cancer and precancerous conditions among 101,761 villagers in Mahareishtra, India. Int J Cancer 10:134–141, 1972.
42. OMS Rapport épidémologique et démographique. Rapp Epidém Démogr 12:171, 1959.
43. Tuyns A, Pequignot G, Jensen O, et al.: La consommation individuelle de boissons alcoolisées et de tabac dans un échantillon de la population en Ille-et-Vilaine. Revue de l'alcol 21:105–150, 1975.
44. McMichael AJ, Hetzel BS: Time trends in upper alimentary tract cancer mortality and alcohol consumption in Australia. Comm Hlth Stud 1:43–47, 1978.
45. Rankin DW: The epidemiology of epithelionia of the mouth and tongue. Austral Dent J 14:236–240, 1969.
46. Malowalla AM, Silverman S Jr, Mani NJ, et al.: Oral cancer in 57,518 industrial workers of Gujorat, India. Cancer 37:1882–1886, 1976.
47. Ramulu C, Raju MV, Venkatarathnam G, et al.: Nicotine stomatitis and its relation to carcinoma of the hard palate in reverse smoker of chuttas. J Dent Res 52:711–718, 1973.
48. Smart CR, Lyon CR, Skolnick M, et al.: Cancer of the head and neck in Utah. Am J Surg 128:463–465, 1974.
49. Pindborg JJ: Epidemiological studies of oral cancer. Int Dent J 27:172–178, 1977.
50. Keller AZ: Cellular types, survival, race, nativity, occupations, habits and associated disease in the pathogenesis of lip cancer. Am J Epidemiol 91:486–499, 1970.
51. Lindquist C, Teppo L: Risk factors lip cancer. Am J Epidemiol 109:521–530, 1979.
52. Lindquist C, Teppo L: Epidemiological evaluation of sunlight as a risk factor of lip cancer. Br J Cancer 37:983–989, 1978.
53. Ringertz N (ed): Cancer incidence in Finland, Iceland, Norway, and Sweden. A comparative study. Acta Path Microbiol, Sect A, Suppl 224, 1971.
54. Tan KN: Cancers of the lip in Australia: Austral Dent J 15: 179–184, 1970.
55. Cancer Registry of Norway: Trends in cancer incidence in Norway 1955–1967. Oslo: Univsitetsforlaget, 1972.
56. Cancer Registry of Norway: Cancer registration in Norway: The incidence of cancer in Norway 1969–1971. Oslo: The Norwegian Cancer Society, 1973.
57. The Cancer Registry of Norway: The incidence of cancers in Norway 1953–1958. Oslo: The Norwegian Cancer Society, 1961.
58. The Cancer Registry of Norway: The incidence of cancer in Norway 1959–1961. Oslo: The Norwegian Cancer Society, 1961.
59. Cancer in New South Wales. Incidence and mortality 1973. Sydney: New South Wales Central Cancer Registry, Health Commission of NSW, 1978.
60. Cancer in New South Wales. Incidence and mortality 1974. Sydney: New South Wales Central Cancer Registry, Health Commission of NSW, 1979.
61. Cancer incidence in Finland 1973. Publ No 23. Helsinki: Finnish Cancer Registry – The Institute for Statistical and Epidemiological Cancer Research, 1976.
62. Szpak CA, Stone MJ, Frenkel EP: Some observations concerning the demographic and geographic incidence of carcinoma of the lip and buccal cancer. Cancer 40:343–348, 1977.
63. Jones JH: Squamous carsinoma of the lip and mouth in Northern Ireland. Br J Cancer 22:502–505, 1968.
64. Segi M, Noye H, Segi R, et al.: Countries of high death rates for cancer (1970–1972). Nagoya, Japan, 1977.

65. Eneroth CM: Salivary gland tumors in the parotid gland, submandibular gland, and the palate region. Cancer 27:1415–1418, 1971.
66. Nielsen NH, Mikkelsen F, Hansen JP: Incidence of salivary gland neoplasms in Greenland with special reference to an anaplastic carcinoma. Act path Microbiol Scand (Sect A) 86: 185–193, 1978.
67. Belsky JL, Takiuhi N, Yamamoto T, et al.: Salivary gland neoplasms following atomic radiation: Additional cases and reanalysis of combined data in a fixed population, 1957–1970. Cancer 35: 555–559, 1975.
68. Hirayama T: Descriptive and analytical epidemiology of nasopharyngeal cancer. In: de Thé G, Ito Y (eds): Nasopharyngeal carcinoma: Etiology and control. IARC, Publ No 20. Lyon, France, 1978, pp 167–189.
69. Buell P: Nasopharyngeal cancer in Chinese of California. Br J Cancer 19:459–470, 1965.
70. Zippin C, Tekawa IS, Bragg KU, et al.: Studies on heredity and environment in cancer of the nasopharynx. J Natl Cancer Inst 29:483–490, 1962.
71. Quisenberry WB, Reimann-Jasinski D: Ethnic differences in nasopharyngeal cancer in Hawaii. In: Muir CS, Shanmugaratnam K (eds): Cancer of the nasopharynx. UICC Monogr No 17. Copenhagen: Munksgaard, 1967, pp 64–72.
72. Worth RM, Valentine R: Nasopharyngeal carcinoma in New South Wales, Australia. In: Muir CS, Shanmugaratnam K (eds): Cancer of the nasopharynx. UICC Monogr No 1. Copenhagen: Munksgaard, 1967, pp 73–76.
73. Buell P: The effect of migration on the risk of nasopharyngeal cancer among Chinese. Cancer Res 34:1189–1191, 1974.
74. Buell P: Race and place in the etiology of nasopharyngeal cancer. A study based on California death certificates. Int J Cancer 11: 268–272, 1973.
75. Lanier AP, Bender TR, Blot WJ, et al.: Cancer incidence in Alaska natives. Int J Cancer 18:409–412, 1976.
76. Mason TJ, McKay FW, Hoover R, et al.: Atlas of cancer mortality among U.S. non-whites, 1950–1969. DHEW Publ No (NIH) 76-1201, US DHEW. Washington, DC: US Govt Print Off, 1976.
77. Lin TM, Chem KP, Lin CC, et al.: Retrospective study on nasopharyngeal carcinoma. J Natl Cancer Inst 51:1403–1408, 1973.
78. Lin TM, Yang CS, Tu SM, et al.: Interaction of factors associated with cancer of the nasopharynx. Cancer 44:1419–1423, 1979.
79. Heule W, Henle G, Ho H, et al.: Antibodies to Epstein-Barr virus in nasopharyngeal carcinoma, other head and neck neoplasms and control groups. J Natl Cancer Inst 44:225–231, 1970.
80. Muir CS, Oakley WF: Nasopharyngeal cancer in Sarawak (Borneo). J Laryn 81:197–207, 1967.
81. Neveo S, Meyer W, Altman M: Carcinoma of nasopharynx in twins. Cancer 28:807–809, 1971.
82. de-Thé G, Ablashi DV, Liabeuf A, et al.: Nasopharyngeal carcinoma (NPC). VI. Presence of an EBV nuclear antigen in fresh tumor biopsies – Prelimimary results. Biomedicine 19: 349–352, 1973.
83. Klein G, Giovanella BC, Lindahl T, et al.: Direct evidence for the presence of Epstein-Barr virus DNA and nuclear antigen in malignant epithelial cells from patients with anaplastic carcinoma of the nasopharynx. In: Proceedings of Natl Cancer Inst. Washington, DC: US Govt Print Off, 1974.
84. Tarjussen W, Solberg LA, Hogetveit AC: Histopathologic changes of nasal mucosa in nickel workers. A pilot study. Cancer 44: 963–974, 1979.
85. Shanmugaratnam K: In: de Thè G, Ito Y (eds): Nasopharyngeal carcinoma: Etiology and control. IARC Publ No 20. Lyon, France, 1978.
86. Hu MS, Huang HL: Retrospective study on the etiological factors of nasopharyngeal carcinoma. New Med (Chinese) 12:10, 1972.
87. Fong YY, Chan WC: Dinethylnitrosamine in Chinese marine salt fish. Food Cosmet Toxicol 11:841–845, 1973.
88. Henderson BE, Louie E: Discussion of risk factors for nasopharyngeal carcinoma. In: de Thè G, Ito Y (eds): Nasopharyngeal Carcinoma: Etiology and control. IARC Publ No 20. Lyon, France, 1978.

89. Simarak S, de Jong UW, Breslow N, et al.: Cancer of the oral cavity, pharynx/larynx and lung in North Thailand: Case-control study and analysis of cigar smoke. Br J Cancer 36:130–140, 1977.
90. Keller AZ, Terris M: The association of alcohol and tobacco with cancer of the mouth and pharynx. Am J Public Health 55:1578–1585, 1965.
91. Bross ID, Coombs J: Early onset of oral cancer among women who drink and smoke. Oncology 33:136–139, 1976.
92. Nukada A: Urbanization and drinking patterns in Japan. In: Proceedings 31st International Congress on Alcoholism and Drug Dependence, Feb 23–28, 1975, Bangkok, Thailand, pp 523–526.
93. Horie A, Kohchi S, Kuratsune M: Carcinogenesis in the esophagus. II. Experimental production of esophageal cancer by administration of ethanolic solution of carcinogens. Gann 56:429–444, 1965.
94. Haenszel W (ed): Epidemiological approaches to the study of cancer and other chronic diseases. NCI Washington DC: US Govt Print Off, 1966.
95. Graham S, Dayal H, Rohrer T, et al.: Dentition, diet, tobacco, and alcohol in the epidemiology of oral cancer. J Natl Cancer Inst 59:1611–1617, 1977.
96. Williams RR, Horn JW: Association of cancer sites with tobacco and alcohol consumption and socioeconomic status of patients: Interview study from the Third National Cancer Survey. J Natl Cancer Inst 58:525–547, 1977.
97. Muir CS, Kirk R: Betel, tobacco, and cancer of the mouth. Br J Cancer 14:597–608, 1960.
98. Jussawalla DJ, Haenszel W, Deshpande VA, et al.: Cancer incidence in greater Bombay: Assessment of the cancer risk by age. Br J Cancer 22:623–636, 1968.
99. Jussawalla DJ, Deshpande VA: Evaluation of cancer risk in tobacco chewers and smokers: An Epidemiologic assessment. Cancer 28: 244–252, 1971.
100. Jussawalla DJ, Deshpande VA, Haenszel W, Natekar MV: Differences observed in the site incidence of cancer, between the Parsi community and the total population of Greater Bombay: A critical appraisal. Br J Cancer 24:56–66, 1970.
101. Paymaster JC, Gangadharan P: Cancer in the Parsi community of Bombay. Int J Cancer 5:426–431, 1970.
102. Reddy CR, Kaneswari VR, Chandramouli KB, et al.: Evaluation of oral, pharyngeal, laryngeal, and esophageal cancer risk in reverse smokers of chutta. Int Surg 60:266–269, 1975.
103. Wahi PN, Lahiri B, Kehar U, et al.: Oral and oropharyngeal cancers in North India. Br J Cancer 14:627–641, 1965.
104. Jayant K, Balakrishnan V, Sanghvi LD: A note on the distribution of cancer in some endogamous groups in Western India. Br J Cancer 25:611–619, 1971.
105. Ramulu C, Reddy CR: Carcinoma of the hard palate and its relation to reverse smoking. Int Surg 57:636–641, 1972.
106. Muir CS, Evans MD, Roche PJ: Cancer in Sabah (Borneo). Br J Cancer 22:637–645, 1968.
107. Menakant W, Muir CS, Jain DK: Cancer in Chiang Mai, North Thailand. A relative frequency study. Br J Cancer 25:225–236, 1971.
108. Hirayama T: An epidemiological study of oral and pharyngeal cancer in Central and Southeast Asia. Bull WHO 34:41–69, 1966.
109. Kwan H: A statistical study on oral carcinomas in Taiwan with emphasis on the relationsip with betal nut chewing: A preliminary report. J Formosan Med Assoc 75:497–505, 1976.
110. Winn D, Blot WJ, Shy CL, Pickle L, Toledo A, Fraumeni J: Snuff dipping and oral cancer among women in the southern United States. New Engl J Med 304:745–749, 1981.
111. Brown RL, Suh JM, Scarborough JE, et al.: Snuff dippers' intra-oral cancer: clinical characteristics and response to therapy. Cancer 18:2–13, 1965.
112. Smith JF, Mincer HA, Hopkins KP, et al.: Snuff-dippers lesion: A cytological and pathological study in a large population. Arch Otolaryngeal 92:450–456, 1970.
113. Brenner MH: Trends in alcohol consumption and associated illnesses. Am J Pub Health 65:1279–1292, 1975.
114. Junod B, Pasche R: Etio-épidémiologie des cancers de la bouche et du pharynx en Suisse. Schweiz Med Wochen Schr 108:882–887, 1978.

115. Tuyns AJ: Cancer of the esophagus: Further evidence of the relation to drinking habits in France. Int J Cancer 5:152–156, 1970.
116. Breslow NE, Enstrom JE: Geographic correlations between cancer mortality rates and alcohol-tobacco consumption in the United States. J Natl Cancer Inst 53:631–639, 1974.
117. Martìnez I, Torres R, Frìas Z: Cancer incidence in the US and Puerto Rico. Cancer Res 35(Part 2):3265–3271, 1975.
118. Schwartz D, Lellouch J, Flamant R, et al.: Alcohol et cancer. Résultats d'une enquête rétrospective. Rev Franc Etudes Clin et Biol 7:590–604, 1962.
119. Spring JA, Buss DH: Three centuries of alcohol in the British diet. Nature 270:567–572, 1977.
120. McKenzie JC: Social implications of alcohol consumption. Proc Nutr Soc 31:99–106, 1972.
121. Terris M: Epidemiology of cirrhosis of the liver: National mortality data. Am J Pub Health 57:2076–2088, 1967.
122. DeLint J, Schmidt W: Consumption averages and alcoholism prevalence. A brief review of epidemiological investigations. Br J Addict 66:97–107, 1971.
123. Segi M: Age-adjusted death rates for selected sites of cancer in Japan (1950–51/1970–71). Mimeo, 1973.
124. Smith EM: An analysis of cohort mortality from tongue cancer in Japan, England and Wales, and the United States. Unpublished data.
125. Ikeda M, Miyata, Masaki et al.: Multiple cancer involving esophagus and other organs. Clinics of cancer (Gan no Rinsho) 25:84–88, 1979.
126. Council on the Population Problems. The trends of population in Japan. Tokyo: Ministry of Finance, Bureau of Printing, 1974, pp 278–281.
127. Kono S, Ikeda M: Correlation between cancer mortality and alcoholic beverage in Japan. Br J Cancer 40:449–455, 1979.
128. Schoenberg BS, Bailar JC, III, Fraumeni JF, Jr: Certain mortality patterns of esophageal cancer in the United States, 1930–1967. J Natl Cancer Inst 46:63–73, 1971.
129. Hirayama T: Smoking and cancer: A prospective study on cancer epidemiology based on a census population in Japan. In: Proceedings of the 3rd World Conference on Smoking and Health. NYC, June, 1975. USDHEW Publ No 77-1413. Washington, DC, 1977, pp 65–72.
130. Wynder EL, Bross IJ, Feldman RM: A study of the etiologic factors in cancer of the mouth. Cancer 10:1300–1323, 1957.
131. Kuratsune M, Kohchi S, Horie A, et al.: Test of alcoholic beverages and ethanol solutions for carcinogenicity and tumor-promoting activity. GANN 62:395–405, 1971.
132. Tuyns AJ: Cancer of the oesophagus: Further evidence of relation to drinking habits in France. Int J Cancer 5:152–156, 1970.
133. Vogler WR, Lloyd JW, Milmore BK: A retrospective study of etiologic factors in cancer of the mouth, pharynx, and larynx. Cancer 15:246–258, 1962.
134. Nelson JF, Ship II: Intraoral carcinoma: Predisposition factors and their frequency of incidence as related to age at onset. J Am Dent Assoc 82:564–568, 1971.
135. Einhorn J, Wersâtt J: Incidence of oral carcinoma in patients with leukoplakia of the oral mucosa. Cancer 29:2189–2193, 1967.
136. Mashberg A, Meyers H: Anatomical site and size of 222 early ssymptomatic oral squamous cell carcinomas. A continuing prospective study of oral cancer. II. Cancer 37:2149–2157, 1976.
137. Greenberg M: A proportional mortality study of a group of newspaper workers. Br J Indus Med 29:15–20, 1972.
138. Moss E: Oral and pharyngeal cancer in textile workers. Ann NY Acad Sci 271:301–307, 1976.
139. Moss E, Lee WR: Occurrence of oral and pharyngeal cancers in textile workers. Br J Indus Med 31:224–232, 1974.
140. Whitaker CJ, Moss E, Lee WR, et al.: Oral and pharyngeal cancer in the Northwest and West Yorkshire regions of England, and occupations. Br J Indus Med 36:292–298, 1979.
141. Browne RM, Cainsey MC, Waterhouse JA, et al.: Etiological factors in squamous cell carcinoma. Comm Dent Oral Epidemiol 5:301–306, 1977.
142. Fraumeni JF Jr: Geographic distribution of head and neck cancers in the United States. Laryngoscope 88(Suppl 8): 1–4, 1978.

2. Epidemiology of Esophageal Cancer: A Review

NICHOLAS E. DAY, NUBIA MUÑOZ and PARVIZ GHADIRIAN

Introduction

The purpose of studying the epidemiology of a particular cancer is principally twofold. First, to identify factors whose modification may reduce that cancer's incidence and, secondly, a more general aim, to understand better the mechanisms that modify risk for cancer in human populations. For cancer of the esophagus, considerable success has been achieved in attaining both aims. In some areas of the world specific factors have been identified, control of which would eliminate most of the disease. In other areas, particularly where the disease is common, the epidemiological evidence points overwhelmingly to the role of environmental factors in determining risk. It seems, however, that the role of environmental factors is not as simple as, for example, the role of cigarette smoking in lung cancer where a single factor is the major determinant of risk. High risk for esophageal cancer usually results from the interaction of several factors, in particular environmental factors which modify host or tissue susceptibility. Elucidating the mechanism by which these interactions operate should not only provide insight into how practical intervention might be achieved, but also may serve as a more general model for carcinogenesis in humans. The purpose of this chapter is to give the evidence supporting these conclusions, presenting the worldwide occurrence of the disease and reviewing the many analytic epidemiological studies that have been performed.

Descriptive epidemiology

General occurrence

The occurrence of esophageal cancer throughout the world, on a country basis, is reasonably well reflected by the mortality figures since the disease is normally fatal. Table 1 gives the age-standardized rates for a range of countries (1,2). The high rates for both males and females in China is the most noteworthy feature, demonstrating that although relatively rare in the West, esophageal cancer is a major disease for a large proportion of the world's population. The country-wide

Correa, P. and Haenszel, W. (eds.), Epidemiology of Cancer of the Digestive Tract.
© *1982 Martinus Nijhoff Publishers. The Hague/Boston/London. ISBN-13:978-94-009-7504-0*

22

Table 1. Age-standardized mortality rates/10^5 per year for esophageal cancer in selected countries[a] (adjusted to the world standard population).

Country	Males	Females
China[b]	31.7	15.9
Singapore	14.4	2.3
Puerto Rico	13.6	5.2
Chile	9.8	5.0
Switzerland	7.2	0.8
Japan	7.1	1.6
Scotland	7.1	3.7
Ireland	5.8	3.8
England & Wales	5.5	2.9
Costa Rica	5.3	2.0
Paraguay	5.3	1.4
New Zealand	5.2	2.0
Australia	4.4	1.8
USA	4.3	1.1
Belgium	3.9	0.8
Federal Republic of Germany	3.8	0.7
Austria	3.8	0.5
Iceland	3.7	4.1
The Netherlands	3.2	1.2
Sweden	3.1	0.8
Denmark	3.0	1.1
German Democratic Republic	2.8	0.5
Greece	2.0	0.7
Rumania	1.9	0.5

[a] WHO (1).
[b] Li (2).

figures for mortality available globally can be supplemented by incidence figures from 'Cancer Incidence in Five Continents' for within-country comparison for some regions, as shown in Table 2 (3,4,5).

High rates among blacks, particularly males, in the cities of southern Africa are noteworthy. Lower but still relatively high rates are seen among the Chinese in Singapore and the Indians in Bombay, in parts of Japan, of the Caribbean and of Latin America, and among blacks in the United States. Among most of the populations shown in Tables 1 and 2, there is a large male excess of the disease, except among the three Indian populations (Bombay, Singapore, Natal), and parts of Scandinavia and the United Kingdom. In the rest of Europe female rates are extremely low.

Tables 1 and 2 give a general view of the frequency of esophageal cancer, but they do not reveal the remarkable variation in incidence that is exhibited within small areas.

Table 2. Annual incidence rates/10^5 population (adjusted to the world standard population) of esophageal cancer in different populations in the world.

Population	Males	Females
AFRICA		
Mozambique		
Lourenço Marques[a]	4.4	0.0
Nigeria		
Ibadan	1.5	1.1
Rhodesia		
Bulawayo - African	63.8	2.2
South Africa		
Johannesburg - Bantu[a]	12.9	1.2
Cape Province - Bantu[b]	37.5	14.3
Natal - African[b]	40.9	12.3
Cape Province - coloured[b]	10.1	0.0
Natal - Indian[b]	5.5	12.9
Cape Province - white[b]	4.4	1.0
LATIN AMERICA		
Brazil		
Recife	5.2	1.6
Sao Paulo	13.1	2.2
NORTH AMERICA		
USA		
Alameda - black	13.2	2.9
San Francisco Bay area - black	15.2	3.7
Detroit - black	14.1	3.7
San Francisco Bay area - Chinese	9.2	1.8
Detroit - white	4.0	1.1
San Francisco Bay area - white	4.0	1.9
Alameda - white	3.6	1.5
New Mexico - Spanish	2.2	1.1
El Paso - Spanish	6.7	0.9
New Mexico - American Indian	1.4	0.0
Hawaii		
Hawaiian	8.0	1.6
Chinese	4.7	0.0
Philipino	4.5	0.0
Japanese	3.6	0.1
Caucasian	4.7	1.9
ASIA		
India		
Bombay	15.2	10.8
Singapore		
Chinese	20.0	6.4
Malay	2.0	3.7
Indian	5.6	5.9
EUROPE		
Norway		
urban	4.0	0.8
rural	1.9	0.6
OCEANIA		
New Zealand		
European	3.8	1.8
Maori	1.1	0.8

[a] Taken from Cancer Incidence in Five Continents, Volume I (3).
[b] Taken from Cancer Incidence in Five Continents, Volume II (4).
The remaining rates are taken from Cancer Incidence in Five Continents, Volume III (5).

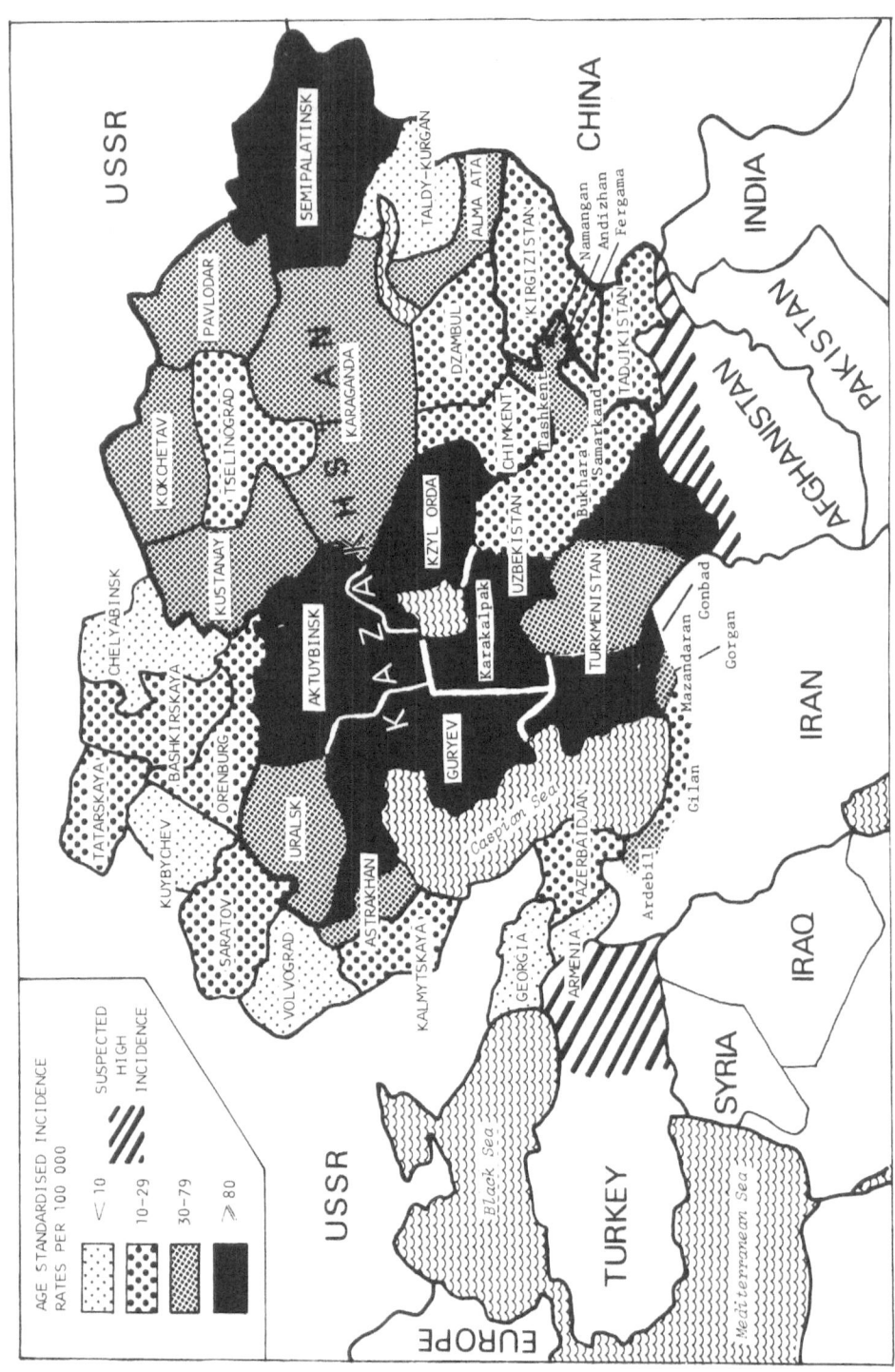

Figure 1. Incidence rates, standardized to the world population, of esophageal cancer among males in Central Asia.

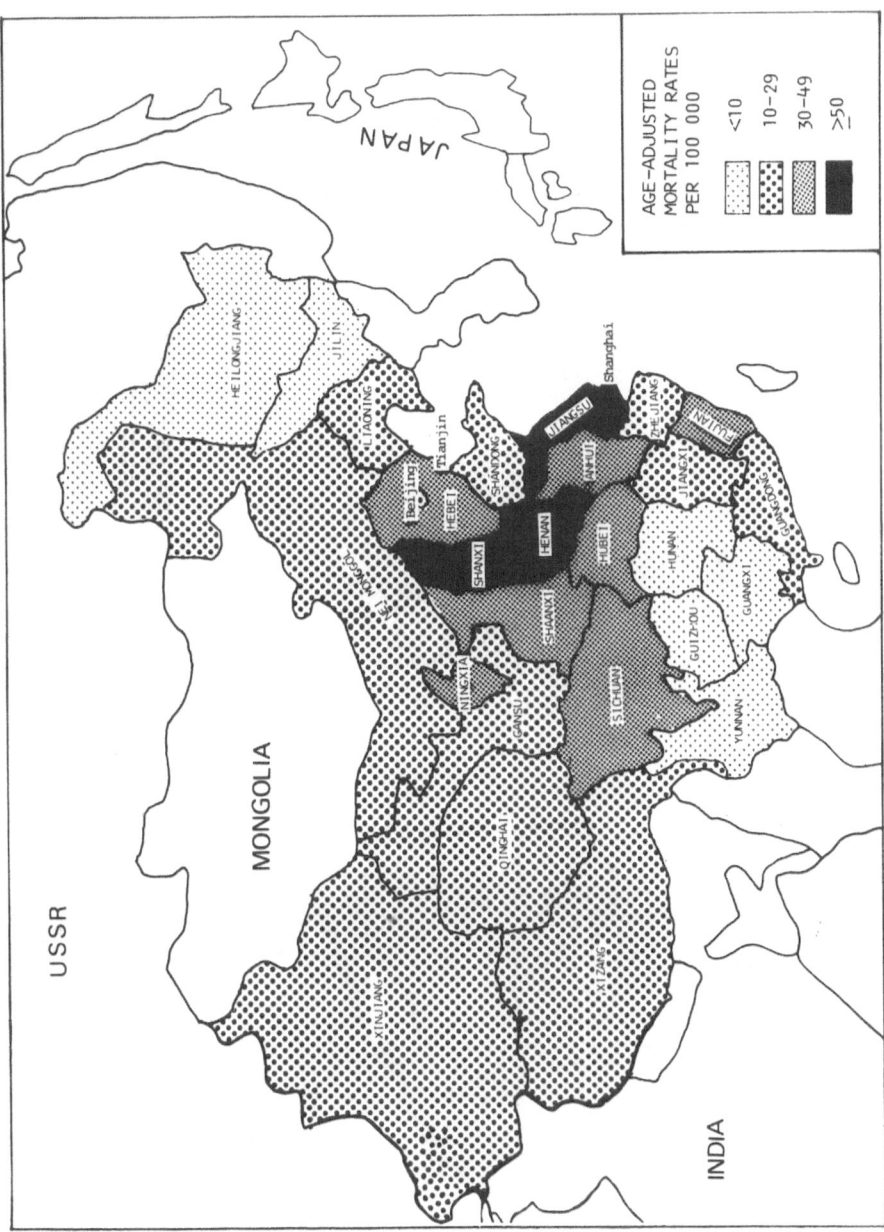

Figure 2. Mortality rates of esophageal cancer, standardized to the world population, among males in China.

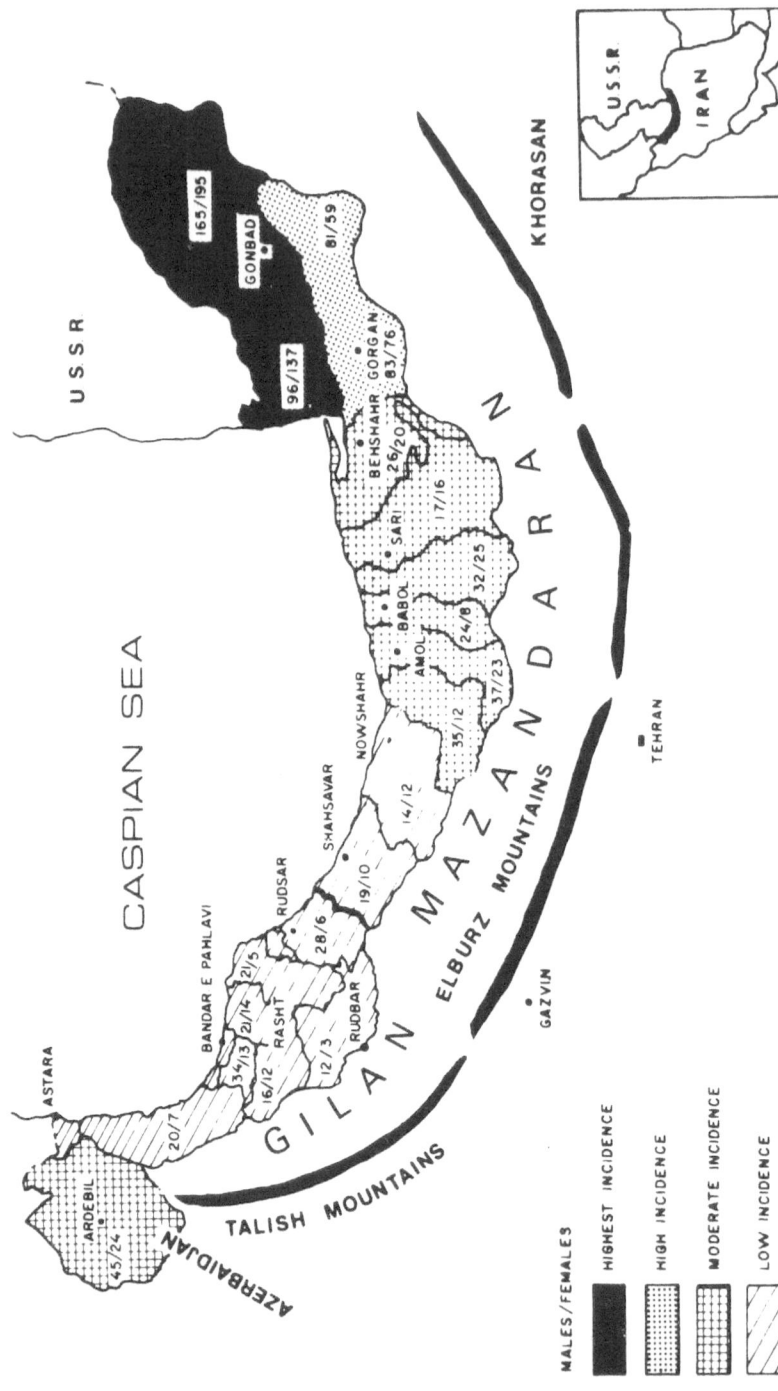

Figure 3. Incidence rates of esophageal cancer, standardized to the world population, among males and females in the Caspian littoral of Iran.

Table 3. Changing sex ratio of esophageal cancer incidence in the Asian cancer belt.

Population	Ratio of male to female incidence[a]	Incidence[a] rate in females
Kazakhstan[b]		
Guryev	0.76	174.3
Kzyl Orda	0.95	99.5
Aktyubinsk	1.44	78.4
Uralsk	1.10	58.7
Semipalatinsk	2.17	40.4
Chimkent	2.45	12.0
Turkmenistan[c]		
West	1.24	92.8
North	2.08	16.9
Tadjikistan	2.75	6.8
Russian SFSR[d]	2.48	4.4
Iran, Caspian region[e]		
South Gonbad	0.85	195.3
South Gorgan	1.09	76.9
Central Mazandaran	1.68	14.3
Gilan	3.59	4.9

[a] Incidence rates, age adjusted to the world population.
[b] Nugmanov & Kolycheva (127).
[c] Nuryagdev (128).
[d] Serenko & Tserkovnogo (129).
[e] Mahboubi et al. (130).

Areas of special interest

Asia. The feature of greatest interest in the occurrence of esophageal cancer is the appearance of very sharp changes in incidence, with the risk in some circumscribed areas rising to rates higher than those seen for almost any other cancer anywhere in the world. Many of these areas are seen in the belt of land running from Turkey to eastern China. Anatolia (6), northeast Iran, the muslim republics of the USSR (7), northern Afghanistan (8) and, in China, the provinces of Xingiang, Henan, Jiansu, Shanxi and Sichuan all lie in this belt (2). Figures 1 and 2 show the overall distribution in the region, the wide range in incidences being apparent. (In this section the words incidence and mortality are used interchangeably, an approximation which may be justified for esophageal cancer since survival is very poor, and in this instance by the fact that for some areas only morbidity figures are available, whereas for others only mortality has been collected.) Within this region, there are foci of special interest, where the change in incidence is especially sharp. The province of Mazandaran in Iran is one (Fig. 3) (9), and in China several such localities have been identified (2), namely: (a) The Tai-Hang mountain area at the border of Henan, Hebei and Shanxi provinces (Fig. 4); (b) Northern Sichuan (Fig. 5); (c) The Da-bie mountain area on

28

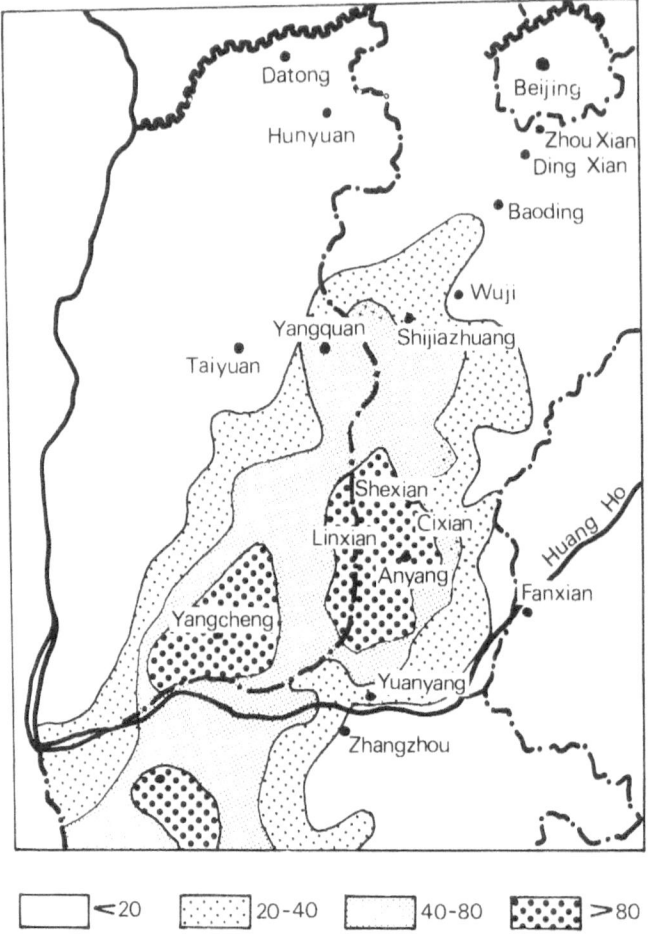

Figure 4. Esophageal cancer mortality rate distribution in areas of the Taihang mountain.

the border of Anhui and Hebei province; (d) South Fukien and regions of northeastern Guangdong; (e) The northern area of Jiansu Province; (f) Northern Xingiang area where the population is mainly of Kazakh nationality.

Throughout Soviet Central Asia, one can see patches of very high incidence, around Guryev and in Turkmenia to the east of the Caspian area close to the Aral sea and further east in Semipalatinsk, north of Mongolia and in northern and eastern Siberia (7).

In most of the area shown in Figs. 1 and 2, the male excess seen in Tables 1 and 2 diminishes as the incidence rises, and in some areas of highest incidence there is even an excess among females. This changing sex ratio is shown in Table 3.

A further noteworthy point is the association with ethnic group. Throughout Iran, Afghanistan, Soviet Central Asia and western China, the highest rates are

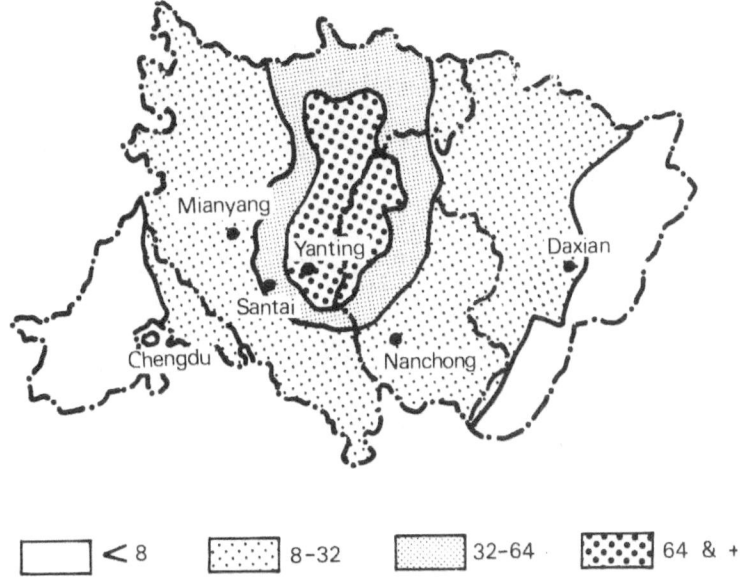

Figure 5. Esophageal cancer mortality rate distribution in North Sichuan.

found among people of Mongol or Turkic origin, such as the Kazakh, Uzbek, Turkoman in northeast Iran, and the Turkoman and Uzbek in Afghanistan. Among neighboring populations of Caucasian origin, Russians or Tadjiks in the Soviet Union, Persians in Iran, much lower rates are seen. In northern and eastern Siberia, the population groups with high rates, the Yakuts, Chukchi, Eskimos, Evenki and Yukagir (7), are again of basic Mongol origin. The related people of Alaska, Greenland and The Aleutian Islands are also reported to have had high rates which are now declining (10, 11).

In Xingiang, the highest rates are seen among the Kazakhs, followed by the Mongols. The Uighurs have considerably lower rates. The pattern seen in southeast China is partially reflected in the incidence rates recorded in Singapore (12). The two dialect groups with high rates, the Hokkien and the Teochew, come respectively from Fukien Province and the Swatow region of Guangdong Province, noted above as a high incidence area in China. The Cantonese-speaking group, by contrast, has low rates, as found in most of Guangdong Province (13).

Africa. Throughout much of eastern and southern Africa, similar sharp changes in incidence are seen, although in west and north Africa the disease appears to be rare. In addition to the urban populations given in Table 2, the central and western areas of Kenya including Nairobi, the southern half of Malawi together with the adjacent regions of Zambia, and the Transkei and the Ciskei to the

30

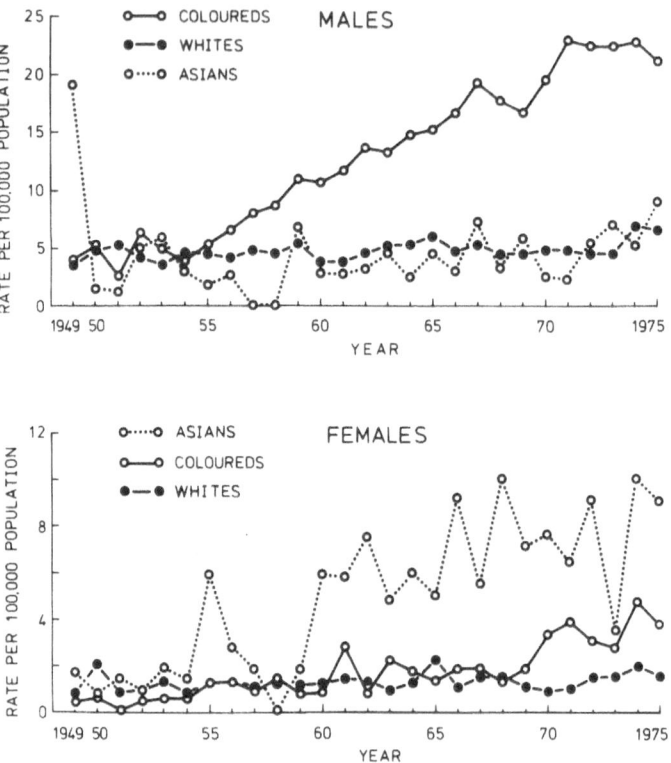

Figure 6. Time trends in mortality rates for esophageal cancer, standardized to the world population, in southern Africa. From Rose (21).

south, all have high relative frequency of the disease (14, 15, 16, 17).

Contiguous with the areas of high incidence are areas where the disease is rare, thus showing changes similar to the steep gradients in incidence seen in central Asia. Throughout most of Tanzania and Uganda, in northern Zambia and northern Malawi, in Mozambique and in most of rural southern Africa and Namibia, the incidence is low (15).

In Kenya, Malawi and Zambia the disease is predominantly one of males, with sex ratios (M:F) over 10:1, but in southern Africa there is a tendency for the sex ratio to fall with increasing incidence. In the Transkei, where the highest incidence rates are found, the M:F ratio approaches 1.5:1 and is lowest where the incidence is highest.

Interest has centered on the Transkei not only because of the high incidence, but also because within its borders, an area less than one hundred and fifty by one hundred miles, the variation in incidence is very marked (18).

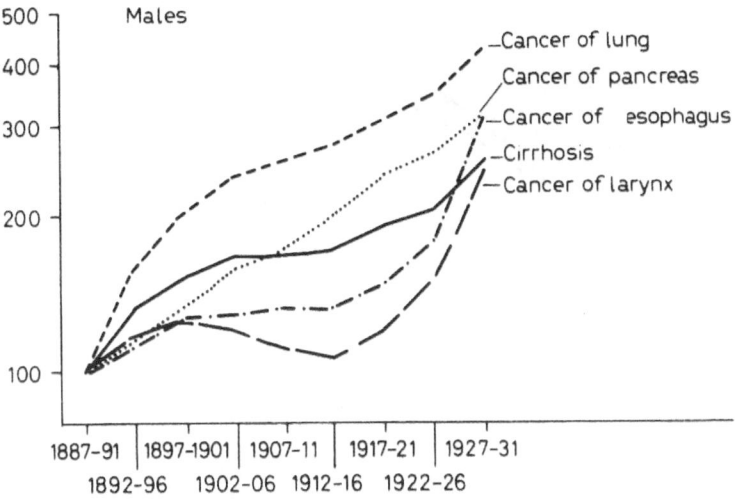

Figure 7. Increasing mortality from various cancers and from liver cirrhosis in successive cohorts in France. From Tuyns & Audigier (22).

France. The other country where very high rates are seen is France, and within France, there is also marked variation in the incidence of esophageal cancer (19). Of even greater interest than the variation between Departments, is the variation observed between the different communes of the high incidence area of Brittany (20). Both the level of risk and the steepness of the variation are striking.

Time trends. In China, the high rates of esophageal cancer do not seem to be of recent origin. Published time trends (2, 13), indicate that the rates have remained stable for at least forty years, and reports from the early medical literature indicate that the disease was common in northern China two thousand years ago. From what is now northeast Iran, the disease was described in the thirteenth century, indicating that it has also been common in that area for a long time.

In southern Africa the disease has been increasing rapidly among blacks (Fig. 6), especially males (16, 21). This increase is particularly well documented in the large cities. A similar increase has been seen among blacks in the United States, especially in the northern cities. In Europe, the rate has been increasing among males in France, where cohorts born since 1910 have experienced a sharply increasing rate (22). A similar increase is seen in the mortality from cancer of the larynx, and from cirrhosis (Fig. 7). In Switzerland, by contrast, the rates have been decreasing, as they have in much of Scandinavia, especially Finland (23). In England and Wales, a large fall in esophageal cancer rates occurred in the first fifty years of this century. Since 1950, however, the decline has reversed and a considerable increase has been observed (24). A similar picture has been described in Australia (Fig. 8) (25).

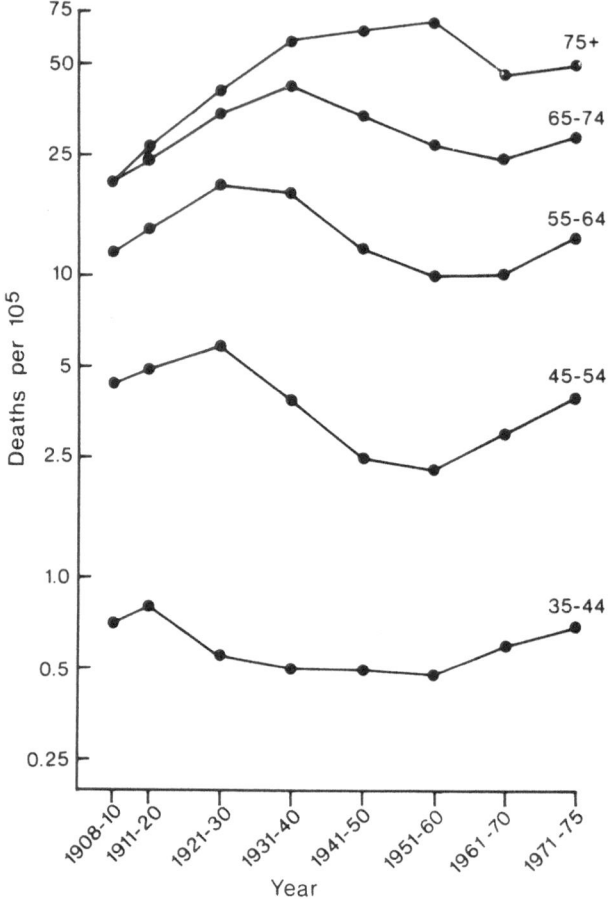

Figure 8. Age-specific death rates, by calendar decade, for cancer of the esophagus: Australian men, 1908–1975. From McMichael (25).

Summary of descriptive epidemiology

In many areas of the world where this cancer is frequent, one sees sharply changing rates. Both the levels that the incidence attains and the rapidity of the changes over short geographic distances are greater than are seen for other cancers. In areas of northern Iran or of China, the cumulative rate to age 75 reaches 20–25%, the same order of magnitude as the rate for lung cancer among heavy cigarette smokers. It is also noteworthy that, apart from special situations such as northwest France or Switzerland where there is high alcohol intake among males, as the rate increases so does the relative proportion of female cases. Most of the areas where the disease is common are poor, and populations among whom rates have risen, such as blacks in southern Africa, have in some way or another suffered preceding impoverishment.

Exogenous causative factors

Alcohol and dietary deprivation appear to be the major determinants of the variation in risk between different populations. Both may act finally by a similar physiological pathway, but in terms of identifiable external factors the two are distinct. To display their full effect, both need to act in conjunction with other factors, which are characteristically carcinogen-mutagens such as tobacco smoke condensates. In Western countries, the main emphasis has been on alcohol and tobacco, but in less developed countries areas of high incidence seem to arise when other particular combinations of exposures and deficiency occur. We shall consider in the following the role of different agents as they have been identified.

Alcohol, tobacco and other smoking and drinking habits

Early studies (26, 27, 28, 29) showed an increase in risk associated with alcohol and tobacco, an association which was studied in some detail in the United States by Wynder & Bross (30). They showed that the two factors combined multiplicatively to increase risk, and that the risk rose smoothly with increasing consumption of either. The total proportion of the risk attributable to the two factors together was some 76%. A considerably higher risk was seen among spirit drinkers than among those who drank beer only.

A similar study in the Department of Ille-et-Vilaine in Brittany (31) arrived at similar results, with multiplicative combined action and high risks associated with high consumption of either. From the Brittany data the joint dose response can be put in the form.

$$\text{Relative risk} = \text{Exp} \, (0.025 \times \text{ALC}) \, (\text{TOB} + 1)^{0.54},$$

where ALC is the average daily ethanol intake, in grams, and TOB is the average quantity of tobacco smoked daily, in grams (32). The exponential increase in risk associated with increasing alcohol intake shows the dominant effect of alcohol at high exposure levels, in contrast to the sub-linear increase in risk with increasing tobacco smoking. Unlike other studies, no difference was seen between the risk induced by different types of drink.

The risk attributable to drinking more than 40 g of alcohol/day and/or smoking 10 g or more/day of tobacco can be estimated in Brittany at some 83%.

Martinez (33) reported a case-control study performed in Puerto Rico. Al-

Table 4. Relative risks[a] of esophageal cancer by daily amount of alcohol consumed, in hard liquor equivalents.

Hard liquor equivalent (fluid ounces per day)	Number of cases	Number of controls	Relative risk
None	5	55	1.0
1.0– 5.9	16	44	4.0
6.0–14.9	25	50	5.5
15.0–29.9	25	36	7.6
30.0–80.6	19	28	7.5

[a] From Pottern et al. (35).

cohol and tobacco are both major risk factors, particularly among males, where the attributable risks are 52% and 47%, respectively, the corresponding values for females being 17% and 39%. Little excess risk is seen among those drinking solely beer; among those drinking spirits, the greatest risk is among those who drink them straight. Although among males the risk attributable to these two factors, when added, approaches 100%, other factors are also of importance, as we shall discuss in later sections.

Hirayama (34) has reported the results of a prospective study conducted in Japan. The excess risk associated with alcohol was highest for whiskey and shochu (a local liqueur) and lowest for beer.

A study (35) has recently been performed among the black male population of Washington DC, whose rate of esophageal cancer is the highest in the United States. The major risk factor was alcohol, heavy consumption being seen even in the controls (Table 4). The attributable risk for alcohol was reported as 81%. Tobacco played a less important role, and even after excluding from the control group those with smoking-related causes of death the relative risk for heavy smoking (two or more packs of cigarettes per day) was only 2.1 after adjusting for alcohol consumption. A higher risk was seen for spirit drinkers than for beer and wine drinkers, within the same range of total alcohol intake, and among spirit drinkers the risk was highest among those who drank their spirits straight.

In view of the risks associated with alcohol and tobacco, it is of interest to look at the esophageal cancer rates among groups who either do not smoke or are presumed neither to smoke nor drink. Several such groups have been studied in the United States. Among US Veterans (males) Rogot & Murray (36) report a risk among non-smokers only 28% of that expected based on general population rates; from the American Cancer Society prospective study (37) Garfinkel reports a standardized mortality ratio (SMR) for non-smokers of 40% for males and 62% for females; Enstrom & Godley (38), from a representative sample of non-smokers in the United States, give corresponding figures of 55% and 80%; for Seventh Day Adventists, SMRs of 36% for males and 30% for females are

Table 5. Relative risks for esophageal cancer among smokers and ex-smokers.

A.	Current smokers (cigarettes only)		
	Number smoked/day	Esophageal cancer[a]	Esophageal cancer[b]
	< 10	3.06	
	10–20	4.34	
	21–40	12.42	
	> 40	9.20	
	All smokers	6.43	6.1
B.	Ex-smokers		
	Interval since quitting	Esophageal cancer[a]	Esophageal cancer[b]
	< 5 years	4.77	2.9
	5–9 years	2.50	
	10–14 years	2.06	1.2
	15–19 years	1.21	
	≥ 20 years	2.48	

[a] Rogot (42).
[b] Doll & Peto (41).

reported (based on only two cases) (39), whereas for Mormons (40) the figures are 45% and 69%, although for active Mormon males a lower figure of 22% has been noted. In general, as we might expect, the SMRs are closer to 1 for females than for males.

For those who give up one or both of the two addictions, only scanty information is available. Among ex-smokers, the prospective studies of British doctors (41) and of US Veterans (42) give similar figures (Table 5), corroborated by the case-control findings of Wynder (43) (Fig. 9). In none of the studies, however, was adjustment made for the drinking habits of the ex-smokers.

The results from Puerto Rico (33) suggest a large reduction in risk ten years or more after giving up alcohol, but neither level of former alcohol consumption nor tobacco consumption is given, rendering the interpretation less clear.

In the United Kingdom (24) and Australia (25), the dominant effect of alcohol is apparent on examining time trends. The steep fall in the rate of esophageal cancer in the two countries that took place in the first half of this century parallels a fall in total alcohol consumption (Fig. 10). Since the mid 1950s, esophageal cancer has been moving up fairly sharply, and a corresponding increase in alcohol consumption began a few years earlier. The trends for spirits in alcohol consumption began a few years earlier. In the United Kingdom a high correlation (0.82 for males, 0.91 for females) has been found between the standardized cohort mortality ratio and per capita ethanol consumption of the general population when the cohort of interest was aged 25–29. If the parallelism of the trends

36

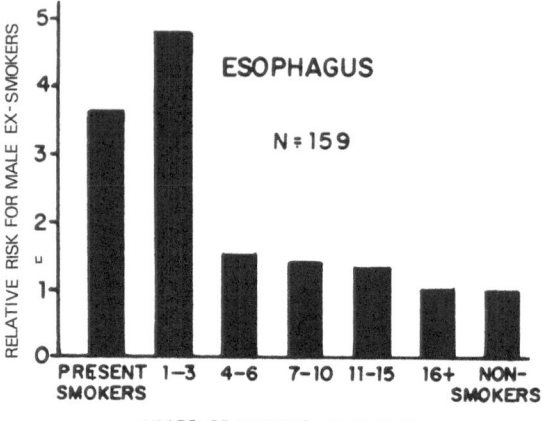

Figure 9. Relative risk of male ex-smokers for esophageal cancer, by years since stopping smoking. From Wynder (43).

between alcohol consumption and esophageal cancer rates reflect a causal relationship, then the immediacy with which changes in alcohol consumption affect the cancer rates would suggest that alcohol has principally an effect on the late stages of carcinogenesis, bearing out a speculation by Boyland that alcohol acts as a promoter.

Outside the industrialized countries, the situation is different. In northern Iran, alcohol and tobacco contribute little to the overall risk (44), no effect being seen for chewing tobacco (nass) (45), a habit sometimes suggested as being of importance in determining the high rates in Soviet Central Asia. Recent work from China (2) does not indicate a substantial role for these factors, nor does a study among the Chinese in Singapore (46), where the incidence is particularly high among those born in China. Alcohol and tobacco hardly play a role, although both were identified as risk factors.

Jussawalla (47) gives a comprehensive review of the role of smoking, chewing and drinking habits in Bombay, where esophageal cancer is about equally common in males and females. A summary of the findings is given in Table 6. Alcohol on its own does not appear to play a role. In conjunction with smoking, drinking local brews containing a high proportion of raw spirits is associated with particularly high risk, as is smoking the local type of cigarette, the bidi. As can be seen, combined exposures lead to particularly high risks. Of great interest is the inability of chewing, smoking or drinking to explain more than a small fraction of the incidence in females, although these factors explain a large fraction of the incidence in males. Few women indulge in more than one of the three different habits, and few drink alcohol. In contrast to the oral cavity, for

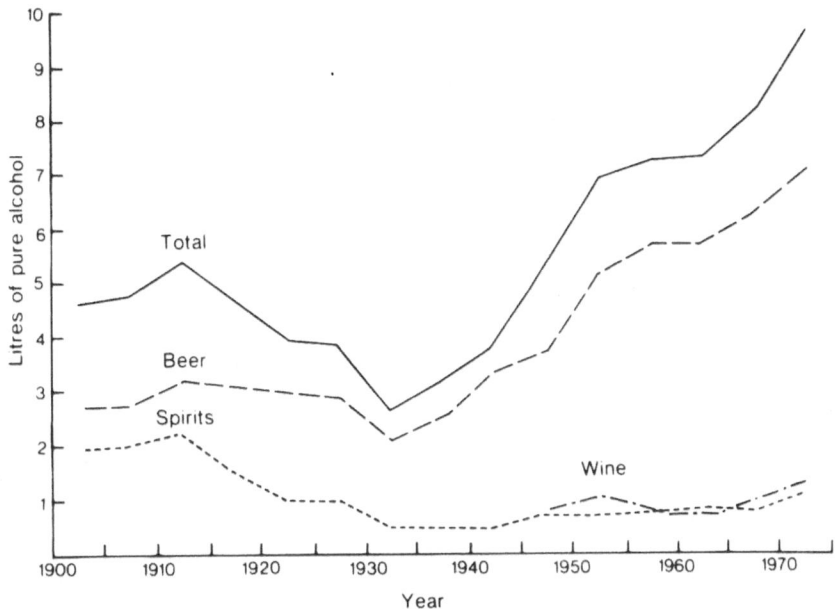

Figure 10. Time trends in per capita consumption of alcohol in beer, wine and spirits, Australia, 1900–1975. From McMichael (25).

which 70% of tumors are attributable to chewing and smoking, the figure for the esophagus is only 50%, both sexes combined (48).

Among Africans in South Africa, in the urban areas, several case-control studies have been reported relating esophageal cancer to tobacco use (17, 49, 50). Alcohol has not been incriminated as an important risk factor, the only alcoholic drink legally available until the last decade being beer (in recent years, spirits have been legalized). Bradshaw & Schonland (49) reported a study of African males from Johannesburg, some results of which are given in Table 7, together with the results of an early study from Durban. The higher risk for pipe tobacco, in contrast to cigarettes, is of note, particularly in view of the more frequent use of pipe tobacco among the Xhosa, coming from the Transkei. In the Transkei itself, the smoking of homegrown tobacco in pipes is more common in cases than controls (51). Tobacco use appears to have a potent carcinogenic effect on the esophagus of Africans in South Africa, and appears to underlie at least part of the variation in incidence in the Transkei.

Unusual practices associated with pipe smoking have been described in the Transkei (52). The residues in the stem (injonga) are sucked out through a straw and swallowed, and the residues in the bowl of the pipe (isixaxa) are scraped out and then chewed. These residues have demonstrated mutagenic activity in the Ames test (53) at a considerably higher level on a weight basis than cigarette

38

Table 6. Relative risk for esophageal cancer associated with combinations of smoking, chewing and drinking, in Bombay.[a]

	Males	Females
Smoking		
Bidi	8.0	7.4
w. cigarettes	2.8	—[b]
both types	37.5	—[b]
Chewing		
betel with tobacco	2.9	1.8
betel without tobacco	15.9	6.3
Alcohol		
foreign brew	2.4	—[b]
local brew	12.0	—[b]
Smoking and chewing		
with tobacco	24.4	4.9
without tobacco	94.2	—
Smoking and alcohol use	18.1	—[b]
Chewing and alcohol use	12.0	—[b]
Smoking alone	4.2	17.8
Chewing alone	4.2	17.8
Alcohol use alone	0.4	—[b]

[a] Based on Jussawalla (47).
[b] Insufficient numbers for a relative risk estimate.

smoke condensates (54). An interesting parallel is seen in northeastern Iran, where the eating of residues from opium pipes is widespread in both sexes. These opium residues have a mutagenic activity in the Ames test at the same level, per unit weight, as that of the Transkei tobacco pyrolysates (53). Unlike other areas of Iran, where opium use is reported to be primarily a male habit (55), in the high incidence population of northern Iran the use among males and females is about equal (56), as also appears to be the case in northern Afghanistan (57) where esophageal cancer is also common in both sexes.

In summary, in Europe and the United States the great majority of cases of esophageal cancer arise from the combined multiplicative effect of alcohol and tobacco. Most of the evidence suggests that the stronger the habitual form of alcohol, the higher will be the risk. It is still unclear whether alcohol on its own has a carcinogenic effect, although the question may not be well posed, since, given the detectable risk for lung cancer among non-smoking passive smokers, all substantial alcohol drinkers may be to some extent smokers. In other areas of the world, the dominant effect of alcohol is not apparent, but smoking or chewing in various forms may be, or has shown to be, important, as in southern Africa, India and Iran.

Table 7. Relative risks associated with various smoking and drinking habits in South Africa.[a]

	Johannesburg	Durban
Tobacco		
none	1.0	1.0
cigarettes	2.3	0.8
pipe tobacco	3.7	2.3
cigarettes and pipe tobacco	5.0	8.5
Alcohol		
none	1.0	1.0
local	1.3	1.0
western	2.0	1.9

[a] Adapted from Bradshaw & Schonland (49).

Dietary insufficiency

A common theme running through the results of many analytic studies of the epidemiology of esophageal cancer is the association of the disease with poverty and a restricted diet (58). Most populations with a high incidence are poor, although not all poor populations have a high incidence and, within such populations, those who develop the disease come from the lower socio-economic groups. In many studies the low economic level is reflected in poor diet.

Wynder & Bross (30) in a study mainly of Caucasians in New York, found a substantially lower intake among cases of green and yellow vegetables, milk, butter and eggs. In a study of US blacks in Washington, DC, Pottern and her coworkers (35) report a lower intake of fresh and frozen meat, dairy products, eggs, and fruit and vegetables. Martinez (33) reports a low intake of fresh vegetables and fruits, with eggs and meat, in the Puerto Rican population at high risk. From Japan, Hirayama (34) reports a lower consumption of fruit and meat among cases than controls in a study conducted in the prefectures of Nara, Wakayama and Mie, where the incidence is high. In the Asian esophageal cancer belt, the areas of high incidence have low rainfall, and cultivation of vegetables is difficult (9). A similar pattern is seen in China (2); in Xingiang, the high risk Kazakhs have much lower consumption of fruit and vegetables than the lower risk Mongols or Uighurs. In Sichuan, the amount of fresh vegetables in the diet is inversely related to the esophageal cancer incidence, and in Hebei Province migrants from high incidence regions eat less vegetables, beans, fish, meat and eggs than the lower risk indigenous population. In northern Iran, the population in the high incidence area has a notably low intake of vegetables and fruit and a much higher proportion of protein intake is derived from the staple food, bread (56). In a case-control study, even in the areas of restricted diet, the cases consumed less fruit and vegetables and generally had a more limited diet, than a control group matched for village of residence (45). In the Soviet Union, Kolicheva (7) refers to the poor diet among the indigenous groups in northern and eastern Siberia, with low intake of fruit and vegetables. By contrast, the case-control study in Brittany did not demonstrate any particular dietary limitation (59) among the cases, but, as discussed later, the nutritional status of those with high alcohol intake cannot be determined solely from their food consumption.

In addition to studies incriminating specific dietary factors, other studies have more generally shown a lower socio-economic level among cases. In the United States, the Ten City Survey of 1947 showed a smooth decrease in risk with income, the poorest group having some two and a half times the incidence of the richest group. The case-control study reported by Wynder & Bross (30) found lower educational status among the cases, as well as a poorer dietary history. Duration of schooling was also found to be inversely related to risk of eso-phageal cancer in a case-control study in Singapore (42). In Puerto Rico, Mar-tinez (33) showed, in addition to the effects of alcohol and tobacco, that the disease was more common in the lower income groups. Farmers and agricultural workers had twice the risk of managerial and professional workers (60).

Thermal irritation

Hot drinks and food have often been linked to esophageal cancer, but the temperature at which food and drink are taken is a difficult variable to study. The unsatisfactory nature of investigations into the temperature at which food or beverages are consumed is demonstrated by a study of the rise in temperature at the lower end of the esophagus subsequent to swallowing measured quantities of coffee kept at a controlled temperature (61). The quantity, rather than the temperature, of the coffee drunk per sip was the determinant factor.

In addition, responses to questions on the temperature at which one takes one's drink or food are necessarily subjective and open to various biases. Never-theless, accepting all the caveats there is a certain accumulation of data suggest-ing an effect.

In Japan, Segi (62) has shown that the prevalence of taking rice gruel cooked in hot tea parallels the mortality from esophageal cancer. In a case-control study in high incidence prefectures, Hirayama confirmed this association at the indi-vidual level, persons taking hot tea gruel (chegayu) at least once a day having twice the risk of those consuming it less frequently (34). Hirayama (60), in his prospective study, also showed an increased risk associated with drinking hot green tea. Martinez (33), in the Puerto Rican study already referred to, found that more esophageal cancer cases than controls claimed to drink their coffee hot rather than warm or cold.

De Jong et al. (46), reporting a study from Singapore, indicate not only an apparently higher frequency among cases of those who claim to drink beverages 'burning hot', but also a higher frequency among Hokkien or Teochew-speaking controls, as opposed to Cantonese-speaking controls. Habitual temperature at which beverages are drunk might thus explain partially the dialect group differences in incidence. In northern Iran, surveys have suggested that inhabitants of the high risk areas drink their tea at hotter temperatures (64), drink more tea per day, and drink less water (56) than do residents of the lower risk area but the differences are not large. Results of a case-control study indicated similar differences between esophageal cancer cases and controls (45), but also between gastric cancer cases and controls. Experimentally, tea extracts have been reported to have a promoting action in mouse skin carcinogenesis (65).

In the Soviet Union, the high rates in the Central Asian Republic are commonly supposed to be related to the high consumption of strong hot tea. The native population of northern and eastern Siberia, with high esophageal cancer rates, are also reported to be heavy drinkers of hot tea (7).

Thus, although the range of evidence from prospective studies, case-control studies and population comparisons, is persuasive that an effect exists, the degree of risk, and the extent to which risk in certain populations is attributable to it, is in doubt.

Other exogenous factors

Like most tissues, the esophagus is susceptible to the carcinogenic effects of ionizing radiation. Data from the A-bomb survivors (66) and from the cohort treated by radiation for ankylosing spondylitis (67) demonstrate the effect.

The follow-up of 17,800 insulation workers in North America (68) suggests that asbestos increases risk for the disease, with 18 cases observed when only 7.01 were expected. Cicatricial strictures of the esophagus due to the ingestion of lye occasionally give rise to malignant tumors. Vinson (69), writing forty years ago, stated that malignancy is rarely, if ever, observed in benign strictures arising from other causes. Lye, however, was formerly responsible for some 60% of strictures, which may also have been more severe. A specific effect for lye is not established.

The eating of bracken fern has been associated with increased risk for esophageal cancer in Japan (34). Daily consumption increases risk two-fold or more compared to less frequent consumption. There has been speculation that the relatively high incidence of the disease in North Wales is in part related to local use of bracken fern.

In the region of Linshien County, in northern China, the consumption of pickled vegetables and of mouldy flour has attracted attention. Both show some degree of mutagenicity in the Ames test (70, 71) and the amount consmed is positively, if rather weakly, associated with esophageal cancer incidence (2). In

Xingiang, mouldy food is also found more frequently in the diet of the Kazakhs than of the Mongols or Uighurs (2).

There is no clear epidemiological evidence that nitrosamines are involved in the etiology of the disease, but this lack may reflect more the limit of present epidemiological and chemical methods, than the underlying biological reality.

The suggestion that syphilis is associated with esophageal cancer was not confirmed by case-control studies (28, 30).

Various occupations have slightly higher risk for the disease, most of which one can assume to have high alcohol consumption (72). Clemmesen also mentions as being elevated risk a group of occupations involving various types of metal work, plumbers, brass and bronze workers, electrical apparatus makers. However, the overall occupational component in the causation of esophageal cancer is probably small.

The use of plants with a high tannin content for infusions, or their consumption by other means, has been mentioned in association with esophageal cancer, particularly in the Caribbean region (73), but no clear analytic results have been published. In northern Iran, silica fibers on seeds which contaminate the wheat have been found in the flour, and their size would indicate a carcinogenic potential (74), but no epidemiological data are available on the actual risk their presence entails.

Host susceptibility

Any hypothesis of carcinogenesis must acknowledge the existence of exogenous carcinogens acting on a host of varying degrees of susceptibility. Most research efforts in the field of esophageal carcinogenesis have been directed towards the identification of environmental carcinogens. As described previously in this chapter, in North America and Western Europe 80% or more of the risk can be attributed to alcohol and tobacco. In the high-risk populations of southern Africa, tobacco use but not alcohol appears the main exogenous risk factor. In Iran, it has been postulated that opium pipe residue may be an important esophageal carcinogen. Specific carcinogens have not yet been identified in the other high-risk populations in Central Asia and in China. In high-risk populations in southern Africa, Central Asia and China, however, it appears that poor diet and an associated increased susceptibility may be the major risk determinants. This susceptibility to esophageal carcinogens is less well understood and could be either genetic or environmentally induced or both.

Environmental susceptibility

A common denominator to high-risk populations for esophageal cancer in many areas of the world is a very restricted diet. It is then possible that specific nutritional deficiencies will increase the susceptibility of the esophagus to known or unknown carcinogens. Lower intake of milk, fruit and fresh vegetables in cancer patients that in controls have been reported in several studies (30, 34, 45). The low intake of these specific food items results in a low intake of vitamins A and C and riboflavin. The association of these vitamin deficiencies with an increased risk of cancer of the upper alimentary tract is illustrated by the Plummer-Vinson or Paterson-Kelly syndrome (75, 76). Although the pathogenesis of this syndrome is not totally clear, deficiencies of iron, riboflavin, thiamin, pyridoxine and vitamin C have been described in these patients (77, 78, 79). These deficiencies are associated with an increased risk of cancer of the hypopharynx and upper esophagus. This condition is now rare, but it used to be common in rural areas of Scandinavia and the United Kingdom (80). The relatively high rates for esophageal cancer in females still seen in northern areas of Norway (81) and rural Wales may be the remnants of a high prevalence of Plummer-Vinson syndrome 40–50 years ago. Among the specific nutritional deficiencies associated with esophageal cancer, riboflavin and zinc deficiencies deserve special attention.

Riboflavin deficiency. This vitamin is an essential factor in maintaining the integrity of the skin and particularly of the squamous epithelium of the esophagus.

The experimental evidence linking riboflavin to cancer is complex. Riboflavin deficiency decreases the rates of growth of some types of spontaneous tumors in experimental animals, specifically mammary tumors and lymphosarcoma in mice and Walker carcinoma in rats (82), but it also causes atrophic changes in the epithelium of the esophagus and fore-stomach of mice. The earliest atrophic changes in the esophagus were observed during the third to fifth week of deficiency and later an epithelial hyperplasia and hyperkeratosis were also noted (83). When mice on a riboflavin-deficient diet for a 3–4 week period were treated with DMBA and croton oil, a strikingly high frequency of skin tumors was observed compared with the two control groups, one on a normal diet and the other on a high riboflavin diet (Fig. 11). Tumors also appeared more rapidly after application of the carcinogen to the skin of animals on a deficient diet than on the control diets (84). Complete riboflavin deficiency in the baboon causes atrophy, ulcers and some hyperplastic esophageal lesions interpreted as precancerous (85, 86). Although the degree of riboflavin deficiency induced experimentally to produce the lesions described in animals has not been documented in man, less extreme deficiencies may contribute the creation of a fertile soil

44

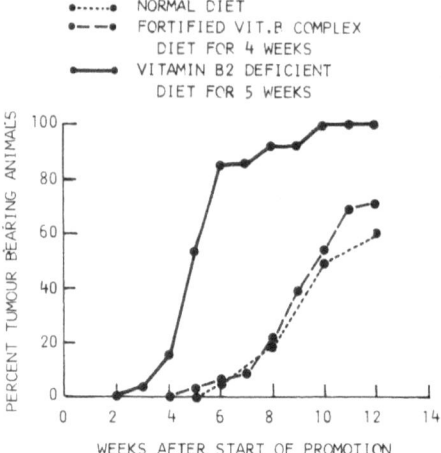

Figure 11. Induction of skin tumors in rats following treatment with DMBA and croton oil, among rats fed a riboflavin deficient diet, a normal diet, and a riboflavin rich diet. From Wynder & Chan (84).

for specific carcinogens.

Clinical and biochemical studies in Iran have confirmed widespread riboflavin deficiency in northern Iran, but this is equally prevalent in the high and low incidence areas for esophageal cancer (87). The earliest instances of angular stomatitis were seen in children aged 2–3 years and the highest frequency and most severe lesions were in schoolchildren and young adults.

Riboflavin deficiency appears to affect both sexes equally and almost all members of the low socio-economic groups of these communities are probably affected for considerable periods during their early years. The strikingly high prevalence (80%) of chronic esophagitis in subjects 15–70 years of age from the high incidence areas of Iran suggests that riboflavin deficiency may be involved in this lesion (88).

Zinc deficiency. Zinc is essential for normal growth and metabolism by virtue of its role in nucleic acid and protein synthesis and its presence in metalloenzymes. Lower concentrations of zinc in blood, hair and esophageal tumor tissue have been reported in patients with esophageal cancer than in matched controls (89), and experimental studies suggest that zinc deficiency enhances the induction of esophageal cancer in rats treated with nitrosobenzylmethylamine (90). It has been demonstrated that high intake of bread high in fiber cases increased fecal excretion of zinc and other minerals, which could lead to zinc deficiencies (91). This observation is of special relevance to the high-incidence populations for esophageal cancer in Iran, whose staple diet is bread. All rural and most urban breads in these regions contain substantial amounts of fiber and phytate. A nutritional survey has revealed that up to 70% of households in these areas receive more than 90% of their protein from bread. However, samples of hair and of nail showed no difference in zinc content between areas of high and low incidence (56).

In the high-risk populations for esophageal cancer in China, low levels of zinc have been reported in the drinking water and in serum, hair and urine specimens of the general population (2).

Genetic susceptibility

A classical example of genetic susceptibility is provided by the segregation of esophageal cancer and *keratosis palmaris et plantaris* (tylosis) observed in some families. The two conditions appear to be due to a single autosomal gene with a dominant effect. This association was originally described in 18 patients with esophageal cancer belonging to two Liverpool families (92). The tylosis in these cases was of the late onset form, appearing after one year of age. The esophageal malignancies have been diagnosed as squamous cell carcinomas arising mostly in the middle and lower thirds of the esophagus. The mean age at onset of cancer was 45 years and the youngest patient was 20 years old. Two additional families with tylosis, in each of which one member has developed esophageal carcinoma, have been reported from Liverpool, in addition to 6 new cases of esophageal cancer in one of the original families (93). In one of them an association between oral leukoplakia and esophageal cancer was also reported (94), which has also been described in a 26-year old patient with esophageal cancer, oral leukoplakia and hyperkeratosis (95). In another family, tylosis has been associated with a congenital esophageal stricture with subsequent development of esophageal carcinoma (96).

This type of genetic susceptibility accounts for only a minimal proportion of esophageal cancers since only a small number of tylosis-associated cancers have been reported. Family studies have also been negative. One of these studies, involving 877 relatives of 101 esophageal cancer patients and 2,572 relatives of control patients, failed to show any influence by hereditary factors, but showed a clear association of this cancer with alcohol abuse (28). Another study from the Soviet Union showed an increase for esophageal cancer among spouses of patients with this cancer, suggesting exposure to common environmental factors rather than a hereditary component (97). In a village in northern Iran, an aggregation of esophageal cancer in one family has been described; the occurrence of 13 cases of esophageal cancer among 19 relatives from 3 generations is striking (95). An unusual proportion of these cases was under age 40, some even being under age 30. Two cousin marriages, plus the remoteness of the village, indicate a high degree of inbreeding in the family.

Case-control studies among the population of northeast Iran, using various genetic markers such as red blood cell enzymes (99) and HLA antigens (100) have, however, yielded negative results. In a recent clinical-endoscopic survey carried out in three villages of the same area, no clear tylosis was detected in 430 individuals examined, although it would be difficult to differentiate it from plantar or palmar hyperkeratosis due to walking barefoot or manual labor (38). As discussed in an earlier section, the populations at high risk in Central Asia and eastern Siberia are of Turkic or Mongol origin. Populations of Caucasian origin in the same region do not suffer the same high rates. The role of genetic factors in this area is in need of further study.

Genetic and environmental susceptibility

Idiopathic steatorrhoea or coeliac disease which seems to result from a combination of genetic and environmental factors has been associated with an increased risk for esophageal cancer. The genetic component is suggested by the familial occurrence with approximately 10% of first-degree relatives affected (101). The mode of inheritance remains to be established but studies of histocompatibility antigens have shown that HLA-B8 and HLA-DW3 are important risk factors for the disease (102, 103). Gluten appears to be the most important environmental factor. Gluten sensitivity which may be dose dependent, will be responsible for the jejunal lesions characterized by villous atrophy resulting in malabsorption. The main symptoms are diarrhea, anemia, weight loss, and some skeletal disorders (104). Since the upper small intestine is the most seriously involved portion of the intestine, deficiencies of iron, folic acid, B12, pyridoxine and vitamins A, C and K have been observed. as well as disturbances of carbohydrate, protein and calcium metabolisms (105). It is of interest to note that severe zinc deficiency has been observed in patients with coeliac disease who do not respond to gluten-free diets (106). Malignant lymphoma of the jejunum has been the most common complication of coeliac disease (107, 108), but an excess of esophageal cancer has also been observed. The patients who developed esophageal cancer have a long history of coeliac disease (mean age 50 years) and the most frequent location of the tumor was middle or lower third (107). An increased incidence of esophageal cancer has also been reported in male relatives of patients with coeliac disease, but no excess of cancer deaths due to lymphoma was observed in relatives of either sex (109).

The increased susceptibility to esophageal cancer in these patients may be the result of both genetic factors and nutritional deficiencies. The long latent period between the onset of coeliac disease and the development of esophageal cancer may favor the nutritional hypothesis.

Precursor lesions

Epithelial dysplasia has been proposed as a precursor lesion of esophageal cancer but little is known about the lesions preceding the dysplasia. The precancerous nature of dysplasia is supported by two types of study: morphological and epidemiological. Morphological studies have shown the presence of dysplasia in the mucosa surrounding in situ or invasive cancers in human surgical specimens (110, 111) and in the esophagus of experimental animals in whom esophageal cancer has been induced following the oral administration of N-nitroso compounds (112, 113). Epidemiological studies have been oriented to determine the prevalence of esophageal dysplasia in low- and high-risk populations for esophageal cancer. They have used post-mortem specimens and cytological smears. Histological examination of the esophagus in 1,000 consecutive autopsies of patients dying from causes unrelated to the esophagus in a low-risk population of the United States revealed a very low frequency of dysplasia (2 cases) and carcinoma in situ (3 cases) (110).

In another post-mortem study, the prevalence of dysplasia in subjects over 40 years of age was compared with the mortality rates of esophageal cancer in three Japanese provinces (114). The prevalence of dysplasia was 37% and did not differ significantly between high- and low-risk provinces, although the severe dysplasia was slightly higher in the high-risk provinces (114).

The low prevalence of esophageal dysplasia (0.2% observed) in the post-mortem study of the United States (110) is not surprising considering the low incidence of esophageal cancer in this population, but the high prevalence (37%) observed in Japan and the lack of correlation with the risk for esophageal cancer are puzzling (114). Possible explanations for these inconsistencies are: (1) there is no clear definition for esophageal dysplasia; (2) irradiation and chemotherapy can produce changes in the esophageal mucosa which resemble dysplastic lesions; patients having received these treatments must therefore be excluded from post-mortem studies (115); lysis post-mortem and poor fixation can also mimic dysplasia.

Preliminary results from a collaborative study including 174 post-mortem specimens from high-risk populations (northern Iran and southern Africa), intermediate-risk (France and Argentina) and low-risk (Mormons from the United States) revealed a prevalence of dysplasia of 15% in the low-risk group, 43% in the intermediate and 55% in the high-risk group (116).

Mass surveys using esophageal cytology have been carried out in the high incidence regions of China. Cytology using an abrasive balloon was obtained in 7,212 subjects over 30 years of age in Linhsien County, Honan Province. In the northern part of the county, where the incidence of esophageal cancer is high, the prevalence rates for mild and severe dysplasia were 26% and 2% respectively and in the south, with lower incidence of esophageal cancer, these rates were 18% and

0.7% respectively (117). In other regions of Honan Province, 21,581 subjects over 30 years of age were examined and the prevalence rates of mild and severe dysplasia were 13% and 1.2%. The prevalence rate of esophageal carcinoma was 0.9%. It was also observed that the frequency of dysplasia increased progressively with age, especially in the case of severe dysplasia. Follow-up studies of 184 individuals with esophageal dysplasia revealed that among the mild dysplasia, 45% regressed to normal, 40% remained unchanged and 15% progressed to severe dysplasia. Out of 79 cases with severe dysplasia 41% regressed to normal or mild dysplasia, 33% remained unchanged and 26% progressed to cancer (118).

Concerning the lesions preceding dysplasia, the information available is very scarce. Although esophageal leukoplakia has been considered as a precursor lesion (119, 120), it is not possible to establish a clear-cut correlation between this lesion and cancer, as there is no agreement in the literature as to its precise definition (121). It has been suggested that the term leukoplakia should be used only when lichen planus, candidiases, white sponge nevus and other specific entities can be excluded (121). Therefore, this term must be used exclusively in a clinical descriptive sense.

In Soviet Central Asia, submucosal fibrosis has been incriminated as a precursor lesion (122), but it has not been reported in other high-risk populations.

To learn about the lesions preceding dysplasia, endoscopic surveys have been carried out in the high-risk populations of northern Iran and central China (88). Esophagoscopy with cytology and biopsies were performed in 430 Iranian subjects aged 15–70 years and 523 Chinese individuals (123). The Iranian findings are summarized in Tables 8 and 9. The endoscopic examination revealed the presence of esophagitis in 85% in Iran and 90% in China. The endoscopic appearance of this lesion is different to that observed in the low-risk populations of Europe and the United States. In low-risk populations, the esophagitis is usually associated with reflux and it is characterized by erosion and ulceration (124, 125). On the other hand, in the high-risk populations of Iran and China, this lesion does not seem to be associated with reflux, as suggested by the low prevalence of incompetent cardias, hiatus hernia and heartburn complaints and by the absence of lesions in the precardial region. Endoscopically this esophagitis was characterized by irregular, swollen and friable mucosa with varying degrees of hyperemia and scattered or confluent leukoplakia but without erosions or ulcerations. Histologically, the lesion was characterized by epithelial changes which include acanthosis with cellular swelling, parakeratosis and desquamation accompanied by varying degrees of lymphoplasmocytic infiltration and vascular proliferation in the lamina propia. In the most severe lesions, epithelial atrophy and dysplasia were observed. These histopathological changes are similar to those observed in rats and non-human primates prior to the induction of esophageal cancer by oral administration of N-nitroso compounds (112, 113). In Iran and China, this chronic esophagitis increases in severity with age and it

Table 8. Endoscopic diagnoses.

Men/age	15–24	25–34	35–44	45–54	≥ 55	Total
Individuals examined	5	17	80	56	60	218
	%	%	%	%	%	%
Normal	40.0	5.9	12.5	7.1	11.7	11.0
Esophagitis						
mild	20.0	52.9	45.0	35.7	26.7	37.6
moderate	40.0	29.4	33.7	39.3	40.0	36.7
severe	0	11.7	7.5	14.3	13.3	11.0
Varices						
single	0	0	6.2	8.9	5.0	5.9
multiple	0	0	8.7	1.8	13.3	7.3
Incompetent cardia	0	5.8	7.5	10.7	5.0	7.3
Hiatal hernia	0	0	2.5	0	0	0.9
Cancer						
suspected	0	0	0	1.8	0	0.5
malignant	0	0	1.3	5.4	1.7	2.3

Women/age	15–24	25–34	35–44	45–54	≥ 55	Total
Individuals examined	5	23	92	61	31	212
	%	%	%	%	%	%
Normal	0	13.0	14.1	3.3	12.9	10.4
Esophagitis						
mild	40.0	65.2	60.8	60.6	54.8	59.9
moderate	60.0	21.7	21.7	21.3	25.8	23.1
severe	0	0	3.3	8.2	6.4	4.7
Varices						
single	0	8.7	4.3	8.2	6.4	6.1
multiple	0	4.3	7.6	24.6	9.6	12.3
Incompetent cardia	0	13.0	6.5	13.1	3.2	8.5
Hiatal hernia	0	0	0	1.6	3.2	0.9
Cancer						
suspected	0	4.3	0	0	0	0.4
malignant	0	0	0	1.6	3.2	0.9

appears to commence early in life, as suggested by the high prevalence even in the age group of 15–20 years. In 90% of the cases it involved the middle and lower thirds of the esophagus, sites most commonly affected by the cancer. The risk factors associated with this chronic esophagitis and in particular its possible association with a deficiency of vitamin A, riboflavin and zinc, are being investigated in ongoing studies in China.

The high prevalence of this lesion in high-risk populations for esophageal cancer in Iran and China suggests that these two lesions are associated with one another. Although the precancerous nature of this chronic esophagitis can only

50

Table 9. Histologic diagnoses.

Men/age	15–24	25–34	35–44	45–54	≥ 55	Total
Individuals examined	5	17	77	54	60	213
	%	%	%	%	%	%
Normal	0	0	5.2	3.7	0	2.8
Esophagitis						
mild	80.0	88.2	58.9	51.8	58.3	58.7
moderate	0	11.8	20.8	29.6	20.0	21.6
severe	0	0	2.6	3.7	3.3	2.8
Acanthosis	80.0	82.4	64.9	55.6	71.7	66.2
Atrophy	0	11.8	10.4	13.0	16.7	12.7
Dysplasia	0	0	5.2	1.9	8.3	4.7
Cancer	0	0	1.3	7.4	1.7	2.8

Women/age	15–24	25–34	35–44	45–54	≥ 55	Total
Individuals examined	5	23	89	59	29	205
	%	%	%	%	%	%
Normal	0	8.7	7.9	3.4	3.4	5.9
Esophagitis						
mild	80.0	69.6	52.8	61.0	51.7	57.6
moderate	0	0	19.1	16.9	31.0	17.6
severe	0	0	1.1	1.7	0	1.0
Acanthosis	80.0	73.9	62.9	67.8	55.2	64.9
Atrophy	20.0	0	9.0	5.1	17.2	8.3
Dysplasia	0	0	4.5	0	6.9	2.9
Cancer	0	0	0	1.7	10.3	2.0

be established by follow-up studies, the following sequence in the natural history of esophageal cancer is proposed: it commences early in life, at least as early as the second decade, with chronic inflammatory changes accompanied by acanthosis, parakeratosis and desquamation of the epithelium, evolving in some cases to epithelial atrophy and dysplasia and finally in a few cases to in situ cancer and later on to invasive cancer.

Summary

The multifactorial nature of the origin of most cancers is widely accepted, but for most cancers little progress has been made in determining what these factors might be, or how they interact. Esophageal cancer appears to provide an excellent model of multifactorial action, where, although not all the components have been unambiguously identified, one can perhaps suggest how different factors take their place in a multistage process of carcinogenesis. One might propose that early stages in carcinogenesis consist of genetic (heritable) damage to the relevant cell, which take place with greater frequency the greater the access to the genetic material of these cells or agents with DNA damaging capability, and that later stages are associated with some form of promoting action. Given the presence of tobacco or opium residues with their mutagenic potential one can then consider the role of modifying agents such as alcohol or dietary deficiency. Alcohol might act in a number of ways. First, as a transport agent in the manner described by Kuratsune (126): alcohol will facilitate the transfer of active agents through the esophageal mucosa to the cells of the basal layer. Secondly, as an irritant: it will lead to an increased turnover of the esophageal epithelium, thereby both increasing the rate at which genetic damage is fixed, and perhaps accelerating the progression through later stages. Thirdly, by inducing nutritional imbalance, since for a number of micronutrients (riboflavin, thiamin, zinc, for example) high alcohol intake will lead to physiological deficiency even though dietary intake appears adequate. The role of these deficiencies has been discussed earlier. Excessively hot food and drink might act, like alcohol, both as a transport agent and as an irritant. Dietary deficiency, acting through dietary-dependent enzyme systems, might alter the rate of activation (or deactivation) of precarcinogens and thus accelerate the early stages; or, as Wynder & Chan (84) showed for riboflavin, their effect on the relevant tissue may be to increase the rate of later stages. The mechanism by which the different factors act is not simply of scientific interest; understanding their nature may lead to practical and effective ways of intervention and primary prevention.

It might be pointed out that the sharp changes in incidence characteristic of the epidemiology of esophageal cancer may be the reflection of multifactor causation. If the joint action of several factors is multiplicative, as is often the case (32), then moderate changes in the distribution of these factors could lead to marked changes in incidence, which only major changes in a single risk factor could bring about. Thus the sharp gradients in incidence seen in central Asia, Brittany or southern Africa may reflect simultaneous changes both in carcinogenic exposure and in susceptibility. It would seem implausible, for example, that a single factor such as cigarette smoking could give rise to the difference between nearby communes in Brittany, and indeed lung cancer which is related mainly to a single factor does not show striking incidence gradients.

References

1. World Health Organization: Age adjusted rates for cancer for selected sites in 46 countries. Segi Institute of Cancer Epidemiology, Nagoya, Japan – 1975–1976.
2. Li JY: The epidemiology of esophageal cancer in China. Proc Third Pacific Rim Conference. 1981.

3. Doll R, Payne P, Waterhouse J (eds): Cancer Incidence in Five Continents. Geneva: International Union Against Cancer, 1966.
4. Doll R, Muir C, Waterhouse J (eds): Cancer Incidence in Five Continents, Vol II. Geneva: International Union Against Cancer, 1970.
5. Waterhouse JAH, Muir CS, Correa P, Powell J (eds): Cancer Incidence in Five Continents, Vol III. IARC Scientific Publications No 15. Lyon: International Agency for Research on Cancer, 1976.
6. Memik F: The possible environmental etiological factors in the carcinoma of esophagus and stomach. Abstracts, 4th Meeting of the European Association for Cancer Research. Lyon, 1977.
7. Kolicheva NI: Epidemiology of esophagus cancer in the USSR. In: Levin DL (ed): Cancer Epidemiology in the USA and USSR. Washington: Department of Health and Human Services, NIH Publication No 80-2044, 1980, pp 191–197.
8. Sobin LH: Cancer in Afghanistan. Cancer 23:678–688, 1969.
9. Kmet J, Mahboubi E: Esophageal cancer in the Caspian littoral of Iran: initial studies. Science 175:846–853, 1972.
10. Lanier AP, Bender TR, Blot WJ, Fraumeni JF, Hurlburt WB: Cancer incidence in Alaska natives. Int J Cancer 18:409–412, 1976.
11. Nielsen NH, Mikkelsen F, Hansen JPH: Esophageal cancer in Greenland. Selected epidemiological and clinical aspects. J Cancer Res Clin Oncol 94:69–80, 1979.
12. Shanmugaratnam K, Wee A: "Dialect group" variations in cancer incidence among Chinese in Singapore. In: Doll R, Vodopija I (eds): Host Environment Interactions in the Etiology of Cancer in Man. IARC Scientific Publications No 7. Lyon: International Agency for Research on Cancer, 1973, pp 67–82.
13. Miller RW: Epidemiology. In: Kaplan HS, Tsuchitani PJ (eds): Cancer in China. New York: Alan R Liss Inc, 1978, pp 39–57.
14. McGlashan N: Esophageal cancer and alcoholic spirits in Central Africa. Gut 10:643–650, 1969.
15. Cook PJ: Cancer of the esophagus in Africa. Br J Cancer 25:853–880, 1971.
16. Rose E: Esophageal cancer in the Transkei. 1955–69. J Natl Cancer Inst 51: 7–16, 1973.
17. Oettlé AG: Cancer in Africa, especially in regions south of the Sahara. J Natl Cancer Inst 33:383–439, 1964.
18. Rose E, McGlashan ND: The spatial distribution of esophageal carcinoma in the Transkei, South Africa. Br J Cancer 31:197–206, 1975.
19. Tuyns AJ: Geographic study on esophageal cancer in Europe. IARC Internal Technical Report 70/007, 1970.
20. Tuyns AJ, Massé LMF: Mortality from cancer of the esophagus in Brittany. Int J Epi 2:242–245, 1973.
21. Rose EF: Epidemiology of esophageal cancer in southern Africa. In: Thatcher N (ed): Advances in Medical Oncology, Research and Education, Vol 9, Digestive Cancer. Oxford: Pergamon Press, 1979, pp 317–326.
22. Tuyns AJ, Audigier JC: Double wave cohort increase for esophageal and laryngeal cancer in France in relation to reduced alcohol consumption during the second world war. Digestion 14:197–208, 1976.
23. Segi M, Kurihara M: Cancer Mortality for Selected Sites in 24 Countries, No 6 (1966–1967). Nagoya: Japan Cancer Society, 1972.
24. Chilvers C, Fraser P, Beral V: Alcohol and esophageal cancer: an assessment of the evidence from routinely collected data. J Epi Commun Hlth 33:127–133, 1979.
25. McMichael AJ: Alimentary tract cancer in Australia in relation to diet and alcohol. Nutr. Cancer 1:82–89, 1979.
26. Young M, Russel WT: An investigation into the statistics of cancer in different trades and professions. Medical Research Council, Special Report Series No 99. London, England: His Majesty's Stationary Office, 1926.
27. Craver LF: Clinical study of etiology of gastric and esophageal cancer. Am J Cancer 16:68–102, 1932.

28. Mosbech J, Videback A: On the etiology of esophageal carcinoma. J Natl Cancer Inst 15: 1665–1673, 1955.
29. Schwartz D, Flamant R, Lellouch J, Denoix PF: Alcool et cancer. Résultats d'une étude rétrospective. Rev Fr Etudes Clin Biol 7:590–604, 1962.
30. Wynder EL, Bross IJ: A study of etiological factors in cancers of the esophagus. Cancer 14:389–413, 1961.
31. Tuyns AJ, Péquignot G, Abbatucci JS: Le cancer de l'oesophage en Ille-et-Vilaine en fonction des niveaux de consommation d'alcool et de tabac. Des risques qui se multiplient. Bull Cancer 64:45–60, 1977.
32. Breslow NE, Day NE: Statistical Methods in Cancer Research. Vol 1 – The Analysis of Case-Control Studies. IARC Scientific Publications No 32. Lyon: International Agency for Research on Cancer, 1980.
33. Martinez I: Factors associated with cancer of the esophagus, mouth and pharynx in Puerto Rico. J Natl Cancer Inst 42:1069–1094, 1969.
34. Hirayama T: Diet and cancer. Nutr Cancer 1:67–81, 1979.
35. Pottern LM, Morris LE, Blot WJ, Ziegler RG, Fraumeni JF: Esophagal cancer among black men in Washington, DC: I. Alcohol, tobacco, and other risk factors. J Natl Cancer Inst (in press).
36. Rogot E, Murray: Cancer mortality among nonsmokers in an insured group of US Veterans. J Natl Cancer Inst 65:1163–1168, 1980.
37. Garfinkel L: Time trends in lung cancer mortality among nonsmokers and a note on passive smoking. J Natl Cancer Inst 65:1169–1174, 1980.
38. Enstrom JE, Godley FH: Cancer mortality among a representative sample of nonsmokers in the United States during 1966–68. J Natl Cancer Inst 65:1175–1183, 1980.
39. Phillips RL: Cancer among Seventh-Day Adventists. J Environm Path Toxicol 3:157–169, 1980.
40. Enstrom JE: Cancer mortality among Mormons in California during 1968–75. J Natl Cancer Inst 65:1073–1082, 1980.
41. Doll R, Peto R: Mortality in relation to smoking: 20 years' observations in male British doctors. Br Med J 2:1525–1536, 1976.
42. Rogot E: Personal communication, 1979.
43. Wynder EL: Role of tobacco in disease development. NY State J Med 80:1238–1245, 1980.
44. Mahboubi E, Day NE, Ghadirian P, Salmasizadeh S: The negligible role of alcohol and tobacco in the etiology of esophageal cancer in Iran: a case-control study. In: Prevention and Detection of Cancer, Part II, Detection, New York: Marcel Dekker Inc, 1978, pp 1149–1159.
45. Cook-Mozaffari PJ, Azordegan F, Day NE, Ressicaud A, Sabai C, Aramesh B: Esophageal cancer studies in the Caspian littoral of Iran: results of a case-control study. Br J Cancer 39:293–309, 1979.
46. de Jong UW, Breslow N, Goh Ewe Hong J, Sridharan M, Sharmugaratnam K: Aetiological factors on esophageal cancer in Singapore Chinese. Int J Cancer 13:291–303, 1974.
47. Jussawalla DJ: Epidemiological assessment of aetiology of esophageal cancer in greater Bombay. Monograph No 1, Int Seminar on Epidemiology of Esophageal Cancer, Bangalore, India, 4 November 1971, pp 20–30.
48. Jayant K, Balakrishnan V, Sanghvi LD, Jussawalla DJ: Quantification of the role of smoking and chewing tobacco in oral, pharyngeal and esophageal cancers. Br J Cancer 35:232–235, 1977.
49. Bradshaw E, Schonland M: Smoking, drinking and esophageal cancer in African males of Johannesburg, South Africa. Br J Cancer 30:157–163, 1974.
50. Rose EF: The role of demographic risk factors in carcinogenesis. In: Nieburgs HE (ed): Prevention and Detection of Cancer, Part 1, Vol 2, Chapter 30, Epidemiology. New York: Marcel Dekker Inc, 1976, pp 25–45.
51. Rose EF: Patterns of occurrence of esophageal cancer with particular reference to the Transkei. In: Silber W (ed): Carcinoma of the Esophagus. Cape Town: Balkema, 1977.
52. Rose EF: Proceedings of the First South African Conference on Carcinoma of the Esophagus, Cape Town, 1977.

53. Hewer T, Rose E, Ghadirian P, Castegnaro M, Bartsch H, Malaveille C, Day NE: Ingested mutagens from opium and tobacco-pyrolysis products and cancer of the esophagus. Lancet ii:494–496, 1978.
54. van Rensburg G: Personal communication, 1979.
55. Sadeghi A, Behmard S, Vesselinovitch SD: Opium: a potential urinary bladder carcinogen in man. Cancer 43:2315–2321, 1979.
56. Iran-IARC Study Group: Esophageal cancer studies in the Caspian littoral of Iran: results of population studies. A prodrome. J Natl Cancer Inst 59:1127–1138, 1977.
57. Gobar AH: L'abus des drogues en Afghanistan. Bull Stupéfiants 28:1–12, 1976.
58. Day NE: Some aspects of the epidemiology of esophageal cancer. Cancer Res 35:3304–3307, 1975.
59. Tuyns AJ, Péquignot G, Jensen OM: Role of diet, alcohol and tobacco in esophageal cancer, as illustrated by two contrasting high-incidence areas in the north of Iran and west of France. Front Gastrointest Res 4:101–110, 1979.
60. Martinez I: Cancer of the esophagus in Puerto Rico – mortality and incidence analysis, 1950–1964. Cancer 17:1279–1288, 1964.
61. de Jong UW, Day NE, Mounier-Kuhn PL, Haguenauer JP: The relationship between the ingestion of hot coffee and intra-esophageal temperature. Gut 13:24–30, 1972.
62. Segi M: Tea-gruel as a possible factor for cancer of the esophagus. Gann 66:199–202, 1975.
63. Hirayama T: An epidemiological study of cancer of the esophagus in Japan, with special reference to the combined effect of selected environmental factors. In: Monograph No 1, Int Seminar on Epidemiology of Esophageal Cancer, Bangalore, India, 4 November 1971, pp 45–60.
64. Mahboubi E, Ghadirian P: Tea-drinking habits and esophageal cancer in adjacent low and high incidence areas of Iran. Cancer Detection and Prevention, Vol 2, 1979.
65. Kaiser HE: Cancer-promoting effects of phenols in tea. Cancer 20:614–616, 1967.
66. Beebe GW, Kato H, Land CE: Mortality experience of atomic bomb survivors 1950–74. Life Span Study Report 8. Radiation Effects Research Foundation, 1977.
67. Smith PG, Doll R: Age- and time-dependent changes in the rates of radiation-induced cancers in patients with ankylosing spondilytis following a single course of x-ray treatment. In: Late Biological Effects of Ionizing Radiation, Vol I. Vienna: International Atomic Energy Agency, 1979, pp 205–218.
68. Selikoff IO, Hammond EC: Asbestos associated disease in United States shipyards. CA: A Cancer Journal for Clinicians 28:87–99, 1978.
69. Vinson PP: Diagnosis and Treatment of Diseases of the Esophagus. London: Baillière, Tindall & Cox, 1940.
70. Lu SH, Camus AM, Tomatis L, Bartsch H: Mutagenicity and carcinogenicity studies on extracts of pickled vegetables collected in Linhsien County, a high incidence area for esophageal cancer in northern China. J Natl Cancer Inst 66:33–36, 1981.
71. Lu SH, Camus AM, Ji C, Wang YL, Wang MY, Bartsch H: Mutagenicity in Salmonella typhimurium of N-3-methylbutyl-N-1-methyl-acetonyl-nitrosamine and N-methyl-N-benzyl-nitrosamine, N-nitrosation products isolated from corn-bread contaminated with commonly occurring moulds in Linhsien County, a high incidence area for esophageal cancer in northern China. Carcinogenesis 1:867–870, 1980.
72. Clemmesen J: Statistical Studies in Malignant Neoplasms. I. Review and Results. Copenhagen: Munksgaard, 1965.
73. Morton JF: Plants associated with esophageal cancer cases in Curaçao. Cancer Res 28:2268–2271, 1968.
74. O'Neill CH, Hodges GM, Riddle PN: Jordan PW, Newman RH, Flood RJ, Toulson EC: A fine fibrous silica contaminant of flour in the high esophageal cancer area of north-east Iran. Int J Cancer 26:617–628, 1980.
75. Vinson PP: Hysterical dysphagia. Minn Med 5:107–108, 1922.
76. Kelly AB: Spasm at the entrance of the aesophagus. J Laryngol Otol 34:285–289, 1919.
77. Jacobs A, Cavill IAJ: Pyridoxine and riboflavin status in the Paterson-Kelly syndrome. Br J Haematol 14:153–160, 1968.

78. Jacobs A, Cavill IAJ: The oral lesions of iron deficiency anaemia: pyridoxine and riboflavin status. Br J Haematol 14:291–295, 1968.
79. Wynder EL, Hultberg S, Jacobsson F, Bross IJ: Environmental factors in cancer of upper alimentary tract: Swedish study with special reference to Plummer-Vinson (Paterson-Kelly) syndrome. Cancer 10:470–487, 1957.
80. Waldenstrom J: Incidence of 'iron deficiency' (sideropenia) in some rural and urban populations. Acta Med Scand 170:252–279, 1946.
81. Norwegian Cancer Society: Geographical Variations in Cancer Incidence in Norway, 1966–1975. Oslo: Norwegian Cancer Society, 1978.
82. Rivlin B: Riboflavin and cancer: a review. Cancer Res. 37:1977–1986, 1973.
83. Wynder EL, Klein UE: The possible role of riboflavin deficiency in epithelial neoplasia. I. Epithelial changes in mice in simple deficiency. Cancer 18:167–180, 1965.
84. Wynder EL, Chan PC: The possible role of riboflavin deficiency in epithelial neoplasia. II. Effect on skin tumor development. Cancer 26:1221–1224, 1970.
85. Foy H, Gillman T, Kondi A: Histological changes in the skin of baboons depried of riboflavin. Medical Primatology 1972. Proc 3rd Conf Exp Med Surg Primates, Lyon 1972, Part II. Basel: Karger, 1972, pp 159–168.
86. Foy H, Mbaya V: Riboflavin. Prog Fd Nutr Sci 2:357–394, 1977.
87. Kmet J, McLaren D, Siassi F: Epidemiology of esophageal cancer with special reference to nutritional studies among the Turkoman of Iran. In: Advances in Modern Human Nutrition,

88. Crespi M, Munoz N, Grassi A, Aramesh B, Amiri G, Mojtabai A, Casale V: Esophageal lesions in northern Iran. A premalignant condition? Lancet ii:217–221, 1979.
89. Lin HJ, Chan WC, Fong JJ, Newberne PM: Zinc levels in serum, hair and tumors from patients with esophageal cancer. Nutr Rep Int, 1977.
90. Fong LYY, Newberne PM: Nitrosobenzylmethylamine zinc deficiency and esophageal cancer. In: Griciute L, Lyle R (eds): Environmental Aspects of N-Nitroso Compounds, IARC Scientific Publications No 19. Lyon: International Agency for Research on Cancer, 1978, pp 503–516.
91. Reinbold JG, Faradje B, Abadi P, Ismail-Beigi F: Decreased absorption of calcium, magnesium, zinc and phosphorus by humans due to increased fiber and phosphorus consumption as wheat bread. J Nutr 106:493–504, 1976.
92. Howel-Evans AW, McConnell RB, Clarke CA, Sheppard PM: Carcinoma of the esophagus with keratosis palmaris et plantaris (tylosis): a study of two families. Quart J Med 27:413–429, 1958.
93. Harper PS, Harper RMJ, Howel-Evans AW: Carcinoma of the esophagus with tylosis. Quart J Med 155:317–333, 1970.
94. Tyldesley WR: Oral leukoplakia associated with tylosis and esophageal cancer. J Oral Pathol 3:62–70, 1974.
95. Ritter SB, Petersen G: Esophageal cancer, hyperkeratosis and oral leukoplakia: occurrence in a 25-year old woman. J Am Med Assoc 235–1723, 1976.
96. Shine I, Allison PR: Carcinoma of the esophagus with tylosis (keratosis palmaris et plantaris). Lancet i:951–953, 1966.
97. Nasipov SN: Esophageal cancer morbidity as evidenced by the genealogy of patients registered in the Gur'ev province. Vop Onkol 23(8):81–85, 1977.
98. Pour P, Ghadirian P: Familial cancer of the esophagus in Iran. Cancer 33:1649–1652, 1974.
99. Kirk RL, Keats B, Blake NM, McDermid EM, Ala F, Karimi M, Nickbin B, Shahbazi H, Kmet J: Genes and people in the Caspian littoral: a population study in northern Iran. Am J Phys Anthropol 46:377–390, 1977.
100. Hashemi S, Dowlatshahi K, Day NE, Kmet J, Takasugi M, Mogagheghpour N, Modabber FZ: Esophageal cancer studies in the Caspian littoral of Iran: introductive assessment of the HLA profile of patients and controls. Tissue Antigens 14:422–425, 1979.
101. Stokes PL, Asquith P, Cooke WT: Genetics of coeliac disease. In: Clinics in Gastroenterology. London: Saunders, 1973, p 547.
102. Falchuk ZM, Rogentine GN, Strober W: Predominance of histocompatibility antigen HL-A8

in patients with gluten sensitive enteropathy. J Clin Invest 51:1602–1605, 1972.

103. Kenning JJ, Pena AS, van Leeuwen A, van Hooff JP, van Rood JJ: HLA-DW3 associated with coeliac disease. Lancet i:606–608, 1976.
104. Cooke WT, Asquith P: Introduction and definition. In: Coeliac Disease. Clinics in Gastroenterology 3, 1974, pp 3–11.
105. Hoffbrand AV: Anaemia in adult coeliac disease. In: Coeliac Disease. Clinics in Gastroenterology 3, 1974, pp 71–90.
106. Love AHG, Elmes M, Golden NK, McMaster D: Zinc deficiency and coeliac disease. In: McNicholl B, McCarthy CF, Fottrell PF (eds): Perspectives in Coeliac Disease. MTP Press Limited, 1978, pp 335–342.
107. Harris OD, Cooke WT, Thompson H, Waterhouse JA: Malignancy in adult coeliac disease and idiopathic steatorrhoea. Am J Med 42:899–912, 1967.
108. Holmes GKT, Stokes PL, Sorahan TM, Prior P, WAterhouse JAH, Cooke WT: Coeliac disease, gluten-free diet, and malignancy. Gut 17:612–619, 1976.
109. Stokes PL, Prior P, Sorahan TM, McWalter RJ, Waterhouse JAH, Cooke WT: Malignancy in relatives of patients with coeliac disease. Brit J Prev Soc Med 30:17–21, 1976.
110. Postlethwait RW, Wendell Musser A: Changes in the esophagus in 1,000 autopsy specimens. J Thorac Cardiovasc Surg 68:953–956, 1974.
111. Ushigome S, Spjut HJ, Noon GP: Extensive dysplasia and carcinoma in situ of esophageal epithellium. Cancer 20:1023–1034, 1967.
112. Napalkov NP, Pozharisski K: Morphogenesis of experimental tumors of the esophagus. J Natl Cancer Inst 42:922–940, 1969.
113. Adamson RH, Krolikowski FJ, Correa P, et al.: Carcinogenicity of 1-methyl-1-nitrosourea in non-human primates. J Natl Cancer Inst 59:415–422, 1977.
114. Mukada T, Sato E, Sasano N: Comparative studies on dysplasia of esophageal epithelium in four prefectures of Japan (Miyagi, Nara, Wakayama and Aomori) with reference to risk of carcinoma. Tohoku J Exp Med 119:51–63, 1976.
115. Mandard AM, Chasle J, Marnay J: Cancer of the esophagus and dysplasias (preliminary results). Europ J Cancer (suppl) 15–26, 1978.
116. Munoz N, Torres O, Castalleto R, Rc.. E, Mandard AM: Precancerous lesions of the esophagus in high, intermediate and low risk areas. Unpublished material.
117. Coordinating Group for the Research of Esophageal Carcinoma: Studies in the relationship between epithelial dysplasia and carcinoma of the esophagus. Peking: Chinese Academy of Medical Sciences, 1974.
118. Coordinating Groups for the Research of Esophageal Carcinoma, Honan Province and Chinese Academy of Medical Sciences: Studies on relationship between epithelial dysplasia and carcinoma of the esophagus. Chinese Med J 1:110–116, 1975.
119. Sharp GS: Leukoplakia of the esophagus. Am J Cancer 15:2029–2043, 1931.
120. Etienne JP, Delavierre PH, Petite JP, Sauleau P: Les leucoplasies esophagiennes au cours des cirrhoses. Sem Hôp Paris 45:1589–1598, 1969.
121. WHO Collaborating Centre for Oral Precancerous Lesions: Definition of leukoplakia and related lesions: an aid to studies on oral precancers. Oral Surgery 46:518–539, 1978.
122. Kolicheva VJ: Data on the epidemiology and morphology of precancerous changes and of cancer of the esophagus in Kazakhstan, USSR. Thesis, Alma Ata, 1974.
123. Munoz N: Personal communication, 1981.
124. Savary M, Guignard G: Adenocarcinogenesis of the lower esophagus. Acta Endoscop Radiocii 7:217, 1977.
125. Ismail-Beigi F, Horton P, Pope CE: Histological consequences of gastroesophageal reflux in man. Gastroenterology 58:163, 1970.
126. Kuratsune M, Kohchi S, Horie A: Carcinogenesis in the esophagus. I. Penetration of benzo-(a)pyrene and other hydrocarbons into the esophageal mucosa. Gann 56:177–187, 1965.
127. Nugmanov SN, Kolycheva NI: Age, sex and ethnic characteristics of patients with esophageal carcinoma in Kazakhstan. In: Epidemiology of Malignant Tumors. Alma Ata, 1970, pp 272–276.
128. Nuryagdev SN: Epidemiology of malignant tumors in Kazakhstan. In: Epidemiology of

Malignant Tumors. Alma Ata, 1970, pp 308–310.

129. Serenko AF, Tserkovnogo GF: Malignant Tumors (Statistical Data from the USSR). Moscow: Medizina, 1974.

130. Mahboubi E, Kmet J. Cook PJ, Day NE, Ghadirian P, Salmasizadeh S: Esophageal cancer studies in the Caspian littoral of Iran: The Caspian Cancer Registry. Br J Cancer 28:197–214, 1973.

3. Epidemiology of Gastric Cancer

PELAYO CORREA and WILLIAM HAENSZEL

Introduction

For many years the only known outstanding characteristics of gastric cancer epidemiology were its marked inter-population variation in frequency and its declining rates. Studies of migrants from high-risk countries to low-risk countries revealed that the high risk remained after migration, indicating that the experience of the first decades of life determines the outcome. This phenomenon has been explained on the basis of precursor lesions. Diet is suspected to play a major role in gastric cancer etiology but search for carcinogens in the diet has not led to convincing results. Epidemiologic and experimental studies have led to an etiologic hypothesis postulating intragastric synthesis of carcinogens, presently being tested. In this chapter we review the basic data contributing to our knowledge on the epidemiology of gastric cancer.

Demographic factors

Inter-population variation

Mortality rates for gastric cancer have consistently shown a remarkable degree of inter-population variability as seen in Fig. 1, based on data assembled by Segi (1) from recent mortality data published by WHO. The highest rates have consistently been found in Japan; they are over 20 times greater than the lowest rates reported in Fig. 1. Chile and Costa Rica, representing the Andean areas of Central and South America, have consistently shown the second highest rates. Predominantly low-lying hot-humid tropical countries such as Honduras, the Dominican Republic, Thailand and the Philippine islands have the lowest rates on record. East European countries have high rates while western Europe, North America and Australia have average or below-average rates.

A similar geographic pattern is described by incidence rates shown in Fig. 2, based on selected data for males published in 'Cancer incidence in five continents,' Vol. III (except data for Chile which are taken from Vol. I of the same

60

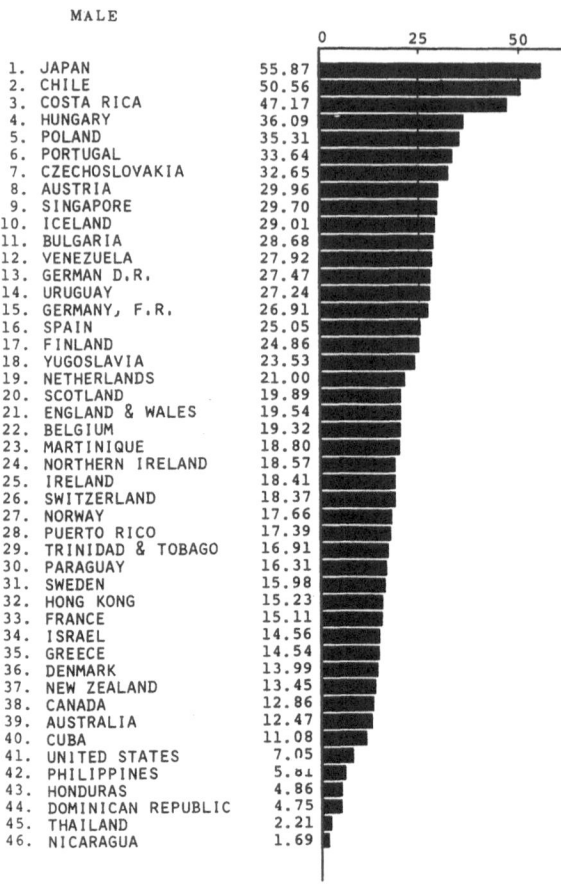

MALE

			0	25	50
1.	JAPAN	55.87			
2.	CHILE	50.56			
3.	COSTA RICA	47.17			
4.	HUNGARY	36.09			
5.	POLAND	35.31			
6.	PORTUGAL	33.64			
7.	CZECHOSLOVAKIA	32.65			
8.	AUSTRIA	29.96			
9.	SINGAPORE	29.70			
10.	ICELAND	29.01			
11.	BULGARIA	28.68			
12.	VENEZUELA	27.92			
13.	GERMAN D.R.	27.47			
14.	URUGUAY	27.24			
15.	GERMANY, F.R.	26.91			
16.	SPAIN	25.05			
17.	FINLAND	24.86			
18.	YUGOSLAVIA	23.53			
19.	NETHERLANDS	21.00			
20.	SCOTLAND	19.89			
21.	ENGLAND & WALES	19.54			
22.	BELGIUM	19.32			
23.	MARTINIQUE	18.80			
24.	NORTHERN IRELAND	18.57			
25.	IRELAND	18.41			
26.	SWITZERLAND	18.37			
27.	NORWAY	17.66			
28.	PUERTO RICO	17.39			
29.	TRINIDAD & TOBAGO	16.91			
30.	PARAGUAY	16.31			
31.	SWEDEN	15.98			
32.	HONG KONG	15.23			
33.	FRANCE	15.11			
34.	ISRAEL	14.56			
35.	GREECE	14.54			
36.	DENMARK	13.99			
37.	NEW ZEALAND	13.45			
38.	CANADA	12.86			
39.	AUSTRALIA	12.47			
40.	CUBA	11.08			
41.	UNITED STATES	7.05			
42.	PHILIPPINES	5.81			
43.	HONDURAS	4.86			
44.	DOMINICAN REPUBLIC	4.75			
45.	THAILAND	2.21			
46.	NICARAGUA	1.69			

Figure 1. Age-adjusted (world population) death rates for malignant neoplasm of the stomach, 1975.

series) (2, 3). The numbers in Fig. 2 refer to the rank order of risk in this selected series as shown in Table 1.

The incidence data are consistent with the mortality findings in pinpointing Japan as the country with the highest risk, followed by the mountainous areas of South America. Marked contrasts are observed between different ethnic groups in the same country: Chinese vs Malays in Singapore, Maori vs whites in New Zealand, blacks vs whites in California and Detroit, Indians vs whites in New Mexico. This seems to indicate that geography per se does not play an unqualified role in gastric cancer causation. Nor does race by itself seem to play an important role in cancer causation as observed by the contrasts provided in Fig. 2: sedentary Japanese have more than twice the rates of Japanese migrants to Hawaii; whites in eastern and northern Europe have considerably higher rates

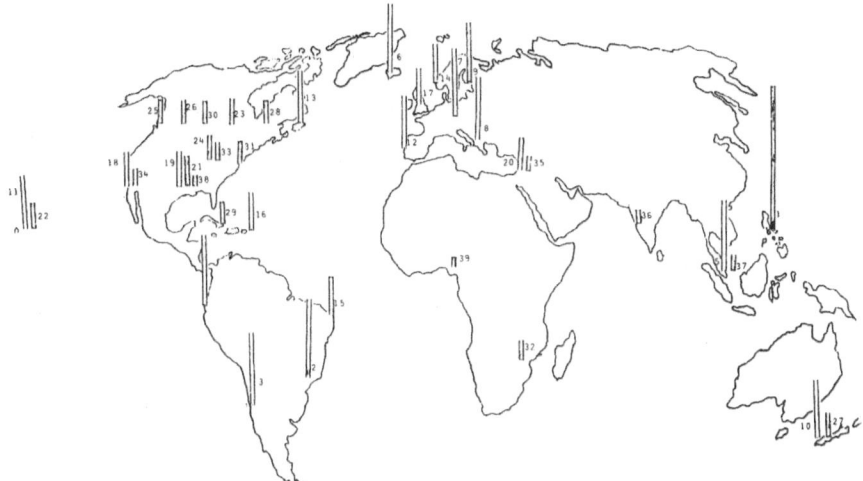

Figure 2. Rank order of age-adjusted (world population) death rates for stomach cancer. Selected registries.

than whites in New Zealand and the United States; Chinese in Singapore have rates approximately 5 times greater than Chinese in Hawaii (rate 8.7, not shown in graph). Blacks represented in the graph all have low rates, Jamaican blacks with considerably higher rates appear to be an outlier: 25.2 (not shown in graph) compared to 7.2 in Nigeria.

Intra-country comparisons have uncovered marked contrasts in risk. In the United States death rates for whites are higher in some regions around the Great Lakes where considerable immigration from Russia and northern Europe took place. In blacks a definite cluster is present in southern Louisiana (4). In Japan the southern areas tend to have lower rates than the north and central areas (5). In Colombia the Andean regions have much higher rates than the coastal or low-lying valleys (6). The rate in northern Brazil is about half the rate in Sao Paulo (2).

Sex ratios

Age-adjusted rates for males and females show a rather constant ratio of 1.6/1 in most populations. This constancy, however, hides a pattern reported by Griffith (7) which seems peculiar to gastric cancer and whose dynamics have not been satisfactorily explained. In younger persons (ages 25–29) the sex ratio is around one; it then raises steadily to a maximum of about 2.2 reached at 55–59 years and thereafter declines progressively to about 1.4 in the oldest age groups (Fig. 3).

Table 1. Average annual age-adjusted incidence rates (world population) per 100,000 males in selected registries (2).

1. Osaka, Japan	91.4	20. Israel, all Jews	21.0
2. Sao Paulo, Brazil	49.5	21. New Mexico, Spanish, USA	18.6
3. Chile (ref. 3)	45.9	22. Hawaii, Caucasian, USA	17.4
4. Cali, Colombia	44.5	23. Manitoba, Canada	16.3
5. Singapore, Chinese	44.3	24. Detroit, black, USA	16.1
6. Iceland	43.0	25. British Columbia, Canada	15.8
7. Cracow, Poland	42.8	26. Alberta, Canada	15.4
8. Slovenia, Yugoslavia	39.5	27. New Zealand, non-Maori	15.3
9. Finland	37.5	28. Quebec, Canada	14.5
10. New Zealand, Maori	36.2	29. Cuba	14.3
11. Hawaii, Japanese, USA	34.9	30. Saskatchewan, Canada	13.9
12. Zaragoza, Spain	33.8	31. Connecticut, USA	13.5
13. Newfoundland, Canada	33.6	32. Bulawayo, African	12.4
14. Norway	24.6	33. Detroit, white, USA	11.7
15. Recife, Brazil	24.3	34. Bay Area, white, California, USA	11.4
16. Puerto Rico	23.3	35. Israel, non-Jews	9.8
17. Birmingham, UK	23.3	36. Bombay, India	9.3
18. Bay Area, black, California, USA	22.6	37. Singapore, Malay	9.2
19. New Mexico, Indian, USA	22.2	38. New Mexico, other white, USA	7.3
		39. Ibadan, Nigeria	7.2

Griffith has called attention to the fact that the total calorie intake, and therefore the amount of food, is similar in both sexes during childhood and early adolescence; increased consumption is noticed in young to middle-aged males, as compared to females, and at old age the sex disparity in consumption becomes smaller. The correspondence in changes with time for the two phenomena led him to propose the hypothesis that a carcinogen in food, whose dose is proportional to the amount of food ingested, could be a causal factor in gastric cancer. The age-dependency of sex ratios may also reflect the fact that gastric carcinoma involves at least two biologic entities with distinct age and sex-specific incidence curves: the so-called 'intestinal' and the so-called 'diffuse' types, described in detail below (8). Geographic comparisons of histologic types of gastric cancer showed that the intestinal type accounted for most of the excissive incidence in high-risk populations (9).

Time trends

The decline in mortality rates for gastric cancer has been a poorly understood phenomenon in most countries. It was first noticed and best expressed in the United States (10) but it has also been evident in most other countries (2, 3, 5, 11). In Norway the decline in mortality rates started in the 1930 decade, leveled off

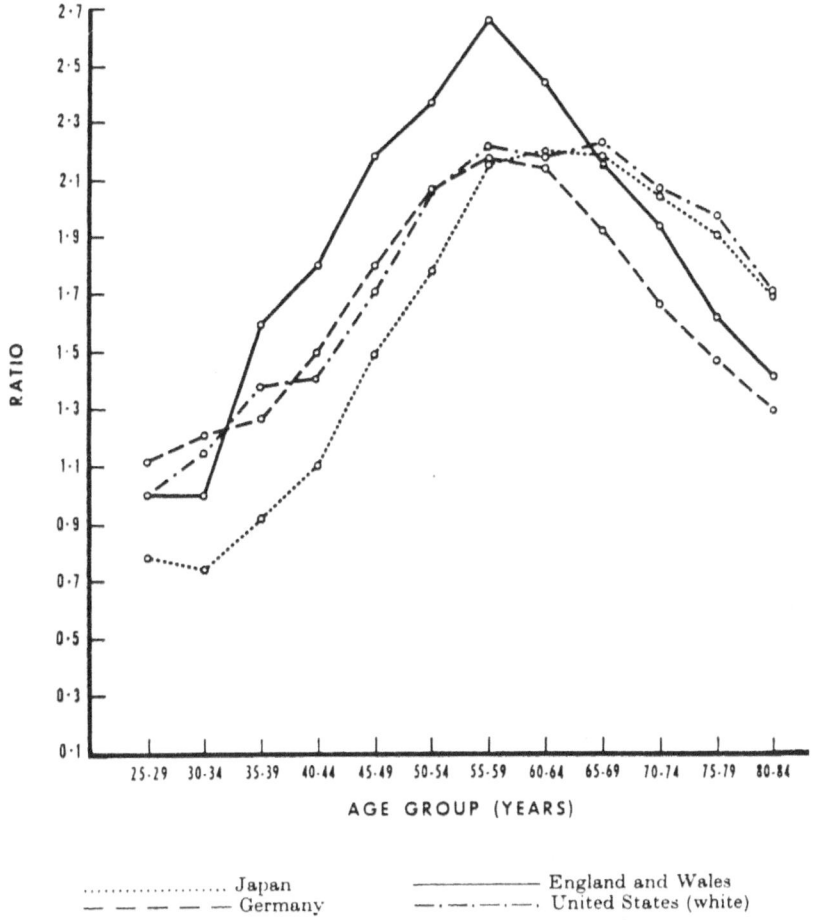

Figure 3. Ratio of male to female death rates from gastric cancer at ages 25–84 years in four countries, 1958–63. (7)

during the war years and resumed its decline after 1951 (Fig. 4). Trends in food consumption which had started before the war were reversed during the war and resumed after the war thus showing an apparent correlation with cancer trends (12). The study cited showed that in Norway the greater decline had been in the intestinal type. This resulted in a reversal of the relative frequencies of histologic types: the intestinal type was markedly excessive in the 1940s and the diffuse type modestly excessive in the 1960s, as seen in Fig. 5. Similar tendencies have been reported in the United States (13). Recent data from Japan showed a decrease in rates of intestinal type tumors, most pronounced in the younger cohorts (14).

64

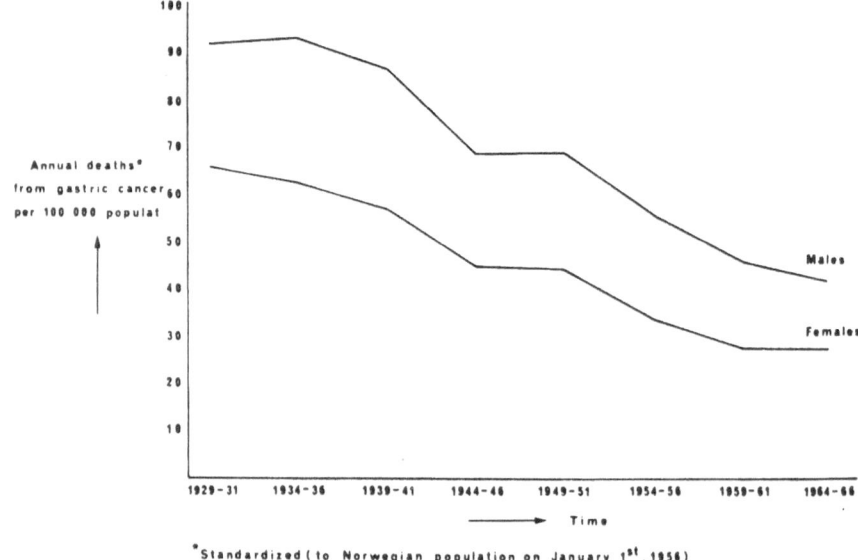

Figure 4. Time trends in age-adjusted cancer death rates per 100,000 in Norway, by sex. (12)

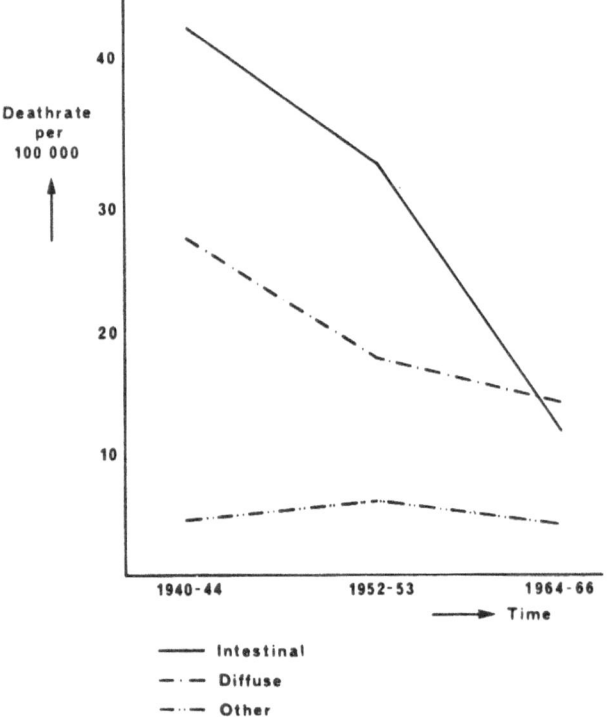

Figure 5. Time trends in age-adjusted gastric cancer death rates per 100,000 in Norway, by histologic type (males only). (12)

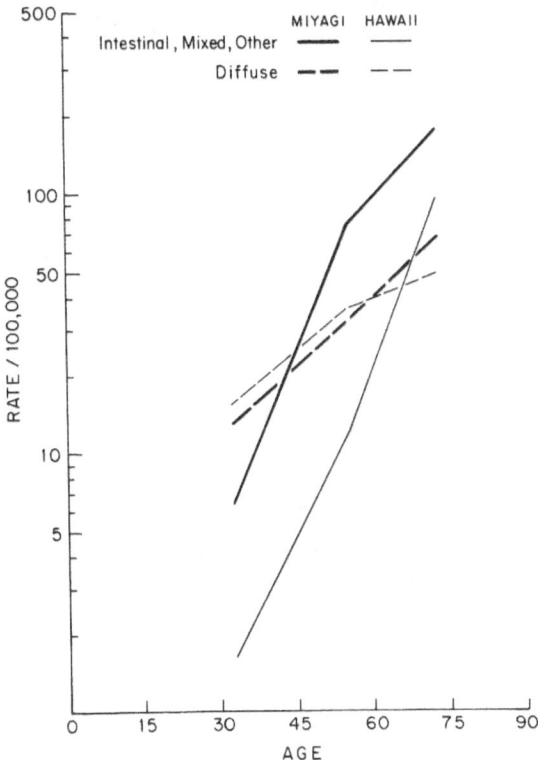

ESTIMATED INCIDENCE RATES OF STOMACH CANCER
BY HISTOLOGIC TYPE - MIYAGI AND HAWAII FEMALES

Figure 6. Estimated incidence rates of stomach cancer, by histologic type, Miyagi and Hawaiian females.

Migration effects

Migrants to the United States who were born in countries with high gastric cancer risks continue to experience high risks in spite of their removal to a low-risk environment (15, 16). Detailed studies of Japanese migrants revealed that the high risk was the first generation of migrants. Their US-born offspring displayed rates similar to those of the adopted country. When the migration effects were correlated with histology it was apparent that the dynamics of the process was quite different for each major histologic type (Fig. 6). The intestinal type accounted for most of the decline in rates, the incidence of the diffuse type remained unchanged. Each type, moreover, kept the same slope in the age-specific incidence curves in Japan and Hawaii (17). This appears to indicate that the forces responsible for the diffuse carcinomas are the same in Japan and

Hawaii. Such forces are different from those operating for intestinal carcinoma. The expression of the latter is delayed (age-specific incidence curves displaced to the right) in Hawaii as compared to Japan, but once the process begins the similar slope values suggest that it progresses at the same speed in both countries (17).

Socio-economic class and occupation

A marked inverse socio-economic gradient in risk has been noted in many countries with lower classes having approximately 2.5 times the risk of the upper classes. This has not been accompanied by a consistent pattern of excess risk in specific occupations, although miners, fishermen and agricultural workers have been considered to be at higher risk than other occupations (18). An urban-rural gradient has been described in some studies but is not a constant feature of the epidemiology of the disease. In general, urbanization is associated with lower risk. Urban-rural differences however, may be determined by migration patterns. In some countries high risk has been observed in some rural areas but not in others (6). Since the first generation migrants maintain their original risk, the risk of the population of any given city will be equivalent to a weighted average of the risks of the native and migrant populations. A city with heavy migration from high-risk areas may, therefore, display a risk much greater than expected on the basis of the native population aɩone. If, on the other hand, the migration is predominantly from low-risk areas, the risk of the city would be depressed. In populations with heavy in-migration it has been possible to demonstrate a strong correlation between the gastric cancer risk of the immigrants and that prevailing in their place of birth (6).

Host factors

Blood groups

A modest excess representation of blood group A has been reported in gastric cancer patients when compared to the general population (1.2:1) (11). When blood group frequencies were correlated with histology it was found that the group A excess was restricted to the diffuse histologic type in populations of different ethnic roots (Colombians, Norwegians, Japanese) (17, 19, 20). Table 2 shows the data for Colombian and Japanese populations.

These findings suggest that the expression of genetic susceptibility might be limited primarily to diffuse carcinoma. Genetic factors alone can account only for a small fraction of the inter-population variability in gastric cancer risk.

Table 2. Percent distribution of blood groups in gastric cancer patients.

	Blood group		
	A	O	B + AB
Colombia			
general population	18	69	13
intestinal-type carcinoma	22	70	8
diffuse-type carcinoma	35	55	10
Japan (and Hawaii Japanese)			
general population	38	31	31
intestinal-type carcinoma	39	29	32
diffuse-type carcinoma	49	29	22

Pernicious anemia

This familial disease is associated with an excessive risk to gastric cancer, again pointing to some genetic susceptibility (21). Blood group A is also excessively represented in pernicious anemia patients but most gastric carcinomas in patients with that disease are of the intestinal type. Such carcinomas are predominantly found in the body and the fundus of the stomach and originate in areas of marked intestinal metaplasia. It would appear that in this situation, contrary to diffuse carcinoma, the susceptibility leads to gastritis and the histologic type of carcinoma is determined more by the gastritis than by other hypothetical blood group A-linked susceptibility factors.

Familial aggregation

There have been several reports of familial aggregation of gastric cancer (22, 23), as well as reports of gastric cancer in twins (24). Most family studies indicate that close relatives of gastric cancer patients have a significantly elevated risk, but exposure to a common carcinogenic environment has not been ruled out. Familial aggregation has been linked to immunologic abnormalities which include antiparietal cell antibodies among other immunological deficiencies (25). It is not clear to what extent these immunologic abnormalities may be associated with the chronic gastritis which precedes cancer.

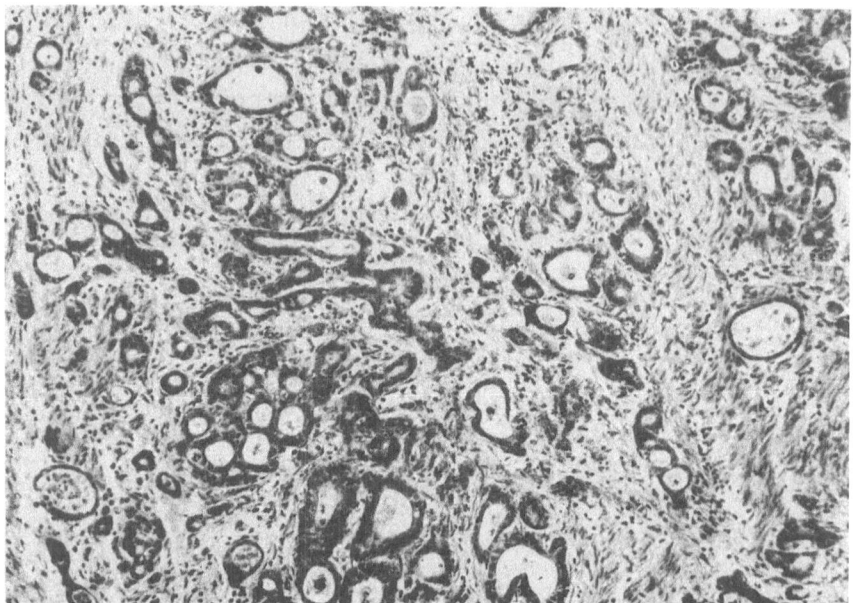

Figure 7. Microphotograph of gastric carcinoma of intestinal type showing well-formed glandular elements.

Pathology

Histology types

Investigators have gradually realized that gastric cancer is not a homogeneous histologic entity. Some rare tumors have been recognized for many years as separate entities, especially malignant lymphomas and leiomyosarcomas. The notion that even carcinomas may not represent a unique homogeneous entity developed in part from the observation by Jarvi that some carcinomas apparently evolved from gastric mucosa with abnormal morphologic characteristics (26). The abnormal features conveyed to the gastric mucosa an intestinal appearance and the tumors originating there resembled those usually found in the intestine. The mucosal changes were interpreted by Morson as intestinal metaplasia (27) and the tumors labeled 'intestinal type' (Fig. 7). Other tumors did not show the cellular cohesiveness needed to form glandular structures and invaded the gastric wall in a diffuse fashion and for this reason have been labeled 'diffuse type' (Fig. 8). The male–female ratio for intestinal type tumors is higher than observed for the diffuse types. The ratio of intestinal to diffuse types increases with age (8). These early indications of the epidemiological value of this classification have been corroborated by later findings discussed below.

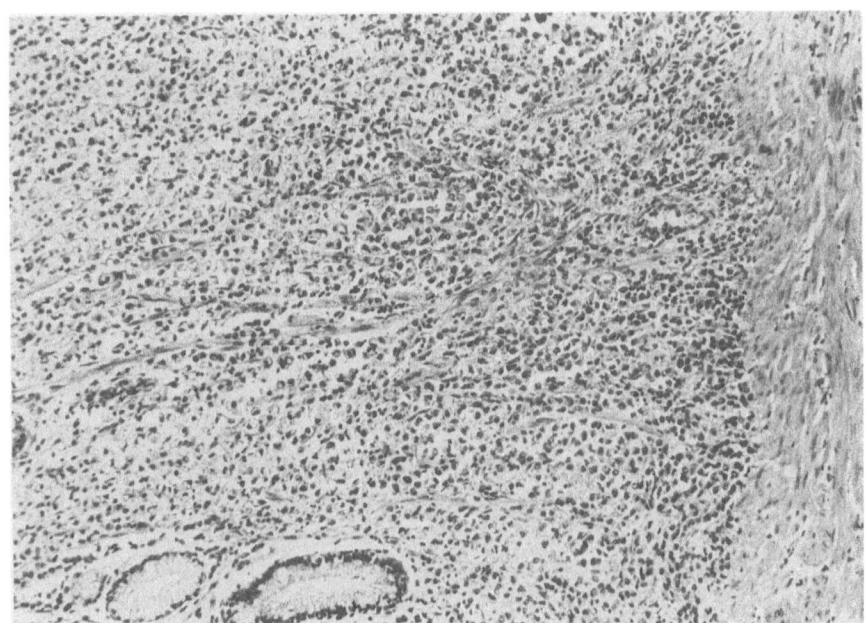

Figure 8. Microphotograph of diffuse gastric carcinoma showing lack of cohesion of cells.

Precursor lesions

The concept of gastric cancer precursors has evolved from a series of observations of the pathology and epidemiology of the disease. Its origins date back to
1883 when Kupfer described islets of intestinal glands in the gastric mucosa (28).
According to the then prevailing concepts of pathogenesis, they were interpreted
as misplaced embryonal rests and duly labeled 'heterotopias'. Not much consideration seems to have been given to the possibility that these heterotopias may
have pathologic significance until Bonne et al. in 1938 described that Chinese
immigrants had a high frequency of gastric carcinoma and atrophic gastritis with
'goblet cell metaplasia', which is equivalent to the so-called heterotopias (29). By
contrast, the native Malays had a low frequency of carcinoma and a low prevalence of metaplasia. Jarvi and Lauren in 1951 described carcinomas resembl-
ing those of the intestine originating in such areas of 'heterotopia' (26). The
nature of these heterotopias began to be reevaluated and the idea that they were
not embryonic rests but rather a change from the gastric to intestinal mucosa,
'metaplasia', began to find some supporters. Morson in 1955 described small
gastric carcinomas originating in areas of intestinal metaplasia (27). Siurala did
repeated biopsies in individuals followed over a period of years and described
progression from atrophic gastritis to gastric carcinoma (30).

The epidemiology of precursor lesions has been studied intensively in Colombia where a cancer registry in the city of Cali reported that immigrants from the Andean mountains of Nariño had a very high incidence of gastric carcinoma, especially of the intestinal type (6). A systematic search for intestinal metaplasia in autopsy material from 6 groups of immigrants, as well as from the local natives, revealed a close correlation between gastric cancer incidence, especially of the intestinal type, and the prevalence of metaplasia (31). Imai et al. reported a similar positive correlation between metaplasia and carcinoma while comparing Japanese and US populations (32). The association with metaplasia is largely limited to intestinal-type carcinoma. In surgical specimens, carcinomas of the intestinal type are usually surrounded by severe intestinal metaplasia. The prevalence of intestinal metaplasia in specimens with diffuse carcinoma is about the same as in the general population under study (9). In low-risk populations, diffuse carcinomas are usually surrounded by normally appearing mucosa.

Detailed studies of the gastric mucosa in high-risk populations have described a series of lesions which apparently represent a continuum of change from normal to carcinoma (33). The complete process is believed to take a long time: 16 to 24 years in cell kinetics studies (34).

The mildest and, therefore, probably the earliest lesion observed is superficial gastritis, characterized by infiltration of lymphocytes, plasma cells and polymorphonuclear leukocytes in the superficial portion of the lamina propria. It is usually accompanied by necrosis of epithelial cells and regenerative changes in the glandular neck region. It is widely believed that this type of gastritis can be produced by a variety of injuries and that it may be repaired ad-integrum. The lesion considered to be next in the severity scale is chronic atrophic gastritis, characterized by loss of glands as determined by the visualization of areas of lamina propria devoid of glands and occupied only by connective tissue and white blood cells (Fig. 9). There are varying degrees of atrophy. On this atrophic background the process of intestinal metaplasia sets in with the appearance of glands lined by cells normally present only in the intestine: absorptive cells, goblet cells, argentaffin cells and Paneth's cells. These cells are distinguished by their morphologic characteristics, as well as by the abnormal set of enzymes they contain: alkaline phosphatase, leucine aminopeptidase, sucrase. When all of the morphologic and enzymatic characteristics expressed in the phenotype of these cells correspond to those of the normal intestine, the metaplasia is usually labeled mature and, insofar as it remains mature, the probability of transformation to neoplastic cells appears remote (Fig. 10). In some patients, however, there are metaplastic cells which appear less mature and do not show the complete set of intestinal enzymes, suggesting that they lose that phenotypic expression and that their intestinalization, as expressed by this set of enzymes, is incomplete. In specimens with gastric carcinomas surrounded by metaplasia, the set of intestinal enzymes is frequently incomplete (35). These same metaplastic cells show abnormalities of the nuclear morphology characterized by increased size, hyper-

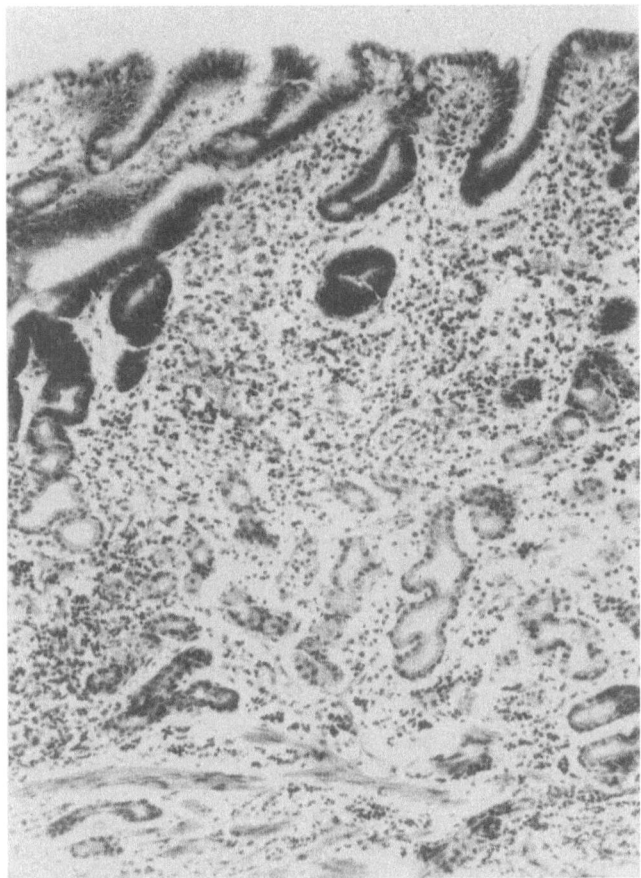

Figure 9. Chronic atrophic gastritis, loss of antral glands.

chromatism and irregular shape. In pathology terminology these changes are known as 'dysplasia', which also implies distortion of the glandular architecture. These architectural changes have been divided in 2 groups: when they resemble hormonally-induced proliferations of glandular tissue they are called 'hyperplastic dysplasia', and when they resemble a benign proliferation of tubular glands they are called 'adenomatous' or 'villous' dysplasia (Fig. 11). Dysplasias are believed to carry an increased risk of transformation into invasive carcinomas. Although gastric cancer is more frequent in males than in females, studies in Finland and Colombia have found equal prevalence of atrophic gastritis in both sexes. Dysplastic changes, on the other hand, are more common in men, indicating that the promotional stages of the carcinogenic process are expressed more strongly in men (36).

Atrophic gastritis and intestinal metaplasia increase with age in both sexes,

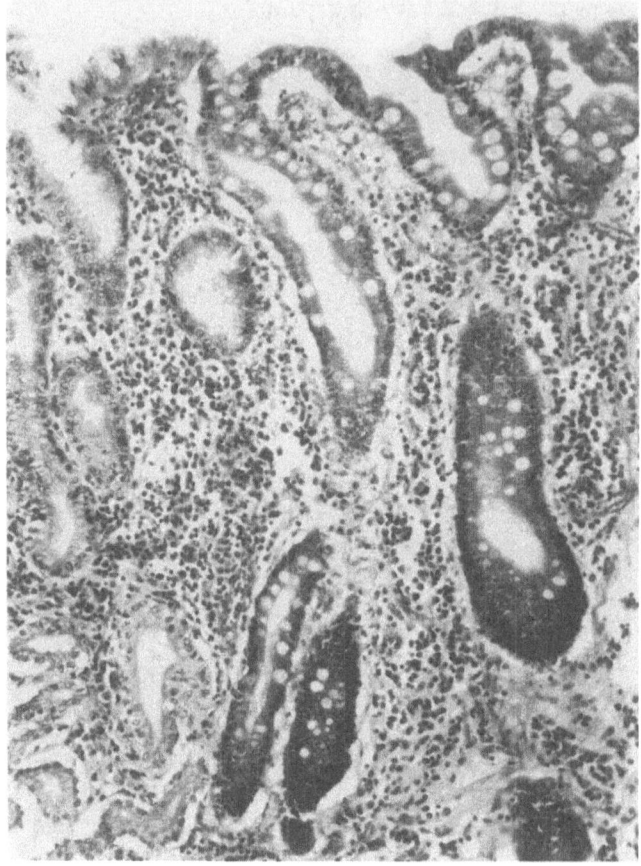

Figure 10. Mature intestinal metaplasia of gastric mucosa with multiple goblet cells.

not only in prevalence but also in surface area covered. Studies of the dynamics and rate of conversion from one stage of the precursor lesions to the next, reveal that the entrance of individuals in a given community into the precursor lesion cycle occurs at a rather early stage. Population surveys in Nariño have shown that after age 30 the proportion of individuals with some of the precursor lesions remains constant, suggesting that the selection of the members of the community who will (or will not) enter the cycle of precursor lesions is determined by that age. The proportion of individuals in the later stages, characterized by increase in the surface area covered by metaplasia and by dysplasia, rises with age (36).

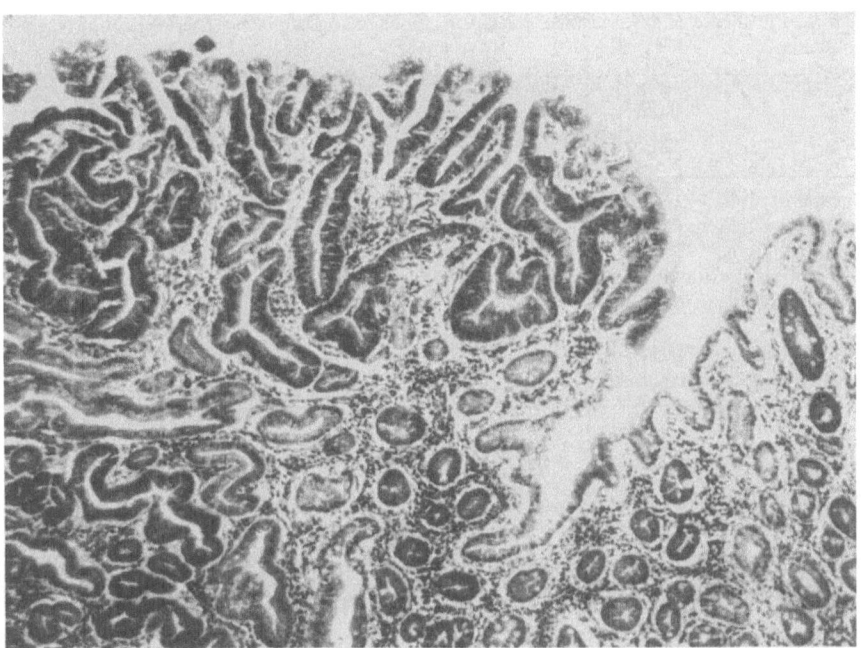

Figure 11. Marked adenomatous dysplasia in gastric mucosa with intestinal metaplasia.

Chronic gastritis

There are basic differences between the types of chronic gastritis and their relationship to carcinoma. Strickland has proposed the term Type A gastritis for those cases presenting positive antiparietal cells antibodies and Type B gastritis for those not associated with such antibodies (37). Type B gastritis, however, is a heterogeneous group. At least 3 types of chronic gastritis can be defined on the basis of etiopathogenic considerations, as shown in Table 4: autoimmune (ACG), hypersecretory (HCG) and environmental (ECG) (38).

All gastritis appear to result from repeated injuries to the mucosa which cannot be adequately dealt with by normal defense and repair mechanisms. The nature of the injury determines the topography of the lesion (Fig. 12). In the case of HCG the injurious agent appears to be an exaggeration of the normal acid-pepsin secretion, to the point of overriding the defense mechanisms of the antrum. In ACG the injurious agents act via immune mechanisms. The injury in ECG is probably based on dietary toxins and irritants. Only ACG and ECG lead to mucosal atrophy, metaplasia and dysplasia, thus involving a high risk for gastric carcinoma.

74

Table 3. Prevalence of gastric cancer precursor lesions in consecutive gastric biopsies of Nariño, Colombia.

	Males		Females	
	≤49 yrs	50+ yrs	≤49 yrs	50+ yrs
Number of cases	45	31	35	12
Prevalence of lesions (%)				
normal	0	0	11.4	0
superficial gastritis	6.7	9.7	0	0
Chronic atrophic gastritis				
simple	35.5	16.1	40..0	41.7
with mature metaplasia	28.9	29.0	34.3	25.0
with dysplastic metaplasia	28.9	45.0	14.3	33.3

Stump carcinoma

It has been recently documented that gastrectomy for benign conditions conveys an increased risk of carcinoma of the remaining gastric stump (19, 39). The increased risk is expressed about 10 years post-gastrectomy but increases with time thereafter. Several series of gastrectomized patients summarized in Table 5, prepared from data published by Nichols (39), have shown that, if the original reason for gastrectomy was gastric ulcer the risk of developing stump carcinoma is greater than when gastrectomy was performed for duodenal ulcer. The interpretation of the finding is open to question because there is a possibility that in gastrectomy for gastric ulcer a small carcinoma could have been present in the

CHRONIC GASTRITIS

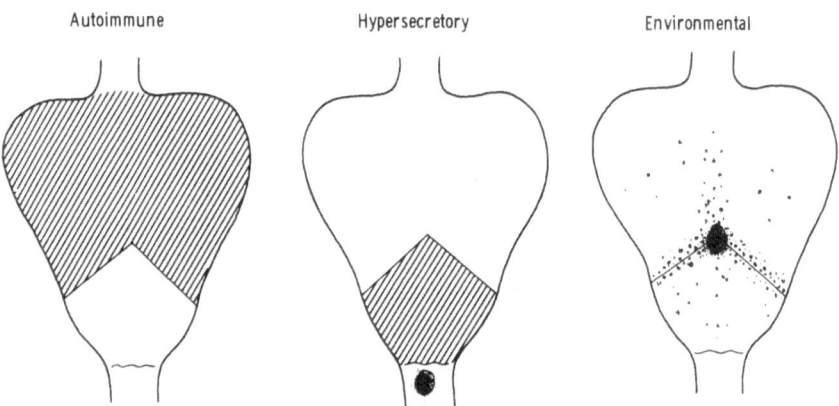

Figure 12. Diagrammatic representation of the topography of chronic gastritis. The shaded areas represent the area involved by each type of gastritis. (38)

Table 4. Characteristics of types of chronic gastritis.

	Autoimmune	Hypersecretory	Environmental
Topography	Diffuse in corpus and fundus only	Diffuse in antrum only	Multifocal, antrum, corpus and fundus
Histology	Atrophy, metaplasia, dysplasia	Regenerative hyperplasia, lymphoid infiltrate	Atrophy, metaplasia, dysplasia
Genetic predisposition	Yes	Probable	No indication
Blood group	Group A overrepresented	Group O overrepresented?	Same as general population
Geographic distribution	Northern Europeans – rare in other groups	Urban centers	Same as epidemic gastric cancer: rural childhood. Mountains.
Peptic ulcer	No	Yes, duodenal or pre-pyloric	Yes, high, mostly near incisura angularis
Etiology	Genetic – autoantibodies to intrinsic factor and parietal cells	Stress. Psychosomatic. Neurogenic	Diet rich in abrasives and irritants, low in protectors (milk, antioxidants?)
Acid-pepsin secretion	Normal to gradually decreasing	Excessive	Normal to gradually decreasing
Gastrinemia	High	Normal	Usually normal to gradually lower (depends on antral atrophy)
Cancer precursor	Yes – in corpus, intestinal type	No	Yes, any location, mostly near the incisura, intestinal type

ulcer (19). Although there may be some truth in this statement, there is no evidence that it could account for all of the observed excess. The impression conveyed by the several reports on the subject is that gastrectomy per se increases the risk of stump cancer which is accentuated in the case of gastric ulcer, perhaps because the latter is often accompanied by preexistent precursor lesions.

Environmental factors

Geochemistry

There have been suggestions that gastric cancer is related to occupations involving close contact with the soil. Soil composition has been associated with gastric cancer risk but the nature of the association varies from place to place. Most findings are based on a search for coincidences in maps of geological formations

Table 5. Stump carcinoma by previous diagnosis of disease leading to gastrectomy.

	Duodenal ulcer	Gastric ulcer	Gastric duodenal ulcer	Other	Total
Number of cases	2594	1672	484	365	5115
Carcinoma	3	22	1	2	28
% ca. in gastrectomy	0.11	1.31	0.21	0.54	

Source: Nichols (39).

and soil contents and maps of stomach cancer risk. Soils with high content of peat and other organic matter have been incriminated in Great Britain, peat and clay soils in the Netherlands, ill-defined and alluvial soils in Japan (18). Acidic soils are generally found in areas of high risk to stomach cancer. Soil of volcanic origin in Japan, Chile, Costa Rica and Iceland are consistently associated with high gastric cancer risk. Soft drinking water has consistently been associated with enhanced risk (11). Attempts to correlate the distribution of trace elements with stomach cancer risk have reported excesses of chromium and deficiency of nickel, vanadium and lead in Wales; by contrast, in Devonshire nearly all trace elements were excessive in high cancer risk areas, especially cobalt, nickel and iron. In Wales chromium, cobalt and zinc values were lower in the gardens of families whose members had gastric cancer than in controls (40).

Diet

We have noted that the remarkable inter-population variation in gastric cancer risk cannot be explained solely on the basis of race or geography, but these factors can influence dietary habits and in so doing have an indirect effect on gastric cancer risk. This, together with the fact that the gastric mucosa stays in sustained contact with food, were the basis for etiologic hypotheses pointing to dietary habits. It has been speculated that diet may play a carcinogenic role in a number of ways: (a) food items may be carcinogenic; (b) they may be vehicles for carcinogens; (c) they may contain precursors of carcinogens; (d) they may be converted to carcinogens in the food preparation process; (e) they may contain promoters of carcinogens; and (f) they may lack inhibitors of carcinogens. The above characteristics are not mutually exclusive and there may be other unknown ways by which diet may influence carcinogenesis (18).

Descriptions of dietary habits of populations at high risk have suggested possible associations between gastric cancer and a variety of food items: rice in Japan, fried foods in Wales, potatoes in Slovenia, grain products in Finland, spices in Java, and smoked fish in Iceland. Starchy foods were the most fre-

Table 6. Prevalence (%) of gastric cancer precursor lesions (chronic atrophic gastritis and intestinal metaplasia) by level of use of dietary itms, Nariño, Colombia (47).

Level of use		Level of use of lettuce	
		high	low
Corn	high	54	51
	low	28	53
Blackberries	high	55	52
	low	29	35

quently implicated items in any descriptive studies (18).

In the United States it has been observed that the decline in cancer mortality coincided with the decrease in the consumption of cabbage and the increase in consumption of lettuce and citric fruits (10). A number of case-control studies have focused on dietary items in several parts of the world. Wynder et al. (41) found no noteworthy differences between cases and controls in Iceland, Slovenia and the United States. Meinsma reported higher frequency of bacon and lower frequency of citric fruits in cases than in controls in The Netherlands (42). Acheson and Doll found no significant case-control differences in England (43). Higginson reported more frequent use of fried foods in cases in Kansas City (44). Graham et al. found smaller proportions of cases using raw vegetables (lettuce, tomatoes, coleslaw) in Buffalo (45). Hirayama reported that cases in Japan consume less milk and more salted foods than controls (46). Although no universally observed association can be found to implicate any food as linked with gastric cancer risk, a number of studies have reported that green leafy vegetables such as lettuce, as well as citric fruits, are associated with lower risk. Bjelke has interpreted his findings in Norway and the United States as showing an independent protective effect of vitamin C (21). There is speculation, therefore, that vitamin C may play an inhibitory role in gastric carcinogenesis. Bjelke has pointed out that some items such as salted fish and vitamin C may interact with respect to histologic expression of the carcinoma. It thus appears that the effect of any specific item might depend on the presence of other items and that a very complex interaction of a variety of foods may determine whether potential dietary carcinogens are expressed or remain inactive.

Few studies of diet in patients with suspect precursor lesions (atrophic gastritis, intestinal metaplasia) have been done. Since the prevalence of precursors is high in areas at high risk to stomach cancer, it may be assumed that the same dietary patterns described for stomach cancer are applicable to its precursors. Studies conducted in the high-risk area of Nariño, Colombia show an excessive consumption of corn, wheat and cabbage (47). An inverse relationship (less use of these items in the high-risk area) was found for lettuce and other green leafy

78

Table 7. Percent of individuals using well water for cooking and average NO$_3$-content of wells (ppm), Nariño, Colombia.

Area	Percent of individuals using well water	Average nitrate content (ppm) of wells
High risk		
A	39	12.5
B	73	39.0
Low risk	23	1.7

vegetabels. With respect to food preparation, salting of foods for preservation was generally more used in high-risk areas. In a case-control study individuals identified by gastroscopy and biopsy to have atrophic gastritis reported higher consumption of corn and fava beans and lower consumption of lettuce and other green leafy vegetables than the controls (persons with normal gastric mucosa). These data shown in Table 6 suggest a peculiar interaction of food items: lettuce seems to prevent the association between atrophic gastritis and corn consumption only when the amount of corn eaten was not excessive.

An overview of the studies of the relationship between diet and gastric cancer, conducted in a variety of countries and cultures, leads to the following general impression: the diet in high-risk populations is low in fat, low in animal proteins and rich in vegetables which provide ˜n abundance of starch and a moderate amount of protein but insufficient amounts of green leafy vegetables. In addition, salt use is frequently excessive in such populations. Nitrate may play a role as discussed below.

Nitrates and nitrites

Interest in nitrates and nitrites increased recently because of a series of reports from different disciplines which converged on the idea that they may have a role on gastric carcinogenesis (48). Druckrey (49) showed that N-nitroso compounds (many of which are known carcinogens for a wide variety of experimental animals) can be formed in the gastric cavity of rats after feeding nitrites and amines. Sander induced esophageal carcinomas in rats fed nitrites and amines (50). Nitroso-guanidines are strong experimental carcinogens (51). Several epidemiologic studies have reported a positive association between nitrates supply and gastric cancer rates (48). In the Worksop area of England the death rate for gastric cancer was abnormally high at a time when the nitrate content of the water supply averaged 90 mg/liter (52), compared with average levels of less than 10 mg in towns at lower risk. In Chile a strong positive correlation was found

79

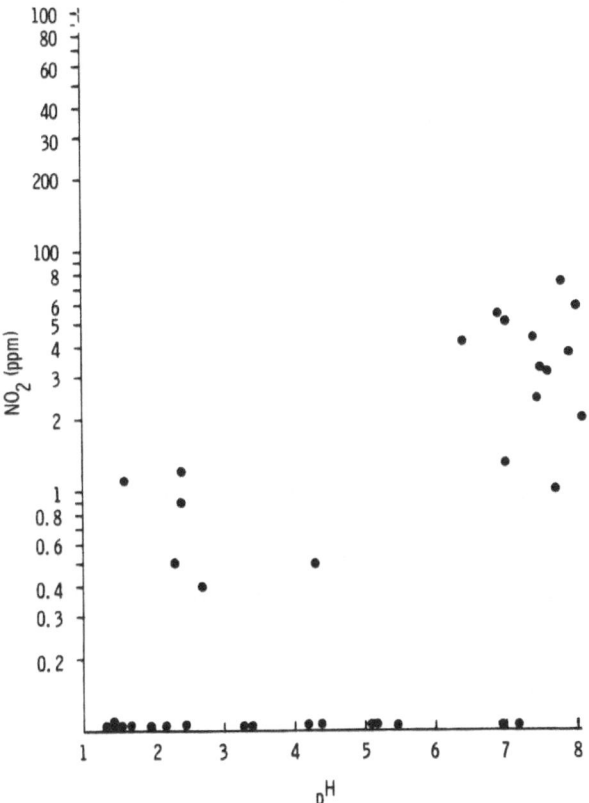

Figure 13. Correlation between pH and nitrite content of gastric juice, Nariño, Colombia.

between gastric cancer rates and the use of sodium nitrate as fertilizer (53, 54). In Colombia areas with high gastric cancer risk reported a high frequency of use of water from dug wells for their drinking and cooking needs (31). Similar findings were reported from Japan (55). In Nariño (Colombia) the nitrate content of water from dug wells was significantly greater in areas of high risk (Table 7).

Nitrate by itself will not react with other nitrogen-containing compounds to form carcinogens. It has to be reduced to nitrite. The conversion of nitrate to nitrite can occur in nonrefrigerated foods (56), in the oral cavity (57), or in the stomach or bladder, and is mostly dependent on reductases supplied by the bacteria.

Microenvironment

The accumulated evidence pertaining gastric cancer etiology has led to close

Table 8. Fasting gastric microenvironment in normal and high gastric cancer risk patients.

Microenvironmental component	Normal	High risk
Histology	Normal	Atrophic gastritis
pH	Below 5	Above 5
Thyocyanate	Present	Present
Nitrate	Present	Present
Nitrite	Absent or minimal	Usually elevated
Bacteria	Sterile	Abundant
Trace elements	Present	Present

scrutiny of the microenvironment of the gastric cavity. The precursor lesions of the mucosa, and especially the multiple foci of intestinal metaplasia, result in a mixture of acid-producing areas alternating with atrophic areas which are hypo- or achlorhydric and may allow bacterial proliferation. The gastric juice is a composite environment which represents the secretion of all areas of the mucosa. Comparative studies in normal subjects and patients with precursor lesions have shown the pattern described in Table 8.

As seen in the table, the key elements in this microenvironment are the presence of atrophic gastritis, bacteria, elevated pH and high levels of nitrite. Figure 13 shows the correlation between pH and nitrite content of gastric juice. To this set of factors we should add those provided by food, as reviewed above: high salt content, abundant complex carbohydrates, low levels of fat and animal protein. The findings on stump carcinoma and some experimental work also raise the possibility of a role for biliary reflux.

Etiologic hypothesis

The prevailing hypothesis on gastric cancer etiology has been expressed as follows (58):

'It is postulated that one major subtype of gastric carcinoma ('intestinal type') is the end result of a series of mutations and cell transformation begun in the first decade of life. The mutagen could be a nitroso compound synthesized in the upper gastrointestinal tract by the action of nitrite (i.e., from food or saliva) on naturally occurring nitrogen compounds. Under normal conditions these nitroso compounds do not reach the gastric epithelial cell, presumably because their synthesis is inhibited by antioxidants present in food or because of their inability to pass the mucosal barrier. The barrier may be overcome by abrasives or irritants such as hard grains, food with high sodium chloride concentration, or surfactants. Once the first mutation occurs, the glandular gastric epithelium is gradually changed to intestinal-type epithelium, the mucosal barrier altered and the pH elevated. Under these conditions, bacteria proliferate in the gastric cavity and facilitate the conversion of nitrates to nitrites, thereby increasing the nitrite pool and the probability of formation of mutagenic-carcinogenic nitroso compounds. This process of gastric atrophy and intestinal metaplasia goes on for 30 to 50 years until some of the individuals affected have the final mutation or cell transformation which allows the cell to become autonomous and invade other tissues.'

Research bearing on the hypothesis continues in several countries and its results have been supportive of the central theme. One of the central questions has been the identification of the substrate for nitrosation, which of course will determine the chemical structure of the putative carcinogen. Since the great majority of nitrosamines require metabolic activation, it is not surprising that in experimental animals they induce cancer of the liver and other internal organs but not in the stomach mucosa. The search is then for direct-acting carcinogens. Nitroso-guanidines have been studied by Endo (59) mostly following the clue provided by findings of Sugimura (51) that MNNG (n-methyl-N^1-nitroso-N-guanidine) is a potent carcinogen for the glandular gastric mucosa of rodents and dogs. Endo found that methyl-guanidine can be nitrosated to form mutagens detectable with the Ames Salmonella test and identified as probably due to methyl-nitroso-cyanamide. It has not been determined, howevei, that this reaction takes place after nitrosation of human food.

In search for similarities in the diet of high-risk populations we noted that spermidine was present in beans eaten in South America and in fish eaten in Japan. Nitrosation of spermidine resulted in direct-acting mutagens (60). This reaction may be blocked by ascorbic acid. There is no evidence to date that this reaction takes place in actual human situations.

Some of the high-risk populations of Colombia consume large amounts of fava beans as their staple food. Mutagens have been found in their gastric juice (61). Tannenbaum (62) and Montes (63) have found that nitrosation of Colombian fava beans results in the formation of potent direct-acting mutagens as seen in Table 9.

Marquardt et al. found that nitrosation of Japanese fish results in potent direct-acting mutagens (64). Lower levels of direct-acting mutagens were also reported after nitrosation of other foods frequently consumed by other high-risk populations: beans and borsh. An extract of Japanese fish treated with nitrite at pH 3 administered to a small number of Wistar rats led to the induction of glandular stomach carcinoma and some precursor lesions such as intestinal metaplasia (65).

It thus seems that nitrosation of foods stands out as a possible source of gastric

Table 9. Mutation ratio (extract/background) of extracts of fava beans after nitrosation Ames test. Salmonella typhimurium TA100 (63).

	Mutation ratio	
	Beans	Beans + NO_2
Complete beans	1.1	1.9
Germs	1.0	2.1

carcinogens and this may explain why such different dietary items as fish and beans may play a similar role in gastric cancer etiology.

References

1. Segi M: Age-adjusted death rates for cancer for selected sites (A-classification) in 46 countries in 1975. Segi Institute of Cancer Epidemiology, Nagoya, Japan.
2. Waterhouse J, Muir C, Correa P, Powell J (eds): Cancer incidence in five continents, Vol. III. International Agency for Research on Cancer Scientific Publication No 15, Lyon, France, 1976.
3. Doll R, Payne P, Waterhouse J (eds): Cancer incidence in five continents. A technical report. International Union Against Cancer, Geneva, 1966, pp 78–83.
4. Mason TJ, McKay FW, Hoover R, Blot WJ, Fraumeni JF: Atlas of cancer mortality for US countries: 1950–1969. DHEW Publication No (NIH) 75–780, 1975.
5. Hirayama T: Epidemiology of stomach cancer. Gann Monograph on Cancer Research 11:3–19, 1971.
6. Correa P, Cuello C, Duque E: Carcinoma and intestinal metaplasia of the stomach in Colombian migrants. J Natl Cancer Inst 44:297–306, 1970.
7. Griffith GW: The sex ratio in gastric cancer and hypothetical considerations relative to aetiology. Br J Cancer 22:163–172, 1968.
8. Lauren P: The two histological main types of gastric carcinoma: diffuse and so-called intestinal-type carcinoma. An attempt at a histo-clinical classification. Acta Pathol Microbiol Scand 64:31–49, 1965.
9. Muñoz N, Correa P, Cuello C, Duque E: Histologic types of gastric carcinoma in high- and low-risk areas. Int J Cancer 3:809–818, 1968.
10. Haenszel W: Variation in incidence of and mortality from stomach cancer, with particular reference to the United States. J Natl Cancer Inst 21:213–262, 1958.
11. Piper DW: Stomach cancer. International Union Against Cancer. Technical Report Series, Vol 34, Geneva, 1974.
12. Muñoz N, Asvall J: Time trends of intestinal and diffuse types of gastric cancer in Norway. Int J Cancer 8:144–157, 1971.
13. Muñoz N, Connelly R: Time trends of intestinal and diffuse types of gastric cancer in the United States. Int J Cancer 8:158–164, 1971.
14. Hanai A, Fujimoto I: Trends of stomach cancer incidence and histological types in Osaka. Symposium on trends in cancer incidence, Oslo, 1980. In press: UICC, Geneva, 1981.
15. Haenszel W: Cancer mortality among the foreign-born in the United States. J Natl Cancer Inst 26:37–132, 1961.
16. Haenszel W, Kurihara M, Segi M, Lee RKC: Stomach cancer among Japanese in Hawaii. J Natl Cancer Inst 49:969–988, 1972.
17. Correa P, Sasano N, Stemmerman GN, Haenszel W: Pathology of gastric carcinoma in

Japanese populations: comparisons between Miyagi Prefecture, Japan and Hawaii. J Natl Cancer Inst 51:1449–1459, 1973.

18. Haenszel W, Correa P: Developments in the epidemiology of stomach cancer over the past decade. Cancer Res 35:3452–3459, 1975.
19. Taksdal S, Stalsberg H: Histology of gastric carcinoma occurring after gastric surgery for benign conditions. Cancer 32:162–166, 1973.
20. Correa P: IAP Maude Abbott Lecture. Geographic pathology of cancer in Colombia. Int Pathol 11:16–22, 1970.
21. Bjelke E: Epidemiologic studies of cancer of the stomach, colon, and rectum. Scand J Gastroenterol 9(31), 1974.
22. Macklin MT: Inheritance of cancer of the stomach and large intestine in man. J Natl Cancer Inst 24:551–571, 1960.
23. Woolf CM: A further study on the familial aspects of carcinoma of the stomach. Am J Human Genet 8:102–109, 1956.
24. Harvald B, Nauge M: Catamnestic investigation of Danish twins: preliminary report. Danish Med Bull 3:150–158, 1956.
25. Creagan ET, Fraumeni JF: Familial gastric cancer and immunologic abnormalities. Cancer 32:1325–1331, 1973.
26. Jarvi O, Lauren P: On the role of heteropias of the intestinal epithelium in the pathogenesis of gastric cancer. Acta Pathol Microbiol Scand 29:26–44, 1951.
27. Morson BC: Carcinoma arising from areas of intestinal metaplasia in the gastric mucosa. Br J Cancer 9:377–385, 1955.
28. Kupfer C: Festschrift. Arz Verein Munch, p 7, 1883.
29. Bonne C, Hartz PH, Klerks JV, et al.: Morphology of the stomach and gastric secretion in Malays and Chinese and the different incidence of gastric ulcer and cancer in these races. Am J Cancer 33:265–279, 1938.
30. Siurala M, Varis K, Wiljasalo M: Studies of patients with atrophic gastritis: a 10–15 year follow-up. Scand J Gastroenterol 1:40–48, 1966.
31. Cuello C, Correa P, Haenszel W, Gordillo G, Brown C, Archer M, Tannenbaum S: Gastric cancer in Colombia. I. Cancer risk and suspect environmental agents. J Natl Cancer Inst 57:1015–1020, 1976.
32. Imai T, Kubo T, Watanabe H: Chronic gastritis in Japanese with reference to high incidence of gastric carcinoma. J Natl Cancer Inst 47:179–195, 1971.
33. Correa P, Cuello C, Duque E, Burbano LC, García FT, Bolaños O, Brown C, Haenszel W: Gastric cancer in Colombia. III. Natural history of precursor lesions. J Natl Cancer Inst 57:1027–1035, 1976.
34. Fujita S, Hattori I: Cell proliferation, differentiation and migration in the gastric mucosa: a study on the background of carcinogenesis. In: Farber E, Nagayo T, Sugano H, Sugimura T, Weisburger JH (eds): Physiopathology of carcinogenesis in digestive organs. Baltimore: University of Tokyo Press/Univ. Park Press, 1977, pp 21–36.
35. Matsukura N, Kinebuchi M, Kawachi T, Sato S, Sugimura T: Quantitative measurement of intestinal marker enzymes in intestinal metaplasia from human stomach with cancer. Gann 70:509–513, 1979.
36. Cuello C, Correa P, Zarama G, López J, Murray J, Gordillo G: Histopathology of gastric dysplasias. Am J Surg Pathol 3:491–500, 1979.
37. Strickland RC, Mackay IR: A reappraisal of the nature and significance of chronic atrophic gastritis. Digestive Diseases 18:426–440, 1973.
38. Correa P: The epidemiology and pathogenesis of chronic gastritis: three etiologic entities. Front Gastrointest Res 6:98–108, 1980.
39. Nicholls JC: Stump cancer following gastric surgery. World J Surg 3:731–736, 1979.
40. Stocks P, Davies RI: Epidemiological evidence from chemical and spectrographical analysis that soil is concerned in the causation of cancer. Br J Cancer 14:8–22, 1960.
41. Wynder EL, Kmet J, Dungal N, Segi M: An epidemiologic investigation of gastric cancer. Cancer 16:1461–1496, 1963.
42. Meinsma L: Voeding en kanker. Voeding 25:357–365, 1964.

84

43. Acheson ED, Doll R: Dietary factors in carcinoma of the stomach: a study of 100 cases and 200 controls. Gut 5:126–131, 1964.
44. Higginson J: Etiological factors in gastro-intestinal cancer in man. J Natl Cancer Inst 37: 527–545, 1966.
45. Graham S, Schotz W, Martino P: Alimentary factors in the epidemiology of gastric cancer. Cancer 30:927–938, 1972.
46. Hirayama T: The epidemiology of cancer of the stomach in Japan with special reference to the role of diet. Unio Intern Contra Cancrum Monograph Ser, 10:37–48, 1967.
47. Haenszel W, Correa P, Cuello C, Guzmán N, Burbano LC, Lores H, Muñoz J: Gastric cancer in Colombia. II. Case-control epidemiologic· study of precursor lesions. J Natl Cancer Inst 57: 1021–1026, 1976.
48. Fraser P, Chilvers C, Beral V, Hill M: Nitrate and human cancer: a review of the evidence. Int J Epidemiol 9:3–11, 1980.
49. Druckrey H, Steinhoff D, Beuthner H, Schneider H, Klarner P: Prufung von nitrit and chronish toxische wirkung an ratten. Arzneim-Forsch 13:320–325, 1963.
50. Sander J: Weitere versuche zur tumor-induktion durch orale application niederer dosen von N-methylbenzylamine und natrium-nitrit. Z Krebsforsch 76:93–96, 1971.
51. Sugimura T, Fujimura S, Baha T: Tumor production in the glandular stomach and alimentary tract of the rat by N-Methyl-N^1-nitro-N-nitrosoguanidine. Cancer Res 30:455–465, 1970.
52. Hill MJ, Hawksworth GM, Tattersall G: Bacteria, nitrosamines and cancer of the stomach. Br J Cancer 28:562–567, 1973.
53. Zalvidar R, Robinson H: Epidemiological investigation of stomach cancer mortality in Chileans: association with nitrate fertilizer. Zeitschrift für Kirchsforschung 80:289–295, 1973.
54. Armijo R, Coulson AH: Epidemiology of stomach cancer in Chile: the role of nitrogen fertilizers. Int J Epidemiol 4:301–309, 1975.
55. Haenszel W, Kurihara M, Segi M, Lee RKC: Stomach cancer among Japanese in Hawaii. J Natl Cancer Inst 56:265–274, 1976.
56. Weisburger J, Raineri R: Assessment of human exposure and response to N-nitroso compounds. A new view in the etiology of digestive tract cancers. Toxicol Appl Pharmacol 31: 369–374, 1975.
57. Tannenbaum SR, Weisman N, Fett D: The effects of nitrate intake on nitrite formation in human saliva. Food Cosmet Toxicol 14:549–552, 1976.
58. Correa P, Haenszel W, Cuello C, Tannenbaum S, Archer M: A model for gastric cancer epidemiology. Lancet 2:50–60, 1975.
59. Endo H, Ishizawa M, Endo K, Takahashi K, Utsinomiya T, Kinochita N, Hidaka K, Baha T: A possible process of conversion of food components to gastric carcinogens. In: Origins of human cancer. New York: Cold Spring Harbor Laboratories, 1977, pp 1591–1609.
60. Kokatnur M, Murray ML, Correa P: Mutagenic properties of nitrosated spermidine. Proc Soc Exp Biol Med 158:85–88, 1978.
61. Montes G, Cuello C, Gordillo G, Pelon W, Johnson W, Correa P: Mutagenic activity of gastric juice. Cancer Letters 7:307–312, 1979.
62. Tannenbaum S: Personal communication.
63. Montes G: Personal communication.
64. Marquardt H, Rufino R, Weisburger JH: On the etiology of gastric cancer: mutagenicity of food extracts after incubation with nitrite. Food Cosmet Toxicol 15:97–100, 1977.
65. Weisburger JH, Marquardt H, Hirota 'N, Mori H, Williams G: Induction of cancer of the glandular stomach in rats by an extract of nitrite-treated fish. J Natl Cancer Inst 64:163–167, 1980.

4. Epidemiology of Large Bowel Cancer

WILLIAM HAENSZEL and PELAYO CORREA

Introduction

Prior to the 1960s, large-bowel cancer received little attention from epidemiologists. The turning point in the epidemiology of large-bowel cancer came with the systematic compilation of incidence data from cancer registries throughout the world. While these efforts were antedated by Segi's compilations of cancer mortality statistics beginning with 1950, which described sizable gradients in large-bowel cancer death rates, the mortality data had been discounted on the grounds that the contrasts were inflated by intercountry differences in diagnostic and treatment facilities and death certification practices. This attitude began to change when the data in the first edition of 'Cancer incidence in five continents' (1) proved to be consistent with the mortality findings. Within a short time span, the concept of substantial intercountry variation in large-bowel cancer risk gained wide acceptance as a prime epidemiologic characteristic of this disease. This feature was stressed at the meeting of the International Working Party of the World Organization of Gastroenterology in 1963, which also noted differences in the presentation of tumors by anatomical segment in high- and low-risk populations (2). The international comparisons pointing to environmental factors as important risk determinants have been reinforced by observations that showed migrants coming to the United States from low-risk European countries and Japan to acquire within their lifetime the high risks characteristic of the host population of US whites (3, 4). The contrasts of high- and low-risk populations revived some earlier work on associated pathologies. Helwig's autopsy studies in St. Louis on the distribution of polyps had identified adenomatous polyps as a possible precursor lesion (5). Correa et al. (6) stressed the need for comparative autopsy studies of polyps in populations at high risk and low risk to large-bowel cancer. This approach established striking differences in prevalence between the two types of populations and strengthened the case for intestinal polyps (or certain subtypes) as precursors of large-bowel carcinomas. The polyp findings raise the possibility of transforming the epidemiology of large-bowel cancer into the epidemiology of intestinal polyps and other suspect antecendent conditions, a step that would facilitate investigations of dietary factors.

Correa, P. and Haenszel, W. (eds.), Epidemiology of Cancer of the Digestive Tract.
© 1982 Martinus Nijhoff Publishers. The Hague/Boston/London. ISBN-13:978-94-009-7504-0

Wynder et al. (7) reviewed the literature up to 1966. Haenszel and Correa (8) later considered the epidemiological findings on magnitude of incidence rates, the sex-age patterns of incidence, and the anatomic localization of tumors in relation to the findings from autopsy studies on the distribution of intestinal polyps. The most comprehensive review of the epidemiological literature bearing on large-bowel cancer has been carried out by Bjelke as part of his studies of digestive tract cancers among Norwegian 'sedentes' and migrants (9). An assessment of animal studies and the development of animal models to test and elaborate mechanisms for the production of large-bowel tumors, which have been stimulated by the epidemiological findings, is outside the scope of this review. We do attempt to identify profitable areas for epidemiological studies that are suggested by findings from animal work, since a review of this rapidly expanding field requires one to place past and current events in context of their implications for future work.

Intercountry variation

'Cancer incidence in five continents,' third edition (10) is the primary source of information on interpopulation variation in risk of large-bowel cancer. Figure 1 summarizes the incidence rates, age-adjusted to the world population standard, for selected registries contributing to that publication. The conventional subdivision of large bowel into colon and rectum is arbitrary and differences in classification may have introduced incomparabilities into the results for the two anatomical segments. For this reason the presentation in Fig. 1 emphasizes the incidence rates for total large bowel, although the separate contributions for colon and rectum are indicated. The presentation has been organized by regions of the world to highlight the interregional variation which has been and remains a distinctive epidemiological characteristic of this cancer site.

For males the ratios in risk between populations at the two extremes of the disease spectrum are on the order of 6–8 to 1; a similar relationship prevails for females. Both sexes yield essentially similar rankings of countries by order of large-bowel cancer risk. The highest incidence is reported by registries in North America and Oceania (United States, Canada, New Zealand). The European registries assume an intermediate position and can be further subdivided into western Europe and Scandinavia and eastern Europe and the Balkans, the first group of countries having generally higher rates. The lowest rates are found in Asia, Africa, and Latin America.

Not all populations are covered by cancer registries, and we have consulted the mortality data for countries with adequate diagnostic and medical care facilities (11) and the relative frequency information from hospital and necropsy sources compiled by Dunham and Bailar (12) to round out the global description of

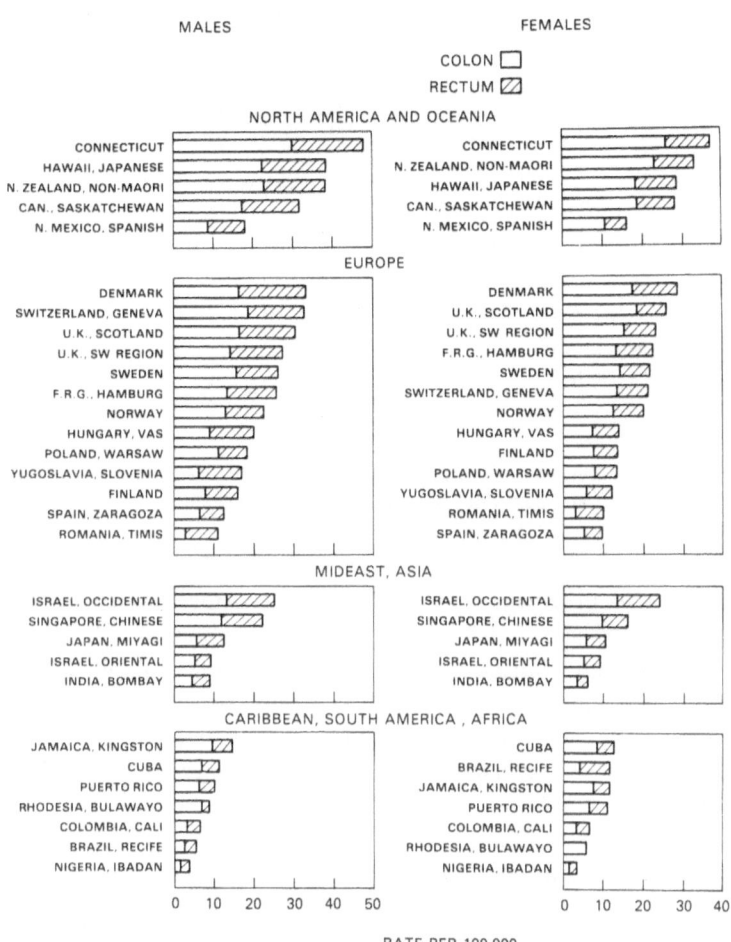

Figure 1. Age-adjusted incidence rates of cancer of the large bowel (colon and rectum), by sex. Selected registries, variable periods close to 1970. *Source:* Reference (10).

large-bowel cancer risk. The findings from these sources agree in most respects with the picture portrayed by the available incidence data.

All tumor registries in Asia have consistently described low incidence rates for large-bowel carcinoma, and the results for selected registries from these continents in Fig. 1 can be viewed as typical. The two African registries in Fig. 1 rank close to the bottom of the list in magnitude of bowel cancer rates and their rates are consistent with those reported for the South African Bantu (13). Latin America presents a more heterogeneous pattern of bowel cancer risks than Africa or Asia. While many Latin American populations (Cali, Colombia; Recife, Brazil) display low rates comparable to those encountered in Africa and

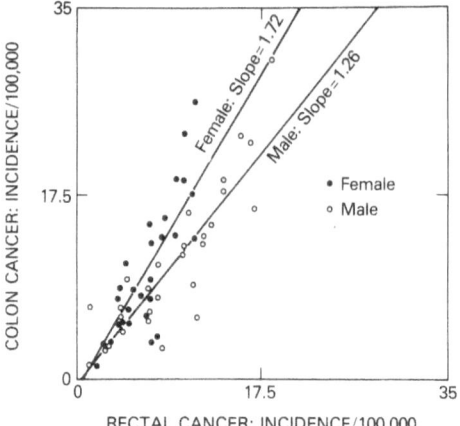

Figure 2. Joint distribution of age-adjusted incidence rates for cancer of the colon and rectum, by sex. Selected registries, variable periods close to 1970. *Source:* Reference (10).

Asia, other populations are at higher risk. The inter-American study of mortality (14) reported bowel cancer mortality in La Plata, Argentina to be only slightly less than that in San Francisco, California and Bristol, England, and the same source described intermediate rates for Sao Paulo and Ribeirão Prêto in Brazil.

While the adequacy of diagnostic and medical care facilities varies among registries, these factors seem unlikely to account for differences of the magnitude observed. Incidence data collected by newly established tumor registries will be important in elaborating and confirming earlier impressions on striking geographical differences in bowel cancer risks.

Colon-rectum ratios

Figure 1 suggests a rough parallelism in population rankings by order of risk for cancer of the colon and rectum, although the ranking for rectum deviates in some respects from the pattern presented for colon. Despite obvious exceptions for individual registries the graph of the joint distribution of rates for colon and rectum for 28 registries in 26 countries (Fig. 2) reveals a strong correlation in the incidence rates for the two conventional subdivisions of the large bowel. A significant feature of Fig. 2 is the sex difference in the relationship between the incidence rates for colon and rectum. Females show the steeper rise in colon incidence for each unit increase in rectum incidence.

Systematic differences in the relationships of incidence for the two localizations can be simply expressed as colon-rectum ratios. The highest colon-rectum ratios of age-adjusted incidence are found in North America and western

Europe. The eastern European registries report distinctly lower colon-rectum ratios that are often below unity. Generally lower colon-rectum ratios prevail in Asian and African populations. The findings for Caribbean and South American countries are more variable. The results for Puerto Rico are representative of the more elevated colon-rectum ratios reported from Cuba and Kingston, Jamaica and deviate markedly from the colon-rectum ratio close to unity reported by the registry in Cali, Colombia.

Part of the variation in colon-rectum ratios presumably arises from different practices in classifying tumors presenting near the rectosigmoid flexure. For example, the colon-rectum ratios in Norway have been inflated in the past by assignment of rectosigmoid tumors to sigmoid colon rather than to rectum (15), the latter being the usual practice. However, the most extreme assumptions on misclassification would not reduce the colon-rectum ratios for North America and western Europe to the values close to or below unity described for Asian and African registries. The sex differences in the behavior of the colon-rectum ratios also argue against an explanation based on classification artifacts, since this would imply sex differences in criteria for tumor localizations in some populations.

Anatomic localization

The variable colon-rectum ratios suggest that colon and rectum may have related, but not identical, etiologies. The greater interpopulation variation in colon cancer risks raises the possibility that the variation may be concentrated in certain segments proximal to the rectosigmoid flexure. Haenszel and Correa (8) collected more detailed data from cancer registries covering high- and low-risk populations and calculated the ratio of sigmoid tumors to those located in the cecum-ascending colon and in the rectum and concluded that the sigmoid-ascending and sigmoid-rectum ratios increased with overall level of colon cancer risk, particularly among males. De Jong et al. (16) investigated this subject in greater detail with similar results. For populations at widely different levels of colon cancer risk, they found differences in the segmental ratios of tumors similar to those described by Haenszel and Correa, but in the intermediate range they found no regular progression in ratios with increasing colon cancer risks.

These studies shared the defect that the basic tumor registry data relied on subjective criteria for tumor location, which vary from country to country and among physicians. Berg and Haenszel (personal communication) attempted to replace the subjective observations with objective measurements based on distance of the lower margin of the tumor from the pectinate line in six populations drawn from the extremes of bowel cancer incidence. For four populations incidence data were available, permitting conversion into estimates of segment-

Table 1. Estimated segment-specific incidence rates per 100,000 population for bowel cancer in Iowa (high risk) and Cali, Colombia (low risk), by sex.

| | Estimated incidence | | | | Difference: Iowa – Cali | | Ratio: Iowa/Cali | |
| | Male | | Female | | | | | |
Segment	Iowa	Cali	Iowa	Cali	Male	Female	Male	Female
Cecum	2.7	0.93	4.7	1.1	1.7	3.6	2.9	4.2
Ascending colon	2.9	0.78	3.8	0.61	2.1	3.2	3.7	6.3
Transverse colon	3.4	0.75	3.9	0.58	2.6	3.4	4.5	6.8
Descending colon	2.4	0.20	1.9	0.22	2.2	1.6	12.	8.5
Sigmoid colon								
≥16 cm	95	0.58	7.3	0.89	8.9	6.4	16.	8.4
8–15 cm	9.2	1.5	6.6	1.3	7.7	5.4	6.1	5.2
6–7 cm	2.7	0.80	2.0	0.48	1.8	1.5	3.3	4.2
4–5 cm	1.9	0.99	1.1	0.70	0.9	0.4	1.9	1.6
2–3 cm	1.3	0.66	0.67	0.64	0.7	0.03	2.0	1.0
0–1 cm	0.39	0.37	0.36	0.47	0.02	–0.1	1.1	0.8

Source: J.W. Berg and W. Haenszel, personal communication (1976).

specific incidence. Table 1 contrasts a high-incidence population (Iowa) with a low-incidence population (Cali, Columbia). The segment-specific incidence rates for regions up to 16 cm distant from the anus are based on direct measurements; for the more proximal colon segments above the reach of a sigmoidoscope, the data still depend on subjective, nonquantitative criteria. The Iowa and Cali comparisons permit some tentative conclusions: (1) in the low-risk population (Cali) the cancer incidence for men and woman was distributed much more uniformly by segments of the bowel; (2) the Iowa-Cali ratios of incidence emphasized the great disparity in risk for the upper sigmoid (≥16 cm from the anus) and for the descending colon in both sexes. Proceeding proximally and distally from this region the ratios become progressively smaller, and within 2–4 cm of the anus the differences between Cali and Iowa were minimal.

These data suggest that in Iowa (and by inference the United States) the hypothesized bowel cancer factor may be exerting its greatest effect distal to the upper sigmoid colon, in the segment 6–15 cm above the anus. In men the most distal 2 cm and in women the most distal 4 cm seem essentially to be unaffected by any bowel cancer factor peculiar to the United States. Such anatomic differences in response could be due to differential sensitivity of the bowel to a carcinogen, but the contrasting locations of cancer in low- and high-risk populations exemplified by Iowa and Cali favor instead different levels of concentration of the responsible factor. The results derived from more precise measurements of tumor location appear to have important epidemiological implications. This information can be considered in the design of case-control

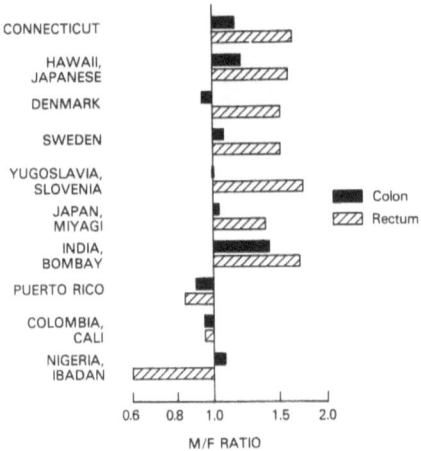

Figure 3. Male–female (M/F) ratios of age-adjusted incidence rates for cancer of the large bowel (colon and rectum). Selected registries, variable periods close to 1970. *Source*: Reference (10).

studies of diet, for example. In the search for case-control differences bowel location may permit separations analogous to those achieved for stomach cancer by the intestinal-diffuse histologic separation made by Jarvi (17) and Lauren (18).

Male–female ratios

Figure 3 describes for colon and rectum the deviations from unity of the male–female ratios of age-adjusted incidence for registries covering high-, intermediate-, and low-risk populations. Colon and rectum appear to have distinctive, rather than common, profiles of variation. Male–female ratios of less than unity are more frequently observed for colon, but each site is characterized by population differences in sex ratios. A more pronounced male excess for rectum is not an invariable rule. Several registries, including Puerto Rico; Kingston, Jamaica; Recife, Brazil; and Ibadan, Nigeria have reported lower sex ratios for colon.

The higher male–female ratios of age-adjusted incidence for rectum than for colon combined with the suggested female excess of colon cancers in low-risk populations raises the possibility of segmental differences in sex ratios for the proximal bowel above the rectosigmoid flexure. The data on incidence specific for tumor location collected in the US Cancer Morbidity Survey of 1969–1971 (19) show the characteristic male excess for rectum to persist in the rectosigmoid and to be present in somewhat attenuated form in the sigmoid colon, while the sex ratios for ascending colon and cecum are close to unity. Documentation of

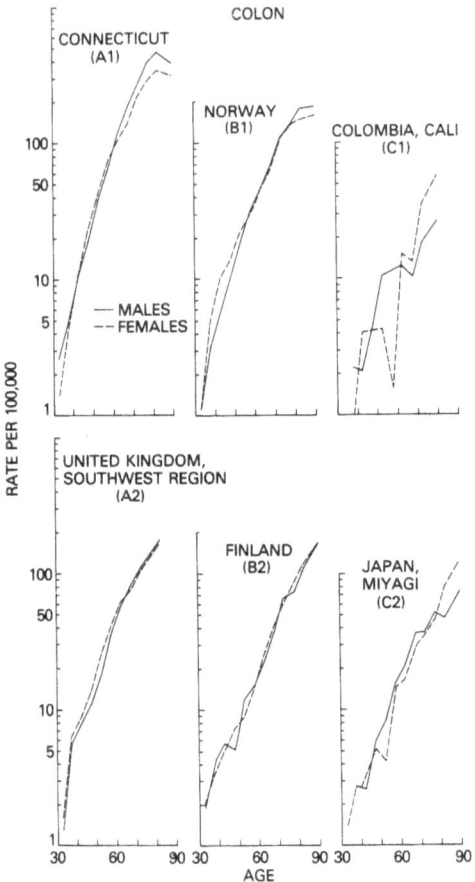

Figure 4. Sex- and age-specific incidence rates for cancer of the colon. Selected registries, variable periods close to 1970. *Source*: Reference (10).

segmental differences in sex ratios from other sources is difficult, because tumor location has not always been precisely specified and recorded by registries.

Sex- and age-specific incidence

Cook et al. (20) computed the slopes of log incidence plotted against log age for 11 cancer registries and showed the slopes of the male curves to be consistently higher for both colon and rectum in all populations studied by them except Finland.

Although the slope values summarize the gross features of the incidence curves, they share with age-adjusted rates the inability to reveal the finer details of age–sex interactions. Haenszel and Correa (8) inspected the sex- and age-specific incidence curves for colon cancer and classified them with respect to absolute magnitude of the rates for the age group 65–74 years, slope, degree of curvature at older ages and the relative positions of the male and female incidence curves. Examination of the most recent incidence data showed all the registries with age-specific incidence at 65–74 years of >100 (type A) to have similar slopes and the only feature differentiating the type A registries was the degree of male dominance in incidence after age 60 or 65. The Connecticut (United States) 1968–1972 excess in male risks after age 60 was pronounced and the results for that registry shown in Fig. 4 are representative of those for Saskatchewan (Canada), 1969–1972; New Zealand, 1968–1971; Birmingham (England), 1968–1972, which we label type A_1. There is another subset of registries with a similar level of incidence, for which the sex differential in risk at the older ages remains minimal, assigned to category A_2. The Southwest Region (England), 1966–1970, typifies the latter group which includes Denmark, 1963–1967; Sweden, 1966–1970; Iowa (United States), 1969–1971.

Registries with age-specific incidence at 65–74 years of 10–40 (low-risk – type C) reveals several examples of higher female rates past age 60. This category, labeled C_1, includes Cali (Colombia), 1962–1971; Cuba, 1968–1972; Timis (Romania), 1970–1972; Oriental Jews (Israel), 1967–1971; Slovenia (Yugoslavia), 1968–1972. Other populations present several crossover points in the male and female incidence curves, giving the impression of a pattern changing from female to male predominance; Miyagi (Japan), 1968–1971 and Puerto Rico, 1968–1972 can be placed in category C_2.

Review of the intermediate B-level registries (rates of 50 to <150) discloses a similar dichotomy. A majority exhibit modest male excesses at the older ages. The results for Norway, 1968–1972, are representative of those for Hamburg (German Federal Republic), 1969–1972, and Vas (Hungary), 1968–1972, placed in category B_1. Finland, 1966–1970, still presents dominant female rates after age 60, type B_2.

A similar classification scheme can be developed for rectal carcinoma.

The magnitude of the intercountry differences suggests the probable presence of intracountry differences as well, at least for countries with large land masses, since political boundaries are often artificial and unrelated to climate, terrain, and other environmental factors that control agricultural and food distribution practices that may influence the level of bowel cancer risk.

This subject has been more intensively pursued in the United States than elsewhere, and elevated risks for both colon and rectum in the Northeast and in North Central regions and a below-average risk in the South have been demonstrated using a variety of source materials and study techniques. The National Cancer Institute morbidity surveys conducted in 1947–1948 and 1969–1971 (19,

21) showed both white and black residents of the northern cities surveyed to have higher incidence than in the South. Burbank (22) in his review of the mortality data for 1950–1967 commented on the cluster of Northeast and Great Lake states with high death rates for colon and rectum among whites and the generally lower rates elsewhere, particularly in the South. His data for blacks also depicted lower risks in a tier of southern states extending from North Carolina to Texas. The higher risks in the North are not explained by the elevated rates for residents of metropolitan areas, which tend to be concentrated in that part of the United States. Haenszel and Dawson (23) studied a sample of deaths from bowel cancer with control for residence and found the deficit in the South to persist in urban and rural areas and metropolitan and nonmetropolitan counties.

The Scandinavian countries present a pattern of gradients in risk with latitude that resembles in certain respects the United States situation. Denmark presents higher bowel cancer risks than the other Scandinavian countries, and it has been observed that the highest rates in Sweden occur in the southwestern part of the country immediately adjacent to Denmark. Data from Finland (24) present a similar geographic configuration. The lowest colon cancer incidence occurs in the northern and eastern regions of the country, and the rates in districts adjacent to Helsinki in the south of Finland are more than 50% above those in the most northern districts. The results for Norway follow closely the pattern described for Sweden and Finland. The highest incidence of large-bowel cancer occurs in Oslo and adjacent counties in southern Norway, and the lowest rates are found in the northern counties.

The status of within-country variation in bowel cancer risk might be summarized as follows. In large countries or in those extending over a wide range of latitudes, regional differences that mimic the international variations in total bowel cancer incidence have been observed. In small, geographically compact countries even if regional differences did exist, the observational situation does not favor their detection.

Information on the variation in bowel cancer risk by counties or small geographical units had been lacking until the publication of US county maps by Mason et al. (25). Since bowel cancer had not been intensively investigated from this point of view, it is not surprising that studies of soil and drinking water content in relation to small area variation for this disease have not been pursued with the same diligence as for stomach cancer and cardiovascular disease. The observations on the role of selenium in inhibiting tumorigenesis (26), coupled with the inverse relationship between selenium occurrence in the soil and forage crops and the death rates for cancer of all sites and of the large bowel in the United States and Canada (27), ensure that environmental geochemistry and the distribution of trace metals in relation to bowel cancer will receive greater attention in the future.

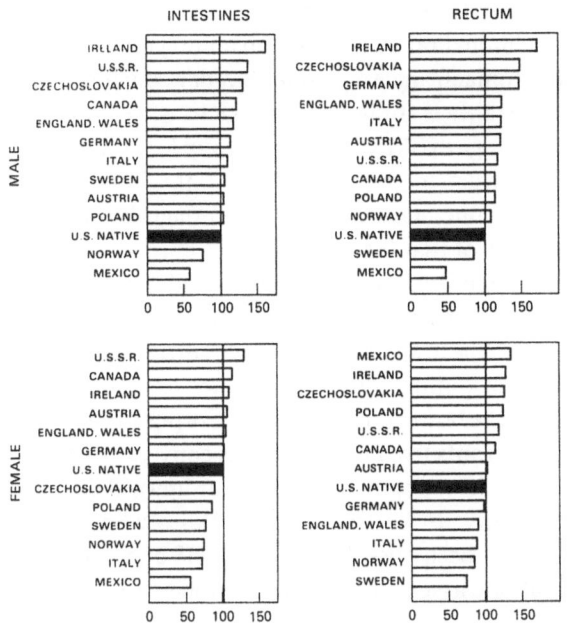

Figure 5. Standardized mortality ratios by country of birth and by sex for cancer of the colon and rectum, United States (35 states), 1950. *Source*: Reference (3).

Migrant populations

Intercountry comparisons of cancer risks confound the effects of diagnostic practices, environmental factors, and host characteristics. With respect to diagnostic artifacts the presumption of true intercountry differences in large-bowel cancer is strengthened by observations on migrant populations. For example, Jews coming to Israel from Yemen and North Africa have experienced in the years immediately after arrival lower bowel cancer incidence than Jews from western Europe and North America (1), a result consistent with global population contrasts for this disease.

Several investigators have recognized the importance of comparing the experience of natives and migrants residing in the same areas to elicit information on the role of environmental and endogenous factors in specific diseases (28) as well as to elaborate the interpretation of intercountry differences in risk. Lombard and Doering (29) reported on site-specific cancer mortality by country of birth in their Boston study and comprehensive coverage of ethnic group variation in large-bowel cancer was provided by Haenszel (3) in his study of 34,000 deaths of foreign-born whites in 35 states as of 1950. The results from that source for intestine (colon) and rectum in the form of standardized mortality ratios

(SMRs) are summarized in Fig. 5. As of 1950, cancer of the colon and rectum was characterized by a limited range of variation among ethnic groups compared to that presented by stomach and esophagus. Similar conclusions were reached by Lilienfeld et al. (30) in their study covering the three years 1959–1961.

The compressed range of SMRs by ethnic group for colon and rectum in Fig. 5 stands in sharp contrast to the magnitude of the international variation in mortality for these same sites. Few of the foreign-born groups had SMRs substantially in excess of that for the US native-born.

When the US foreign-born rates as of 1950 and 1959–1961 were positioned against those in the countries of origin, the mortality from large-bowel cancer among migrants from the low-risk European countries proved to be more closely aligned with the host population of US whites and suggested the following generalization for large bowel (and for breast, corpus uteri, ovary, and prostate as well): rates for migrants from low-risk areas converge during their lifetime to the higher risks of the host population. A similar upward displacement of large-bowel cancer mortality in Australia among Poles who migrated there after World War II has also been observed (31). The US and Australian data suggest that events in adult life associated with migration can visibly affect the level of bowel cancer risk within 2–3 decades.

It has been easy to document the changing large-bowel risk among Japanese in Hawaii and the continental United States. When Smith (32) reviewed the cancer mortality among US Japanese as of 1949–1952, he reported lower death rates from cancer of the colon among US Japanese than for US whites, with a tendency, more pronounced among males, for the US-Japanese rates to be higher than rates for the Japanese in Japan. Haenszel and Kurihara (4) updated the results to 1959–1962. At that time the colon cancer rates for Issei (the original migrants) and Nisei (their US-born offspring) males had risen to closely approximate those for white males; a similar, but smaller, translation had occurred among females. This process of rise to the level of risk in the host population has continued to the present time.

The Japanese experience for colon seems quite consistent with that presented by European migrants although the Issei did not make as complete a transition within one generation as did migrants from Poland (33). The shift to higher US risks has continued in the second-generation Nisei.

One distinction between Japanese and Polish migrants should be noted. The Polish migrants experienced a substantial rise in risk for both colon and rectum, while the Japanese data emphasized selective effects within the intestinal tract. The US-Japan differential in mortality from rectal cancer has never been marked, so that little change in the risk for rectum among Japanese migrants might have been anticipated. However, the relative stability in overall rates for cancer of the rectum has concealed a rise in tumors in the upper rectum and rectosigmoid region among the Hawaiian Japanese.

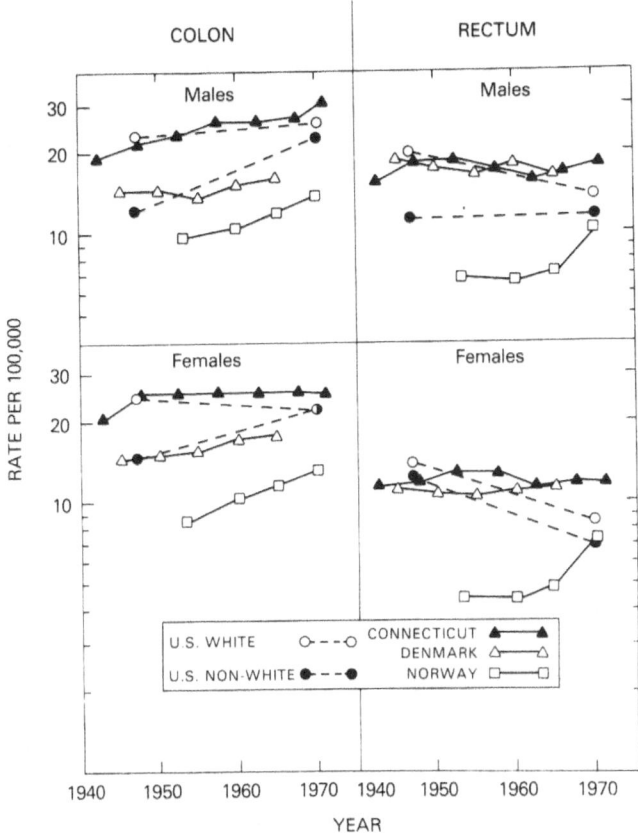

Figure 6. Trends in age-adjusted incidence rates of cancer of the colon and rectum, by sex. Selected countries, 1940–1971. *Source:* References (19, 21, 34–42).

Apart from the Japanese, the possibilities for new studies in the United States on migrants who have come from low-risk areas may be about exhausted. Further work along these lines might be initiated in other countries, such as Canada and Australia, where substantial numbers of migrants arrived after World War II. Another interesting observational situation is presented in Brazil, where there has been recent extensive migration from the poverty-stricken northeastern part of the country (where large-bowel cancer is rare) to Sao Paulo and the south of Brazil, where large-bowel cancer is more frequently seen. The reverse phenomenon – migration from high- to low-risk areas – is not generally available for exploitation, the best possibility from this point of view being Israel.

Time trends

For an overview of time trends one must rely on mortality data. The most

98

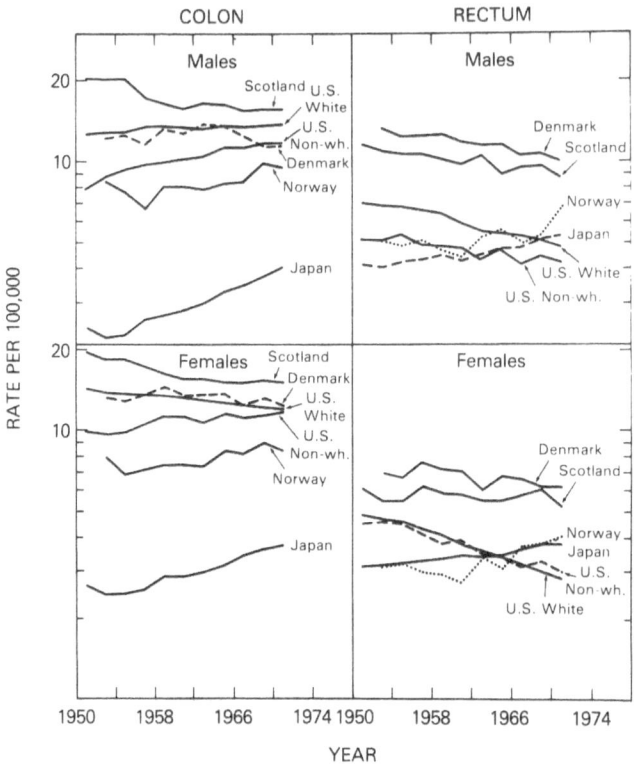

COLON   RECTUM

Figure 7. Trends in age-adjusted mortality rates of cancer of the colon and rectum, by sex. Selected countries, variable time periods, 1950–1972. *Source:* World Health Organization, 1972–1975.

pronounced rise in recorded mortality has occurred in those countries where the risks have been historically low. In certain high-risk populations, such as Scotland and England, the colon cancer rates have declined and there is a group of intermediate-risk countries for which the changes in mortality have been minimal. The differences in time trends between countries at the two extremes of the spectrum of risk are clearly evident.

To illustrate the nature of the changes, Fig. 7 plots curves of age-adjusted mortality for selected populations. Mortality in Japan and Norway has risen almost continuously with few interruptions, while the tendency to lower rates in Scotland, particularly in females, was concentrated in the interval between 1950 and 1965. The companion figure for rectum presents a more consistent pattern of declining mortality than for colon cancer.

Figure 6 presents information on the changes in age-adjusted incidence for cancer of the colon and rectum occurring in 4 areas for which data have been assembled over a substantial time interval. The incidence data for colon cancer

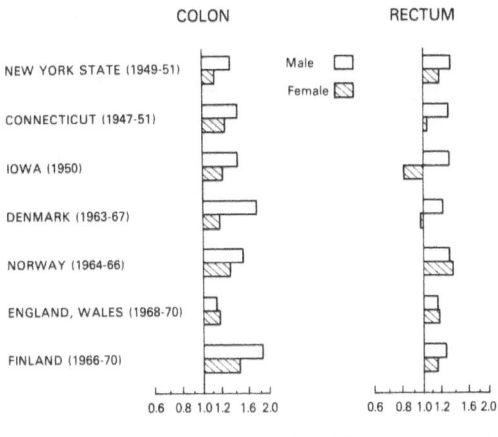

Figure 8. Urban–rural (U/R) ratios of age-adjusted incidence rates for cancer of the colon and rectum. Selected registries, variable time periods. *Source*: References (24, 39, 43–45).

among males show a more pronounced upward trend than that revealed by the corresponding mortality data. The steeper slopes in colon cancer rates for US blacks are the highlight of Fig. 6. The incidence data also reinforce the impression of different time trends for colon and rectum. The curves for rectum display a pattern of declining incidence, particularly among females, as opposed to a pattern of stationary or rising incidence for colon.

The different behavior in incidence trends for colon and rectum raises the more general question about the behavior of the several segments of the large bowel. Data on this point from Connecticut suggest that the upward trend has been most pronounced for both sexes in the proximal colon, with cecum and ascending colon showing the steepest rise.

Urban–rural differences

A higher risk in urban populations is a prominent feature of large-bowel cancer. There is abundant documentation on this point from countries at high-, intermediate-, and low-risk to bowel cancer (24, 39, 43–45).

Figure 8 summarizes the evidence from several sources and indicates a generally more pronounced urban excess for colon than rectum that is better expressed by males.

There is evidence that the urban–rural risk relationships are not constant. In the United States (Iowa) and Norway diminishing urban–rural ratios for colon cancer have been observed for both sexes, attributable to a more rapid rise in rural incidence rates. A similar tendency was present for rectal cancer, except for Iowa females. The pattern of results for Denmark was quite different, where no significant change was observed in the urban–rural ratios for colon; there was a decline in the urban–rural ratios for cancer of the rectum, but the latter was due primarily to a decline in incidence among urban residents.

The nature of the urban–rural gradients in risk have been more extensively investigated in the United States than elsewhere. Mortality tabulations for 1949–1951 (23) showed the US urban excess for large-bowel cancer to persist within each major region of the country. The same pervasive pattern of an urban excess risk has also been described in Norway (46). Detailed residence histories collected for a 10% sample of deaths from cancer of the colon and rectum in the United States for 1958 ruled out the attribution of the excess urban risk to the migration of ill persons to urban centers for medical care (23). In fact, the urban excess risk was enhanced when the contrast was restricted to 'long-term' residents – persons who have resided in the same community for more than 40 years.

The urban–rural ratios should not be interpreted as a measure of the difference in risks between farm and urban populations, since United States farmers account for only a small proportion of the rural population.

Race

The international comparisons have described low risks for large-bowel cancer in Africa, Asia, and Latin Amerika, and the presence of low risk among black and Oriental populations on those continents is beyond dispute. These results, however, confound the effects of race and allied genetic characteristics with those attributable to environmental exposures and different standards of diagnosis and medical care. More precise comparisons of racial differences in risk require that they be made within circumscribed geographic areas, and the available US data can be used for this purpose to good advantage.

The national cancer morbidity surveys in 1947–1948 and 1969–1971 collected incidence data for both white and black populations (19, 21). Within each community and region of the country the white–black differentials are now minimal, a situation that contrasts sharply with 1947–1948, when the incidence of colon cancer among whites in the North and West was almost double that for blacks, and the white excess for rectum was of the order of 50%. In 1947–1948 the same white–black ratio for colon cancer prevailed in the South as in the North, but the racial difference in rectal cancer incidence was even then almost negligible in the South. The changed racial relationship for colon is due primarily to the rise in incidence among blacks; for rectum the narrowing race differential appears traceable to a recorded drop in incidence among whites. The rise in colon

Table 2. Age-adjusted incidence rates per 100,000 population for cancer of the colon and rectum, by race and sex. Hawaii, 1960–1964, 1968–1972.[a]

Race	Colon		Rectum	
	Male	Female	Male	Female
1960–1964				
Caucasian	19.3	27.5	12.6	9.8
Chinese	35.9	23.5	15.8	9.4
Filipino	12.6	14.8	12.4	13.4
Hawaiian	20.2	12.1	6.8	6.9
Japanese	20.7	15.3	11.7	9.8
1968–1972				
Caucasian	23.9	22.9	13.4	12.0
Chinese	28.7	20.9	20.4	5.9
Filipino	16.8	15.3	14.5	0.0
Hawaiian	14.0	16.9	9.4	2.9
Japanese	22.4	18.8	16.3	10.1

[a]*Source*: References (10, 44).

cancer incidence among blacks in the short time span of less than 25 years constitutes one of the strongest pieces of evidence for downplaying the effect of race and allied host factors for this site and for upgrading the role of environmental etiologies.

The best evidence on possible racial differences in risk among the Japanese, Chinese, Filipinos, and Polynesians (Hawaiians) come from the Hawaii Tumor Registry, and Table 2 summarizes the findings from that source. Some of the apparent racial differences in age-adjusted incidence for colon and rectum are probably due to the small numbers of cases observed, particularly for the Chinese, Filipinos, and Hawaiians, and the pertinent point is how small the differences are in that locale when measured on the scale of intercountry variation.

The mortality data for the US Chinese as of 1949–1952 and 1959–1962 (47, 48) reinforce the Hawaii incidence data that describe minimal Chinese–white differences for large bowel and leave open the possibility of slightly elevated colon cancer rates among the US Chinese.

Smith (49) in his review of the American Indian cancer experience as of 1949–1952 reported their risk of large-bowel cancer to be less than half that of US whites. Part of the apparent risk deficit for the American Indian may be attributabel to poor access to medical care and diagnostic facilities due to isolation of several tribes on remote Indian reservations, but this appears unlikely to be the complete explanation. As of 1950, the Mexican-born in the United States (who are of predominantly Indian blood) were also reported to experience lower large-bowel cancer risk (3). The low risks among American Indians still persist (50). The New Mexico Tumor Registry covering the State of New Mexico and the Navajo Indian Reservation in Arizona reports substantially lower incidence rates for Indians than whites (51).

Social class

Most of the information on social-class gradients in cancer risk has come from data collected in England and Wales, Denmark, and the United States. The Registrar General of England and Wales (52) has grouped individual occupations for males into five broad social classes ranging from 'professional' to 'unskilled' on the assumption that mortality is influenced by life-styles associated with different occupational levels as well as by specific occupational hazards and extended this approach to women by classifying female deaths by occupation of the husband. This source of information was exploited once in the United States, when Guralnick (53) reported on occupational mortality among males as of 1950.

In Denmark the Cancer Registry classified all cases reported in Copenhagen during 1943–1947 by district of residence at time of diagnosis and the districts were grouped according to average rental (54), which was stated to be a better indicator of social status than income in the immediate postwar period. A variation of this technique was adopted for the US cancer morbidity survey of 10 metropolitan areas in 1947–1948 (21). All the areas surveyed had been divided into census tracts (areas homogeneous in population characteristics) that were assigned to one of five classes according to median family income. The same relative population distribution by income class was maintained in each area to minimize the confounding of income-class effects with those attributable to other intercity differences.

The composite data on colon from England and Wales suggest a tendency for the highest male risks to occur in the upper social classes; the female results for colon were erratic and inconsistent, and a relationship with social class is not easy to discern for that sex. The findings on rectum from England and Wales portray a weak inverse social-class gradient. The US occupational mortality data for 1950 described an excess colon cancer risk for professional workers, but apart from this little variation was observed among the other social classes. A small deficit in rectal cancer among the same group of professional workers was accompanied by slightly elevated risks for that localization among the lower social classes. The US cancer morbidity survey for 1947–1948 agreed with the mortality data in describing minimal income-class variation in risk for both colon and rectum. The Copenhagen incidence data did not depict a consistent, well-defined social class gradient for total colon among males; the female data suggested a possible elevated risk in the upper classes. A lower risk for cancer of the rectum in the uppermost class of Copenhagen was reported for both sexes, a feature reminiscent of the English male experience.

The composite evidence from populations at relatively high risk to large-bowel cancer leaves some uncertainty as to presence and/or magnitudes of the social-class differences in risk. The absence of clear-cut, consistently observed gradients in the United States, and western Europe, coupled with methodological uncertainties in the analysis of the mortality data, suggest that social-class differences in risk are not an important epidemiological characteristic of the disease in economically developed countries.

The findings from economically developed countries supply no evidence on the situation in low-risk populations. The data from Cali (Colombia) where the overall incidence of large-bowel cancer is one-fifth of that reported by US registries, stand in sharp contrast to those from developed countries (55). The census tract approach, employed in the analysis of data from Denmark and the United States, revealed a marked excess of newly diagnosed cases from the upper socio-economic classes reported to the cancer registry in Cali during 1962–1971. The data tend to overstate the social-class gradient because of underreporting in low-income groups, but the difference is indoubtedly real, and collateral evidence from autopsy studies of adenomatous polyps supports the impression of a minimal risk of large-bowel cancer in the poorest socio-economic class.

What is even more interesting is that the Cali results depict the social-class differences to be concentrated in the segments between the ascending and rectosigmoid colon, a feature that corresponds well with the anatomical specificity in risk gradients noted in international comparisons. Nutritional studies have shown a marked deficit in Cali and throughout Colombia in protein intake, mainly animal protein and a very large socio-economic difference in meat consumption has been reported in Cali (56).

Occupation

The bulk of the evidence on variation in risks by occupation comes from mortality data. The Registrar General of England and Wales in review of 27 broad occupational categories (52) uncovered no consistent pattern of occupational risk for colon and rectum, apart from an above-average risk for colon cancer among professional and administrative workers. The US 1950 results agreed with the English data in singling out professional and white-collar occupations (clergymen, lawyers, managers, accountants, salesmen, etc.) as at high risk to colon cancer.

Recent reports of clusters of colorectal cancer in agricultural workers of the rural area around Memphis, Tennessee, USA, may be related to occupational hazards. The evidence is reviewed by Pratt et al. in another chapter of this monograph (57). Milham reviewed occupational statements on all death certificates for white males filed in the state of Washington for the years 1950–1971 with essentially negative results.

The collective information reinforces impressions of a diffuse, ill-defined excess colon cancer risk among persons in professional and related occupations that may be attributable to general, nonoccupational environmental factors. The failure of the several sources to consistently reproduce findings on individual occupations suggests that any single result for colon or rectal cancer be viewed with reserve. Identification of specific occupational factors for colon and rectum will require long-term prospective observations of employee groups with well-defined exposures along the lines of the follow-up studies of men occupationally exposed to asbestos that have indicated an increased incidence of large-bowel cancer in that group (58).

Religion

Studies of religious groups have been motivated by the search for leads on factors linked to their life-styles that might influence directly or indirectly their site-specific cancer risks. In the United States, MacMahon (59) and later Newill (60) investigated cancer mortality among Catholics, Protestants, and Jews in New York City during the 1950 decade and found minimal variation in total death rate from neoplastic diseases among the three religious groups, but detected some site-specific differences including an excess of large-bowel cancer, confined to the colon, among Jews. Subsequent studies of cancer mortality among Jews were undertaken in New York City (61) and upstate New York (62) utilizing information on religious affiliation of the funeral home and cemetery of burial. The later findings consistently described US Jews to be at higher risk of large-bowel cancer and agreed with Newill in revealing the excess risk to be concentrated in the segments above the rectosigmoid flexure.

The US observations do not mean that elevated colon risks prevail in Jewish populations everywhere. The incidence of large-bowel cancer in Israel is aligned with that for intermediate-risk populations in western Europe (10). Within Israel there is substantial heterogeneity in risk for both colon and rectal cancer, the incidence among Oriental Jews from Asia and Africa being less than half that for persons migrating from Europe and America.

Burbank's review of US mortality data for 1950–1967 identified Utah as the state with the lowest overall cancer death rates for white males and females (22). Since members of the Church of Jesus Christ of Latter-Day Saints (Mormons), a religious group which advocates abstention from use of tobacco, alcohol, tea, and coffee, comprise slightly more than 70% of the Utah population, the reasonable inference was that Mormons have lower cancer risks than other US white populations. Enstrom (63) studied Utah County (approximately 85% Mormon) and demonstrated pronounced deficits in both Utah County and Utah State for cancer of the large bowel and for other sites including buccal cavity, esophagus, lung, and bladder. He also reported that mortality surveillance of a Mormon cohort in California for the years 1970–1972 depicted a deficit in deaths from cancer of the colon and rectum.

This information has recently been amplified by incidence data from the Utah Cancer Registry (64). Since Lyon et al. had access to church membership records, they were able to present cancer incidence rates for the Mormon and non-Mormon populations. Their results showed below-average risks for cancer of the colon and rectum among Mormons and non-Mormons. While the favorable Mormon experience for large-bowel cancer seems to be firmly established, the presence of local environmental factors in Utah and adjacent states that may depress the rates for both Mormons and non-Mormons cannot be ruled out.

Attention was initially directed to the Seventh-Day Adventists because church doctrine proscribes the use of tobacco and alcohol. To utilize this observational situation the cancer mortality experience of a cohort of 35,000 Seventh-Day Adventists in California was monitored for 8 years (1958–1965) with special attention to sites thought to be related etiologically to tobacco use (65, 66). The results indicated the total cancer mortality of the cohort, adjusted for age and sex, to be about 60% of the comparable California rate. Since the Seventh-Day Adventists also possess a distinctive pattern of dietary habits, approximately half adhering to a milk-egg-vegetarian diet, Lemon et al. also investigated colon cancer mortality and reported it to be 60–70% of the California rate. Information on the anatomic distribution of tumors also supports the presumption of lower risks for large-bowel cancer among Adventists. In series from two California hospitals the site of colon-rectal cancers among Adventists were displaced to the right side when compared to non-Adventist controls, the deficit in Adventist patients being concentrated in the descending, sigmoid, and rectosigmoid segments (67).

Other opportunities to observe the experience of religious groups with special characteristics are presented from time to time. For example, the Bombay Cancer Registry has contrasted the site-specific cancer incidence of the local Parsi community (a highly inbred group of about 80,000 survivors of Zoroastrians who left Persia in the seventh century A.D.) with that of the predominantly Hindu population of Bombay and found the Parsis to exhibit a higher incidence of bowel cancer than is typical of Bombay and of many Asian communities (68). The elevated risk for large-bowel cancer among the Parsis is of interest, since this population is known to have a high female breast cancer rate by Asian standards. The Parsis thus conform to the general tendency for breast and large-bowel cancer rates to be closely correlated in interpopulation comparisons.

Tobacco

No important new information on tobacco smoking and large-bowel cancer has been accumulated since this topic was reviewed by Wynder and Shigematsu (69). The findings from three prospective studies on smoking and health (70–72) agree that the association of colon cancer with tobacco use is weak. Nor does the collective evidence demonstrate a regular, consistent gradient in risk by amount smoked for either colon or rectum.

Alcohol

One of the first indications of a possible association between alcohol consumption and large-bowel cancer came from a report by the Registrar General of England and Wales (52) that pinpointed buccal cavity, esophagus, intestines, and rectum (but not stomach) as sites in the digestive tract with excess risks for persons in the alcoholic-beverage trades. This lead has been pursued in systematic geographical correlations of cancer mortality and alcohol consumption. Breslow and Enstrom (73) reported a strong correlation ($r = 0.78$) between beer and rectal cancer in the US male data, which was reproduced in the more heterogeneous data for 24 countries. In both sets of data the relationship appeared to be limited to beer drinking; no association with wine and hard liquors was demonstrable.

These leads have not been consistently confirmed by case-control studies. In studies in England and Wales, Stocks (74) reported large-bowel cancer and beer drinking to be associated, but work elsewhere (75–77) failed to detect a relationship.

Diet

The international variations in risk of large-bowel cancer closely parallel the ranking of countries by stage of economic development. Burkitt (78) felt that no other site was so closely linked to changes in dietary habits that usually accompany economic development. Burkitt recognized the rarity of bowel cancer in most African populations and was impressed by the high fiber and low carbohydrate content of the diet in Africa and other less developed areas of the world in contradistinction to Western countries. In formulating his ideas on the cause of bowel cancer, Burkitt reasoned as follows: reduction in fiber content and bulk favors increased consumption of refined carbohydrates; changes in cellulose content of food alter colonic activity and bowel transit time and excess carbohydrates after the bacterial composition of feces. Carcinogens produced by bacterial action on bile salts or other bile constituents are the probable cause of bowel tumors. Any carcinogen ingested or formed in the gut of refined carbohydrate eaters would be present in a more concentrated form and would be held in contact with the mucosa for a more prolonged period in the constipated colon. Bacterial activity and colonic stasis could account for the anatomical distribution of tumors found maximally in the area where fecal retention is most prolonged and bacterial action most pronounced.

Although Burkitt exercised great ingenuity in developing his hypothesis, there is a weakness. It stems from singling out low-residue diets and refined carbohydrates as the critical differences distinguishing food consumption patterns in high-risk populations from those in populations at low risk to bowel cancer. Individual countries tend to present distinctive configurations of use and non-use which lead to strong positive or negative correlations between specific food items. Under these circumstances international comparisons of per capita food consumption can yield many foods or combinations of foods that appear to discriminate among high- and low-risk populations. For example, Gregor et al. (79) have remarked on the close correlation between national dietary levels of animal protein and mortality from intestinal cancer.

Despite the analytical difficulties, several authors have examined systematically and reported on the correlations between per capita consumption of food items and the incidence and/or mortality of large-bowel cancer (46, 80–82). Their findings are in good agreement, which is not surprising since they all relied on the same primary data sources. Generally speaking, the relationships described were the same for men and women and for colon and rectum. The strongest negative correlations were observed for cereals and pulses and nuts, and the strongest positive correlations were with meat, animal protein, and total fat.

Armstrong and Doll (80) after controlling for associations between foods concluded that the environmental variables most highly correlated with colon cancer rates were meat and animal protein consumption. They noted that control for either of these two variables substantially reduced the correlations with colon cancer for all other food variables and conversely, control for other foods did not reduce the correlation between meat consumption and large-bowel cancer incidence to less than 0.70. Total fat consumption appeared more highly correlated with rectal cancer mortality, but even this correlation was substantially reduced by control for animal protein consumption. The authors also examined their data bearing on the negative association of colon cancer with fiber consumption and found that in their material much of the negative correlation with cereals could be accounted for by control for meat consumption.

Howell (82) pointed out that the vegetable sources of food were independent of or tended to be negatively related to colon cancer and that the associations with the disease were concentrated in the animal sources of food. Total meat protein tended to yield somewhat higher correlations with incidence than did

Table 3. Summary of findings from case-control studies of diet and bowel cancer.

Reference	Study locale	Findings
Stocks (74)	North Wales and Liverpool	Beer drinking positively associated with large-bowel cancer for males. Very weak suggestion of deficit in green vegetable intake by colorectal cancer patients.
Pernu (75)	Finland	No case-control differences found.
Higginson (77)	Kansas City, US	No case-control differences found.
Wynder and Shigematsu (69)	New York City, US	No consistent case-control differences demonstrable for any food items.
Wynder et al. (83)	Japan	Colon cancer patients had diet lower in rice and higher in fruit and milk than controls.
Haenszel et al. (76)	Hawaii, US	Excess bowel cancer risk for Hawaiian Japanese who regularly ate only Western-style meals. Bowel cancer patients ate meats, legumes, and starches more frequently; beef and string beans were major contributors to meat and legume effects.
Bjelke (46)	Norway	Relatively low intake of fish, vegetables, vitamin A and high intake of 'processed' meats by colon and rectal cancer patients. A negative association with coffee was specific for colon cancer. Patients with cancer of the low rectum had diets deficient in fruits, berries, and vitamin C and in this respect closely resembled the diets of stomach cancer patients.
Bjelke (46)	Minnesota, US	Total group of colorectal cancer patients had lower intakes of vegetables, fruits, vitamines A and C, coffee and crude fiber than controls. Lower intake of fruits and vitamin C most marked in patients with low rectum cancer.
Phillips (67)	Seventh-Day Adventists	Higher proportion of colon cancer cases gave history of past use of meat, heavy use of dairy products, except milk, and other high-fat foods compared to Adventist controls. Classification based on current use of meat did not discriminate between cases and controls.

total meat fat, but Howell felt that there was little basis for preferring dietary protein or dietary fat as the more significant association. The problem is that total fat and meat consumption are so highly correlated that it is difficult to estimate separate effects for each factor. Of the meat items, beef was the most strongly associated. The results for pork and poultry were less suggestive, and fish appeared to be an unrelated factor. Howell concluded that the immediate focus for future work should be meat, specifically beef, as the dietary component most likely to be a causative factor in the development of colorectal cancer.

A limited number of studies have searched for case-control differences in the use of foods. One of the earliest was carried out by Stocks (74). The major findings from a series of subsequent investigations are summarized in Table 3. The results from case-control studies up to 1970 were essentially negative, although Wynder's work in Japan (83) did suggest that bowel cancer patients had a more Westernized diet and ate less rice and more fruit and milk than did controls. However, detection of case-control differences is difficult in locales presenting a homogeneous background of diet practices. The study of the Hawaiian Japanese – a population undergoing displacement from low to high colon cancer risk and varying stages of transition from a Japanese to Western-style diet – was the first to uncover important correlations between individual foods and bowel cancer (76). The detection of positive findings was facilitated by the more favorable setting of greater heterogeneity in diet provided by a migrant population.

The Hawaiian Japanese study collected extensive data on individual food items, and reported the relative risks of bowel cancer for individual foods adjusted for other dietary factors. The findings for meats are summarized below:

	Beef	Pork, total	Chicken
Unadjusted	2.2^a	1.5	1.43
Adjusted for			
Beef	–	1.20	1.20
Pork, total	2.1^a	–	1.34
Chicken	2.1^a	1.45	–

[a] Risks significantly different from unity at the 1% level.

Beef exhibited the most pronounced case-control difference and was the only meat that yielded a significantly elevated risk for the summary contrast of above-average vs below-average use. The case-control differences in meat use appeared to be concentrated in some facets of beef consumption.

Other findings were: (1) more bowel cancer patients than controls had abandoned the practice of eating at least one Japanese-style meal daily; (2) patients ate meat, legumes, and starches more frequently, the disparity between patients and controls being less pronounced for starches than for meat and legumes; (3) the case-control differences for meat (beef) and legumes (string beans) persisted among both Issei (migrants) and Nisei (US-born offspring); the excess frequency in consumption of starches was limited to Nisei; (4) the risk differentials, up to 3-fold and greater, compared favorably with those found in case-control studies of other cancer sites and other etiologies (cigarette smoking and lung cancer excepted).

No single case-control study can be viewed as definitive, and the findings must be viewed in the context of other evidence. The interpretation by Haenszel et al. of the Hawaiian-Japanese study relied on collateral evidence from several sources. Their reading of the geographic comparisons was that consumption of meat and refined carbohydrates and mortality from bowel cancer and arteriosclerotic heart disease all appear in relatively affluent populations. In the search for promising lines of investigation they viewed meats (beef) as a more likely etiologic candidate than starches for the following reasons: (1) there is a stronger and more coherent pattern of associations for meat than for starches in the Hawaiian-Japanese data; (2) meat provides a striking example of a change in food practices between Japan and Hawaii – the rise in beef consumption – to parallel the upward displacement of bowel cancer risk among Japanese migrants; (3) an epidemiologic observation exists on an unusual congruence of high meat and low refined carbohydrate consumption; it argues for attention to meat in preference to refined carbohydrates. Argentina has a high meat (beef) intake, and the fraction of calories from refined carbohydrates is relatively low (14). Corresponding to this, Argentina presents a major exception to the usual configuration of a positive association between bowel cancer and atherosclerosis. Mortality from bowel cancer in Argentina is as high as that in the United States, but mortality from arterosclerotic heart disease is moderately low in Argentina. Leveille (84) examined the time trends of colon cancer and food consumption in Connecticut for 1935–1965. He found again the correlation with beef consumption and also called attention to the fact that increases in fat and protein in the diet are accompanied by other changes, notably a reduction in cereal and potatoes in the United States. He found a very strong negative correlation between colon cancer and the consumption of cereals and potatoes.

Enig and collaborators (85) provided a critique of the fat-cancer hypothesis and noted that the increase in fat consumption in the US has been mainly due to an increase in vegetable fat, mostly containing trans double bonds. They suggest that processed vegetable fat should be investigated as possible etiologic agents. It should be noted that the marked increase in vegetable fat consumption has been taking place without a marked reduction in the consumption of other types of fat. This results in an excessive overall fat intake and makes it difficult to assign etiologic roles to one particular type of fat to the exclusion of the other.

Liu and coworkers (86) based their correlation analysis on estimates of the contents of cholesterol, fatty acids and fiber on the items reported in the food consumption tables of FAO. They found that the correlation of colon cancer rates with cholesterol intake remained significant when adjustments were made for fiber and other fats; adjusting for cholesterol, on the other hand, decreased most of the other correlations to nonsignificant levels. In high-risk populations patients with colon cancer tend to have slightly lower levels of blood cholesterol than controls. Two independent studies in Hawaii (87) and Finland (88) have shown that greater stool weight is greater in low-risk populations. Graham and Mettlin (89) reported decreased risk associated with frequent ingestion of vegetables, especially cabbage, brussels sprouts and broccoli. They found some similarity with experimental work showing a reduced risk in animals challenged with a carcinogen and fed indolic compounds of the type found in the above-mentioned vegetables.

The most defensible position to take with respect to dietary factors is that etiologic leads have been generated, but that the evidence does not suffice to choose among them with certainty. New information must be sought either by animal experimentation or by more refined epidemiological studies.

Obesity

Obesity is intimately related to diet and caloric intake, and associations of obesity with large-bowel cancer may arise indirectly via other diet-related factors. For example, while it is true that the Hawaiian Japanese are more obese than people in Japan (90), it does not necessarily follow that obesity per se is implicated in the higher large-bowel cancer rates of the Hawaiian Japanese. The role of body weight has been investigated by a few authors. Sommers (91) reported overweight male and female subjects to be overrepresented in an autopsy series of colon and rectum cancer, when compared with both autopsy controls and data on life insurance policyholders. Wynder and Shigematsu's study in New York City (69) contrasted the weights of patients and controls 2 years prior to diagnosis and found the patient series to have a significant excess of individuals 20% or more overweight.

More recently, Bjelke (46) has examined data from Norway and Minnesota. In Norway no noteworthy differences between colon and rectum patients and controls were found for either sex in weight or weight adjusted for height (bulk index expressed as weight/height^2). In Minnesota the cases displayed higher mean values for weight and bulk index, particularly for males. The case-control study effects are not large, but the consistency between the New York and Minnesota results in describing males to exhibit the stronger relationship between obesity and large-bowel cancer and the failure to detect an effect for either sex in Norway or Japan (83) raise the possibility that the 'obesity' effects may be related to some more specific factors to which American men are more heavily exposed.

Blood group

Vogel and Kruger have made a thorough review of the extensive literature on ABO-blood group and disease. From the composite data, they estimated an 11% excess of colorectal patients of blood group A compared to blood group O. The recent studies in Norway and Minnesota did not detect consistent or marked case-control differences in ABO distribution for large-bowel cancer (46).

Marital status

There is little information on the variation in risk for large-bowel cancer by marital status. Fraumeni et al. (92) examined unpublished 1959–1961 US mortality data and reported that the rates for single women exceeded those for the ever-married at every age for colon and rectum. Studies of women in religious orders offer certain advantages, since they represent well-defined groups who in most orders remain unmarried and celibate throughout life. Such an observational setting minimizes the selective factors that affect the composition of the unmarried general adult female population. Fraumeni et al. (92) analyzed the mortality experience of white, US-born, never-married Sisters in 41 religious communities and found the nuns to have an excess number of colon cancer deaths after age 70 and concluded that the single-married differential for large-bowel cancer presented by the general population experience was consistent with the excess frequency of such cancer in their cohort of nuns.

Reproductive history

Interpopulation comparisons showing a positive correlation between the risks for cancer of the breast and of the large bowel suggest that a review of the epidemiology of large-bowel cancer should touch on the reproductive history parameters investigated with respect to breast cancer. This topic has not been actively pursued, and the only evidence on this point comes from work in Norway and Minnesota (46). These studies found no case-control differences in menarchal or menopausal ages or in age at first childbirth (adjusted for parity). In both the Norwegian and Minnesota series, the relationship with parity differed by anatomical location, with the risk of colonic cancer decreasing and the risk of rectal cancer increasing among women of high parity.

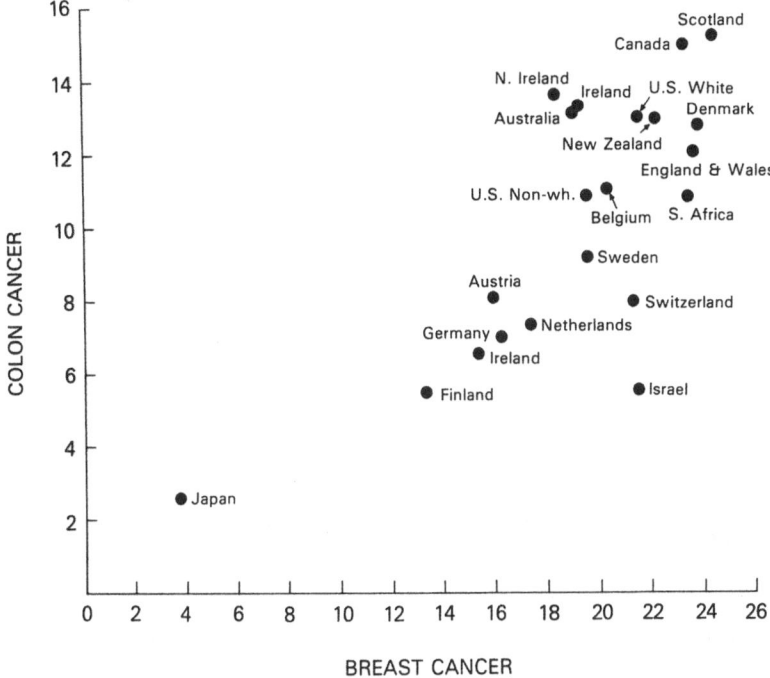

Figure 9. Joint distribution of age-adjusted mortality rates per 100,000 for cancer of the colon and breast. 21 countries, 1960–1961. *Source*: Reference (69).

Association with other diseases

The association of bowel cancer with other diseases has been investigated in a variety of ways. The approach most extensively employed has been to correlate the death rates for specific causes as reported from countries throughout the world. Wynder and Shigematsu (69) have summarized the available mortality data on this subject. A substantial body of data has also been derived from study of the presentation of multiple primary cancer sites in individual patients. Closely allied to the multiple primary approach are autopsy studies on the joint presentation of two or more pathological conditions and the calculation of whether their concordance is greater than expected based on the null hypothesis that the conditions are distributed independently.

Numerous authors have studied the covariation of site-specific cancer mortality among countries, and these efforts have been extended to consider associations with cardiovascular diseases as well. Leaving aside the well-known positive correlation between cancer of the colon and rectum the best-known examples of diseases associated with bowel cancer are: an inverse relationship

114

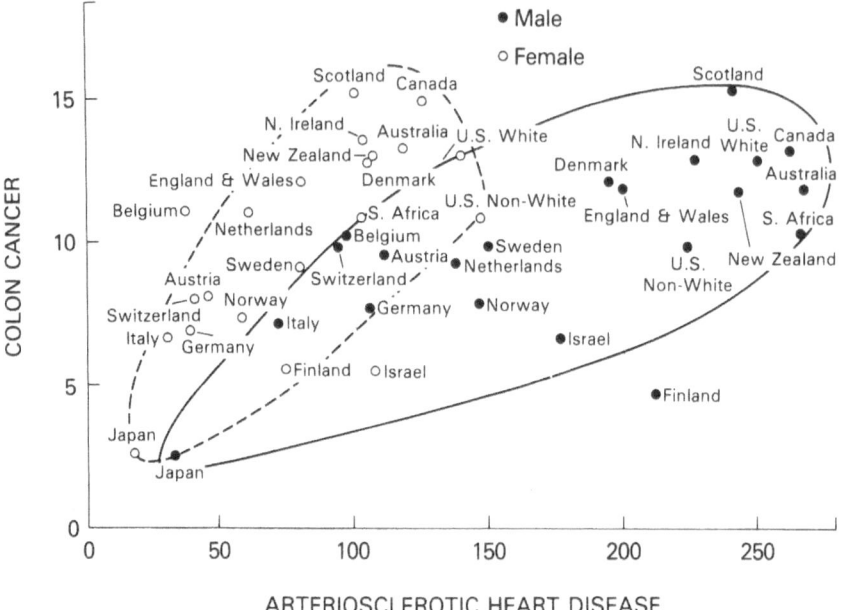

Figure 10. Joint distribution of age-adjusted mortality rates per 100,000 for colon cancer and arteriosclerotic heart disease, by sex. 21 countries, 1960–1961. *Source*: Reference (69).

with stomach cancer, positive associations with cancers of the female breast, endometrium, and ovary, and a positive association with arteriosclerotic heart disease (69). Associations with cancer of the bladder, lung, and pancreas have also been described (46).

The scattergram depicting the joint distribution of mortality from colon and female breast cancer shown in Fig. 9, suggests a rather well-defined, regular relationship. The positive geographical association with breast cancer suggested to Wynder et al. a role for dietary factors, possibly in the terms of fat intake that may influence the internal hormonal environment of the host.

Interest in the association of mortality from colon cancer and arteriosclerotic heart disease arises from the thought that the intake of saturated fats may be implicated in the etiology of the two diseases. The sex-specific nature of the relationships is worth noting. While the two diseases are strongly correlated for each sex (see Fig. 10), the rise in mortality of colon cancer per unit rise in mortality of arteriosclerotic heart disease is greater for females.

The international comparisons also depict an inverse association between cerebrovascular accidents and colon cancer. The attention of Haenszel and Kurihara (4) was drawn to this inverse relationship when they considered the displacement in the mortality of the Japanese migrating to the United States from the prevailing level in Japan to the host population level. They noted a rather complete transition in risks among Issei migrants for cerebrovascular accidents from the high risks in Japan to the characteristic low risks for US whites. Colon cancer also showed a rather complete transition in the opposite direction. The singular aspect of the Japanese migrant experience has been the maintenance of an inverse relationship between colon cancer and cerebrovascular accidents despite the transformation in risks within a single generation from the characteristic level for Japan to that for US whites. The maintenance of the inverse relationship under such radically changed conditions reinforces the belief that the negative association represents a real phenomenon, even though a plausible mechanism for relating the two disease complexes remains to be identified.

The literature on multiple primary cancers has been reviewed by Moertel (93) and Schoenberg et al. (94). The question of interest here is whether the risk of a second primary cancer of a specific site in a defined group of patients is the same, greater, or less than the risk of developing a first cancer at the site in question in the cancer-free population. Utilizing the material from the Connecticut Tumor Registry, Schoenberg et al. found the ratio of observed to expected secondary primaries of the colon to be 1.5 or greater for patients whose primary cancers were located in the breast, corpus uteri, ovary, and cervix uteri. The results of Schoenberg et al. have not been consistently replicated by other investigators. Starting with women whose index cancer presented in the large bowel, Schottenfeld et al. (95) found an excess of second primary cancers of the breast and female genital organs. The ratio of observed to expected cases of breast cancer were 2.1 for the index patients with colon cancer and 1.7 for patients with cancer of the rectum. The corresponding ratios for second primaries of the female genital organs were 2.1 and 0.8 respectively, for the index patients with colon and rectal cancer.

Studies of multiple primaries do not yield definitive results with respect to the association of colorectal tumors with breast and endometrial cancers. One can interpret the studies of second primaries as supporting the site-specific associations revealed by the international comparative studies without accepting the data on second primaries as independent evidence on the presence of site-specific associations.

Familial aggregation

A review of the literature on entities intimately linked to high bowel cancer risks, such as familial adenomatous polyposis coli, an autosomal dominantly inherited disease, is outside the scope of this paper. The epidemiology of bowel cancer suggests that only a minor fraction of bowel cancers can be linked to these and related precursor states, and we confine our attention here to other familial differences in bowel cancer susceptibility for which no obvious mechanisms of inheritance are demonstrable. Observations on familial aggregation are required for studies of both genetic and environmental factors. While studies of familial aggregations of bowel cancer and other diseases are obviously needed, it should be stressed that demonstration of familial aggregation is a necessary, but not sufficient, condition for the presence of genetic variability. Familial aggregation can also reflect common environmental exposures, and for sites in which dietary factors are suspected, a common pattern of dietary habits.

Numerous observations on 'cancer families' strongly suggest a genetic basis for familial aggregation of bowel cancer not related to familial polyposis. Carcinoma of the colon has been reported frequently in 'cancer families,' in association with endometrial carcinoma and multiple primary malignancies (96). Moreover, clusters of bowel cancer cases have been described in other families unaccompanied by malignancies of associated sites (97–99).

Studies to quantitate the degree of familial aggregation have relied on comparisons of the presentation of disease in relatives of affected index patients (probands) with relatives of index controls; sometimes the cases observed among relatives of probands have been contrasted with an expected number calculated from the age- and sex-specific incidence or mortality rates for the population in the area where the families reside. The findings from proband studies of bowel cancer conducted by Macklin (98), Woolf (100), Lovett (101), and Bjelke (46) are in close agreement in describing a 3-fold excess of colorectal cancer risk among relatives of the probands. The excess risk was specific for bowel cancer and was not accompanied by any excess for stomach or other sites.

Proband studies may overestimate the degree of familial aggregation. The bias in such studies arises from the fact that relatives of index cases do not constitute a random sample of families, since they come to the investigator's attention through the presence of an affected individual within the family, so that families with more than one affected individual may have an enhanced probability of being represented in a series of index cases.

Placed in the perspective of the total epidemiological picture of bowel cancer, the results from the proband studies do not suggest genetically determined susceptibility to be of critical importance in determining the level of bowel cancer risk in high-incidence populations.

Polyps

In terms of cancer incidence, the most important condition implicated in colon carcinogenesis is the adenomatous polyp. It is the one entity suspected to be a precursor of the great majority of cases of colon cancer. Other nosologic entities

Table 4. Age-adjusted prevalence rate of colorectal polyps.

Population	Colon cancer incidence	Prevalence rate (%)	
		Hyperplastic	Adenomatous
		Males	
Hawaii-Japanese	Very high	71	63
New Orleans white	High	15	33
New Orleans black	High	14	35
Japan (Akita)	Intermediate	2	35
Japan (Miyagi)	Low	2	13
Colombia (Cali)	Low	11	10
		Females	
Hawaii-Japanese	Very high	51	49
New Orleans white	High	21	19
New Orleans black	High	8	29
Japan (Akita)	Intermediate	4	19
Japan (Miyagi)	Low	1	11
Colombia (Cali)	Low	10	10

– the familial polyposis complex and the chronic idiopathic colitis complex – which, although relatively rare, carry an excessive risk of developing colon cancer will not be reviewed here.

The polyp-cancer relationship constitutes an old medical controversy familiar to many readers. Recent advances have clarified considerably our knowledge of the pathology and epidemiology of polyps. Most investigators of the role of hyperplastic polyps have concluded, mainly on morphological grounds, that they are not precancerous (102, 103). Extensive data on interpopulation variation in prevalence of hyperplastic polyps from autopsy series, summarized in Table 4, also show many inconsistencies in the correlation with colorectal cancer. Interpopulation comparisons of the prevalence of adenomatous polyps correlated much better with the frequency of colorectal cancer (Table 4). People of Japanese extraction living in Hawaii have the highest polyp prevalence on record and very high colon cancer incidence. The Japanese experience indicates that race is not an overriding determinant of the risk of either cancer or adenomatous polyps.

The significance of the geographical associations in the distributions of adenomatous polyps and cancer is enhanced by the greater size and multiplicity of polyps in populations at higher risk to bowel cancer, a feature consistent with the observations that larger and more numerous polyps have a greater tendency to malignant transformation (104).

Epidemiological evidence

The epidemiology of large-bowel cancer is characterized by large intercountry differences in risk, anatomic- and segment-specific patterns of risk, sex-specific patterns of risk, and a disease response modulated by events in adult life linked with migration to a new environment. These features are consistent with a predominant role for environmental factors in the etiology of bowel cancer. The role of genetic factors in the subset of cases linked to familial polyposis is unequivocal, and documentation of familial aggregation for other bowel cancers suggests a genetic basis for individual variability in disease susceptibility. The major point, however, is that the observed magnitude of familial aggregation cannot account for the interpopulation differences in risk without the introduction of extreme, and probably unrealistic, assumptions on population variability in the distribution of 'susceptible' families and individuals.

The concentration of bowel cancer in the economically developed countries of North American and western Europe coincides well with the distribution of high-fat, high-protein diets and suggests large-bowel cancer to be a disease of affluence. This also correlates well with the distribution of endocrine-dependent tumors (breast, endometrium, ovary, prostate) and arteriosclerotic heart disease, which present high risks in affluent populations. The upward displacement of bowel cancer risks, particularly for the segments proximal to the rectosigmoid junction, among Japanese migrants to approximate those of the US white host population argues against racial factors. The results from Israel showing Jews from North America and Europe to have higher risks than Jews from Asia and North Africa provide additional evidence against important racial-genetic determinants.

The features that distinguish colon from rectum include the following points: (1) in high- and intermediate-risk populations colon cancer rates have tended to rise, while those for rectum have remained stationary or declined. The US blacks with a rise of 110% in colon cancer incidence between 1948 and 1970 represents an extreme example of this tendency; (2) the concomitance in geographical distribution of risk with endocrine-dependent tumors and arteriosclerotic heart disease is more clearly defined for colon than rectum.

The segment-specific differences between high- and low-risk populations raise the question whether large-bowel cancer represents a single disease or whether several etiologies are involved. In general, tumor localization appears to be a more promising variable than histology in epidemiological studies. Bowel tumors are predominantly adenocarcinomas, and work to date has not uncovered correlations between histologic characteristics and interpopulation differences in risk.

There are numerous sex differences in the presentation of bowel cancer by geographic area, age, anatomic location, and time periods. Male dominance is firmly established, especially for rectum in the high-risk populations of North America and western Europe. The sex ratios in risk become more variable in Africa, Asia, and Latin America. The US Japanese experience supports the conjecture that the upward trend in male colon cancer is the first response to changed environmental conditions. As of 1960 the colon rates for female Japanese migrants had lagged behind the male rates in making the transition to the elevated risks of the host US white population. Subsequently, the female Japanese rates continued to rise, and now the rates for both male and female Japanese migrants closely approximate the US white experience.

The accumulation of evidence indicates that we can no longer assume that adenomatous polyps are unrelated to large-bowel cancer. From an epidemiologic point of view, the association between adenomatous polyps and colon cancer is supported by the following characteristics: (1) the incidence of colon cancer closely parallels the prevalence of adenomatous polyps in all populations so far studied; (2) whites, blacks, and orientals have a low prevalence of adenomatous polyps while living in areas of low colon cancer frequency, but display high polyp prevalence if they migrate to areas of high colon cancer risk. The difference in adenomatous polyp prevalence between migrant and native Japanese is consistent with the differences in colon cancer incidence in the two groups; (3) in the populations studied, the risk of colon cancer increases with the size and multiplicity of polyps, thus suggesting a dose-effect relationship; (4) the inference of a causal relationship between adenomatous polyps and bowel carcinoma is reinforced by observations on the cancer experience of polyp patients. Prospective studies in Sweden (105) have shown persons with adenomatous polyps to be at higher risk to colon cancer.

Etiologic model

The latest information provided by cancer registries continues to confirm the interactions between risk level, sex ratios, and anatomic localization which led Haenszel and Correa (8) to formulate their epidemiologic model. The components of the model remain valid: (1) in low-risk populations, where the disease is 'endemic,' there is a preponderance of female cases and a relatively uniform distribution of cases throughout the length of the colon with little or no concentration of left-sided tumors in the sigmoid colon; (2) when a new etiologic factor is introduced in a low-risk population, the transition from an 'endemic' to an 'epidemic' phase is first expressed as a rise in sigmoid cancer among older males. This was clearly observed in the data for Japanese migrants to Hawaii as of 1958–1965; (3) a rise in female sigmoid cancer follows later, as shown by the most recent data for Hawaii-Japanese as of 1966–1972; (4) when the epidemic is well established, a rise in cecum and ascending cancer, first noticed in males, is accompanied by similar shifts in the frequency of descending and transverse cancers.

The model postulated could fit a hypothesis based on the presence of a carcinogen in the intestinal contents which become increasingly concentrated as it travels from the ileocecal valve to the rectum. Animal models give ample support for such a hypothesis.

The sex ratio of incidence rates continues to be a puzzling phenomenon since it shows differences among populations, by anatomic localization and between different time periods. Correa and Haenszel postulate that cecum cancer is predominant in females in low-risk populations and that this predominance probably accounts for the female excess in colon cancer in such populations. If the base-line rates of low-risk populations estimate an 'endemic' component present in other populations, the rates for low-risk populations could be subtracted from the latter to estimate the additional 'epidemic' components. The effect of this would be to enhance the estimated male contribution to the 'epidemic' component and to yield the normal male predominance characteristic of most non-sex-related cancers. This, however, falls short of explaining the time trends in the late stages of an epidemic, when females finally attain a high rate of increase. There is a male excess in the prevalence of adenomatous polyps in all populations, including those at low-, intermediate-, and high-risk, but the sex difference in colon cancer incidence is of a lower order of magnitude than that observed for adenomatous polyps. We have, therefore, a male-predominant precursor apparently leading to a sexually more evenly distributed cancer.

We seem, therefore, to be in need of the complementary action of an additional tumorigenic stimulus, a cocarcinogen with preference for females. One possibility in this regard is suggested by the positive correlation between incidence rates for large-bowel cancer and for cancer of the female breast. Large-bowel cancer shares with endocrine-dependent cancers (breast, endometrium, ovary, prostate, testis) several epidemiologic characteristics summarized by Berg (106). It may be suggested that the lack of a pronounced male excess in colon cancer incidence in high-risk populations is due to an extra female component given by response of the colon to endocrine-related carcinogenic factors. It may be that the colon epithelium reponds to the same (or similar) carcinogens responsible for breast cancer, mainly its postmenopausal component. This hypothesis finds some support in experimental carcinogenesis.

Future work

All indications are that we are dealing with direct carcinogens and promoters that come into contact with the large-bowel mucosa and, therefore, are probably carried by the fecal content. Comparative studies of populations at high and low risk to bowel cancer have demonstrated differences in fecal mutagenic activity (107, 108). Mutagens have been found in extracts of fried beef and fried sardines (109, 110); the mutagens from both sources appear to have the same chemical structure which has tentatively been identified as a imidazol-quinoline (IQ) (111). The significance of the latter finding for bowel cancer is debatable since it might be argued that a carcinogen directly ingested with food is not a good prospect for that site, because in that case it should also produce tumors in the upper gastrointestinal tract. The fact that populations at high risk to esophageal and gastric cancer usually do not have a high risk to large-bowel cancer speaks in favor of different etiologies for tumors in the upper and lower digestive tract. The source of the carcinogens and promoters may be chemical precursors found in the bile, or cholesterol excreted with the bile transformed to ultimate carcinogens by bacterial action.

A direct approach to the problem, at the risk of being simplistic, consists of searching for a carcinogen in the stools of patients with cancer or adenomatous polyps. Even better candidates for this approach are the familial polyposis patients. The obvious difficulty with this approach is that the amounts of carcinogen expected are minute, and they may also be unstable. As a short-term goal, Reddy et al. (112) have suggested that identification of chemical or bacterial indicators may discriminate between high- and low-risk populations and between colon cancer patients and controls. Their candidates for possible indicators are β-glucuronidase and 7α-dehydroxylase activities, fecal clostridia, and lithocholic and deoxycholic acid.

Analytical epidemiology has two relatively new options: the identification of a precursor (adenomatous polyps) and the availability of populations at low, intermediate, and high risks. Study of patients with precursor lesions may point to diet and other factors present before habits are changed by the patient as a result of the necrosis and ulceration of the intestinal mucosa brought about by a carcinomatous growth. The study of the diet of cancer and control patients in populations at differing colon cancer risk levels may offer an opportunity to search for items associated with the disease (or with absence of the disease) which may coincide with items that represent additions or deletions to the diet of populations whose cancer risk is changing rapidly (i.e., Hawaiian Japanese) or in populations whose risk is not increasing greatly in spite of changes toward a more affluent type of diet (i.e., Puerto Rico).

The most promising lead identified by epidemiologic studies relates to diet, particularly high-meat, high saturated fat diets. Favorable observational settings with unusual and extreme contrasts in food consumption such as migrants populations and Seventh-Day Adventists should continue to be exploited.

References

1. Doll R, Payne P, Waterhouse J (eds): Cancer incidence in five continents, Vol. I. Tech Rep Int Union Against Cancer. Geneva: UICC, 1966.
2. Boyd J, Landman M, Doll R: The epidemiology of gastrointestinal cancer with special reference to causation. Gut 5:196–200, 1964.
3. Haenszel W: Cancer mortality among the foreign-born in the United States. J Natl Cancer Inst 26:37–132, 1961.
4. Haenszel W, Kurihara M: Mortality from cancer and other diseases among Japanese in the United States. J Natl Cancer Inst 40:43–68, 1968.
5. Helwig EB: The evolution of adenomas of the large intestine and their relation to carcinoma. Surg Gynecol Obstet 84:36–49, 1947.
6. Correa P, Duque E, Cuello C, Haenszel W: Polyps of the colon and rectum in Cali, Colombia. Int J Cancer 9:86–96, 1972.
7. Wynder EL, Hyams L, Shigematsu T: Correlations of international cancer death rates: An epidemiological exercise. Cancer 20:113–126, 1967.
8. Haenszel W, Correa P: Cancer of the colon and rectum and adenomatous polyps: A review of epidemiologic findings. Cancer 28:14–24, 1971.
9. Bjelke E: Epidemiologic studies of cancer of the stomach, colon, and rectum; with special emphasis on the role of diet. Scand J Gastroenterol 9 (13):1–235, 1974.
10. Waterhouse J, Muir C, Correa P, Powell J (eds): Cancer incidence in five continents, Vol. III. International Union Against Cancer. Geneva: UICC, 1976.
11. Segi M, Kurihara M: Cancer mortality for selected sites in 24 countries, No 6(1966–1967). Tokyo: Japan Cancer Society, 1972.
12. Dunham LJ, Bailar JC III: World maps of cancer mortality rates and frequency ratios. J Natl Cancer Inst 41:144–203, 1968.
13. Higginson J, Oettle AG: Cancer incidence in the Bantu and 'Cape Colored' races of South Africa: Report of a cancer survey in the Transvaal (1953–55). J Natl Cancer Inst 24:589–671, 1960.
14. Puffer RR, Griffith GW: Patterns of urban mortality. Sci Publ Pan Am Health Organ 151:45–132, 1967.
15. Eisenberg H, Mork T, Connelly RR: Cancer of the large intestine and rectum: Comparative data from Connecticut and Norway, 1953–1958. Natl Cancer Inst Monogr 15:301–319, 1964.
16. de Jong UW, Day NE, Muir CS, Barclay THC, Bras G, Foster FH, Jussawalla DJ, Kurihara M, Linden G, Martínez I, Payne PM, Pedersen E, Ringertz N, Shanmugaratnam K: The distribution of cancer within the large bowel. Int J Cancer 10:463–477, 1972.
17. Jarvi O: A review of the part played by gastrointestinal heteropias in neoplasmogenesis. Proc Finn Acad Sci Lett 151–187, 1962.
18. Lauren P: The two histological main types of gastric carcinoma: diffuse and so-called intestinal-type carcinoma. Acta Pathol Microbiol Scand 64:31–59, 1965.
19. Cutler SJ, Young JL Jr (eds): Third national cancer survey: Incidence data. Natl Cancer Inst Monogr 41:1–454, 1975.
20. Cook PJ, Doll R, Fellingham SA: A mathematical model for the age distribution of cancer in man. Int J Cancer 4:93–112, 1969.
21. Dorn HF, Cutler SJ: Morbidity from cancer in the United States, Parts I and II. US Department of Health, Education, and Welfare, Public Health Monogr 56. Washington, DC, Supt Doc: US Govt Printing Office, 1959.
22. Burbank F (ed): Patterns in cancer mortality in the United States: 1950–1967. Natl Cancer Inst Monogr 33. Washington, DC, Supt Doc: US Govt Printing Office, 1971.
23. Haenszel W, Dawson EA: A note on mortality from cancer of the colon and rectum in the United States. Cancer 18:265–272, 1965.
24. Teppo L, Hakama M, Hakulinen T, Lehtonen M, Saxén E: Cancer in Finland 1953–1970: Incidence, mortality, prevalence. Copenhagen: Munksgaard, 1975.
25. Mason TJ, McKay FW, Hoover R, Blot WJ, Fraumeni FJ Jr: Atlas of cancer mortality for U.S. counties: 1950–1969. Washington, DC: US Govt Printing Office, 1975.

26. Schwartz MK: Role of trace elements in cancer. Cancer Res 35:3481–3487, 1975.
27. Shamberger RJ, Frost DV: Possible inhibitory effect of selenium on human cancer. Can Med Assoc J 100:682, 1969.
28. Steiner PE: Cancer: Race and geography. Baltimore, Maryland: Williams ? Wilkins, 1954.
29. Lombard HL, Doering CR: Cancer studies in Massachusetts. Cancer mortality in nativity groups. J Prev Med 3:343–361, 1929.
30. Lilienfeld AM, Levin ML, Kessler II: Cancer in the United States. Cambridge, Massachusetts: Harvard Univ Press, 1972.
31. Staszewski J, McCall MG, Stenhouse NS: Cancer mortality in 1962–66 among Polish migrants to Australia. Br J Cancer 25:599–710, 1971.
32. Smith RL: Recorded and expected mortality among Japanese of the United States and Hawaii, with special reference to cancer. J Natl Cancer Inst 17:459–473, 1956.
33. Staszewski J, Haenszel W: Cancer mortality among the Polish-born in the United States. J Natl Cancer Inst 35:291–297, 1965.
34. Norwegian Cancer Society: Cancer Registration in Norway, 1953–1954, 1959.
35. Norwegian Cancer Society: Cancer Registration in Norway, 1959–1961, 1964.
36. Norwegian Cancer Society: Cancer Registration in Norway, 1969–71, 1973.
37. Clemmesen J: Statistical studies in malignant neoplasms, basic tables, Denmark, 1943–1957. Acta Pathol Microbiol Scand, Suppl 174, II, 1965.
38. Clemmesen J: Statistical studies in malignant neoplasms, testis cancer Denmark, 1958–1962. Acta Pathol Microbiol Scand, Suppl 209, III, 1969.
39. Clemmesen J: Statistical studies in malignant neoplasms, lung/bladder ratio, Denmark, 1943–1967. Acta Pathol Microbiol Scand, Suppl 247, IV, 1974.
40. Connecticut State Dept of Health: Cancer in Connecticut – Incidence in rates, 1935–62, 1966.
41. Connecticut State Dept of Health: Annual reports, 1963–1968, 1969.
42. Connecticut State Dept of Health: Conn Health Bull 1–5, 1973.
43. Levin ML, Haenszel W, Carroll BJ, Gerhardt PR, Handy VH, Ingraham SC II: Cancer incidence in urban and rural areas of New York State. J Natl Cancer Inst 24:1243–1257, 1960.
44. Doll R, Muir C, Waterhouse J (eds): Cancer incidence in five continents, Vol. II. New York: Int Union Against Cancer, 1970.
45. Registrar General of England and Wales: Registrar General's statistical review of England and Wales – supplement on cancer, 1965, 1966–1967, 1968–1970. London: HM Stationery Office, 1971.
46. Bjelke E: Epidemiologic studies of cancer of the stomach, colon, and rectum: with special emphasis on the role of diet, 1–5. Ann Arbor, Michigan: University microfilms, 1973.
47. Smith RL: Recorded and expected mortality among the Chinese in Hawaii and the United States with special reference to cancer. J Natl Cancer Inst 17:667–676, 1956.
48. King H, Haenszel W: Cancer mortality among foreign- and native-born Chinese in the United States. J Chron Dis 26:623–646, 1973.
49. Smith RL: Recorded and expected mortality among the Indians of the United States with special reference to cancer. J Natl Cancer Inst 18:385–396, 1957.
50. Creagan ET, Fraumeni JF Jr: Cancer mortality among American Indians, 1950–67. J Natl Cancer Inst 49:959–967, 1972.
51. New Mexico Tumor Registry: Cancer in New Mexico, 1969–72, 1975.
52. Registrar General of England and Wales: The Registrar General's decennial supplement, England and Wales, 1921, 1931, 1951, 1961, Occupational mortality tables. London: HM Stationery Office, 1962.
53. Guralnick L: Vital statistics special reports, Vol 53, No 3. Washington, DC: US Govt Printing Office, 1963.
54. Clemmesen J, Nielsen A: Social distribution of cancer in Copenhagen, 1943. Brit J Cancer 5:159–171, 1951.
55. Haenszel W, Correa P, Cuello C: Social class differences among patients with large-bowel cancer in Cali, Colombia. J Natl Cancer Inst 54:1031–1035, 1975.
56. Aragón LA: Estimación del consumo de algunos alimentos básicos en la ciudad de Cali. Tesis de grado, Cali Universidad del Valle, Facultad de Ciencias Económicas, Cali, Colombia, 1964.

124

57. Pratt CB, Rivera G, Shanks E et al.: Colorectal carcinoma in adolescents: implications regarding etiology. Cancer 40(5) (Suppl):2464–2472, 1977.
58. Selikoff IJ, Hammond EC, Seidman H: Cancer risk of insulation workers in the U.S. IARC Sci Publ 8:209–216, 1973.
59. MacMahon B: The ethnic distribution of cancer mortality in N.Y. City, 1955. Acto Unio Intern. Contra Cancrum 16:1716–1724, 1960.
60. Newill VA: Distribution of cancer mortality among ethnic subgroups of the white population of N.Y. City, 1953–1958. J Natl Cancer Inst 26:405–417.
61. Seidman H: Cancer mortality in N.Y. City for country of birth, religions and socioeconomic groups. Environ Res 4:390–429, 1971.
62. Greenwald P, Korns RF, Nasca PC, Wolfgang PE: Cancer in United States Jews. Cancer Res 35:3507–3512, 1975.
63. Enstrom JE: Cancer mortality among Mormons. Cancer 36:825–841, 1975.
64. Lyon JL, Klauber MR, Gardner JW, Smart CR: Cancer incidence in Mormons and non-Mormons: Utah 1966–1970. N Engl J Med 294:129–133, 1976.
65. Lemon FR, Walden RT, Wood RW: Cancer of the lung and mouth in Seventh-Day Adventists. Cancer 17:486–497, 1964.
66. Lemon FR, Walden RT: Death from respiratory system disease among Seventh-Day Adventist men. J Amer Med Assoc 198:117–126, 1966.
67. Phillips RL: Role of life-style and dietary habits in risk of cancer among Seventh-Day Adventists. Cancer Res 35:3513–3522, 1975.
68. Jussawalla DJ, Jain DK: Cancer incidence in Greater Bombay, 1970–1972. Indian Cancer Society – Bombay Cancer Registry, Bombay, 1976.
69. Wynder EL, Shigematsu T: Environmental factors of cancer of the colon and rectum. Cancer 20:1520–1561, 1967.
70. Doll R, Hill AB: Mortality in relation to smoking – Ten years' observations of British doctors. Brit Med J 1:1399–1410, 1964.
71. Kahn HA: The Dorn study of smoking and mortality among U.S. veterans: Report on eight and one-half years of observation. In: Haenszel WM (ed): Epidemiological study of cancer and other chronic diseases. US. Dept of Healu., Education, and Welfare, National Cancer Institute Monograph No 19. Washington, DC: US Govt Printing Office, 1966, pp 1–126.
72. Hammond EC: Smoking in relation to death rates of one million men and women. In: Haenszel W (ed): Epidemiological study of cancer and other chronic diseases. US Dept of Health, Education, and Welfare, National Cancer Institute Monograph No. 19. Washington DC: US Govt Printing Office, 1966, pp 127–204.
73. Breslow NE, Enstrom JE: Geographic correlations between cancer mortality rates and alcohol-tobacco consumption in the United States. J Natl Cancer Inst 53:631–639, 1974.
74. Stocks P: British Empire Cancer Campaign 35th Annual Report for 1957. Supplement to Part II, 156 pp.
75. Pernu J: An epidemiological study on cancer of the digestive organs and respiratory system – A study based on 7078 cases. Ann Med Intern Fenn 49(33):1–117, 1960.
76. Haenszel W, Berg JW, Segi M, Kurihara M, Locke FB: Large-bowel cancer in Hawaiian Japanese. J Natl Cancer Inst 51:1765–1779, 1973.
77. Higginson J: Etiological factors in gastrointestinal cancer in man. J Natl Cancer Inst 37:527–545, 1966.
78. Burkitt DP: Epidemiology of cancer of the colon and rectum. Cancer 28:3–13, 1971.
79. Gregor O, Toman R, Prusova F: Gastrointestinal cancer and nutrition. Gut 10:1031–1034, 1969.
80. Armstrong B, Doll R: Environmental factors and cancer incidence and mortality in different countries, with special reference to dietary practices. Int J Cancer 15:617–631, 1975.
81. Howell MA: Factor analysis of international cancer mortality data and per capita food consumption. Brit J Cancer 29:328–336, 1974.
82. Howell MA: Diet as an etiological factor in the development of cancers of the colon and rectum. J Chron Dis 28:67–80, 1975.
83. Wynder EL, Kajitani T, Ishakawa S, Dodo H, Takano A: Environmental factors of cancer of

the colon and rectum. II. Japanese epidemiological data. Cancer 23:1210–1220, 1969.

84. Leveille GA: Issues on human nutrition and their probable impact on foods of animal origin. J Anim Sci 4:723–731, 1975.
85. Enig MG, Munn RJ, Keeney M: Dietary fat and cancer trends – a critique. Fed Proc 37:2215–2220, 1978.
86. Liu K, Stamler J, Moss D, Garside D, Persky V, Soltero I: Dietary cholesterol, fat and fiber, and colon cancer mortality. Lancet 2:782–785, 1979.
87. Glober GA, Klein KL, Moore JO, Abba BC: Bowel transit times in two populations experiencing similar colon cancer risks. Lancet 2:80–81, 1974.
88. International Agency for Research on Cancer. Dietary fiber, transit time, fecal bacteria, steroids and colon cancer in 2 Scandinavian populations. Lancet 2:207–211, 1977.
89. Graham S, Mettlin C: Diet and colon cancer. Am J Epidemiol 109:1–20, 1979.
90. Kagan A, Harris BR, Winkelstein W, Johnson KG, Kato H, Syme SL, Rhoads GC, Gay ML, Nichaman MZ, Hamilton HB, Tillotson J: Epidemiologic studies of coronary heart disease and stroke in Japanese living in Japan, Hawaii and California: demographic, physical, dietary and biochemical characteristics. J Chronic Dis 27:345–364, 1974.
91. Sommers SC: Abnormalities accompanying carcinomas of the large intestine. Dis Colon Rectum 7:262–269, 1964.
92. Fraumeni JF Jr, Lloyd JW, Smith EM, Wagoner JK: Cancer mortality among nuns: Role of marital status in etiology of neoplastic disease in women. J Natl Cancer Inst 42:455–468, 1969.
93. Moertel CG: Multiple primary malignant neoplasms: their incidence and significance. Recent Results Cancer Res 7:1–107, 1966.
94. Schoenberg BS, Greenberg RA, Eisenberg H: Occurrence of certain multiple primary cancers in females. J Natl Cancer Inst 43:15–32, 1969.
95. Schottenfeld D, Berg JW, Vitsky B: Incidence of multiple primary cancers. II. Index cancers arising in the stomach and lower digestive system. J Natl Cancer Inst 43:77–86, 1969.
96. Lynch HT, Shaw MW, Magnuson CW, Larsen AL, Krush AJ: Study of two large midwestern kindreds. Arch Intern Med 117:206–212, 1966.
97. Ceulemans G: Incidence familiale multiple du cancer du rectum. J Int Coll Surg 30:649–652, 1958.
98. Macklin MT:Inheritance of cancer of the stomach and large intestine in man. J Natl Cancer Inst 24:551–571, 1960.
99. Peltokallio P, Peltokallio V: Relationship of familial factors to carcinoma of the colon. Dis Colon Rectum 9:367–370, 1966.
100. Woolf CM: A genetic study of carcinoma of the large intestine. Am J Hum Genet 10:42–47, 1958.
101. Lovett E: Family studies in cancer of the colon and rectum. Br J Surg 63:13–18, 1976.
102. Morson BC: Some peculiarities in the histology of intestinal polyps. Dis Colon Rectum 5:337–341, 1962.
103. Lane N, Kaplan H, Pascal R: Minute adenomatous and hyperplastic polyps of the colon: divergent patterns of epithelial growth with specific associated mesenchymal changes. Gastroenterology 60:537–551, 1971.
104. Silverberg SG: Focally malignant adenomatous polyps of the colon and rectum. Surg Gynecol Obstet 131:103–114, 1970.
105. Ekelund G, Lindstrom C: Histopathological analysis of benign polyps in patients with carcinoma of the colon and rectum. Gut 15:654–663, 1974.
106. Berg JW: Can nutrition explain the patterns of international epidemiology of hormone-dependent cancers? Cancer Res 35:3345–3350, 1975.
107. Reddy BS, Sharma C, Darby L, Laakso K, Wynder EL: Metabolic epidemiology of large bowel cancer. Fecal mutagens in high- and low-risk populations for bowel cancer. Mutation Res 72:511–522, 1980.
108. Ehrich M, Aswell JE, Van Tassell RL, Wilkins TD, Walker ARP, Richardson NJ: Mutagens in the feces of 3 South-African populations at different levels of risk for colon cancer. Mutation Res 64:231–240, 1979.
109. Spingarn NE, Weisburger JH: Formation of mutagens in cooked foods. I. Beef. Cancer Letters

7:259–264, 1979.
110. Weisburger JH, Reddy BS, Hill P, Cohen LA, Wynder EL, Spingarn NE: Nutrition and cancer – on the mechanisms bearing on causes of cancer of the colon, breast, prostate, and stomach. Bull NY Acad Med 56:673–696, 1980.
111. Spingarn NE, Kasai H, Vuolo LL, Nishimura S, Yamaizumi Z, Sugimura T, Matsushima T, Weisburger JH: Formation of mutagens in cooked foods. III. Isolation of a potent mutagen from beef. Cancer Letters 9:177–183, 1980.
112. Reddy BS, Mastromarino A, Wynder EL: Further leads on metabolic epidemiology of large-bowel cancer. Cancer Res 35:3403–3406, 1975.

5. Epidemic Colon Cancer in Children and Adolescents?

CHARLES B. PRATT and STEPHEN L. GEORGE

Introduction

Colorectal carcinoma is an unusual form of cancer in children and adolescents (1–7). In the United States, the annual incidence rate, males plus females, all races, as reported by the Third National Cancer Survey, is approximately 2.3 per million persons between the ages of 10 and 19 years (8). Thus, although fewer than 300 cases have been reported in the literature (1–7), an estimated 90 cases will occur in the US in 1980.

At St. Jude Children's Research Hospital (SJCRH), 26 adolescents with this rare form of cancer have been admitted with this diagnosis between March, 1964 and August, 1980. Twenty-two of these subjects were referred after September, 1974. Single patients were referred in 1964, 1966, 1969 and 1973. Three patients were admitted in 1974, 6 in 1975, 4 in 1976, 1 in 1977, 2 in 1978, 3 in 1979 and 3 in 1980.

By place of residence at the time of referral, 9 were from Mississippi, 5 each from Tennessee and Arkansas, 2 from Alabama, and one each was from Louisiana, Missouri, Indiana, Wisconsin and Texas (Table 1). The place of residence was rural for 19 patients: the remaining 7 patients were referred from urban population centers (i.e., with greater than 25,000 persons within the fixed population area).

The purpose of this communication is to review the experience at SJCRH with respect to patient characteristics, results of treatment and epidemiology of colorectal carcinoma in children and adolescents. In addition, the possibility of an increased incidence rate or disease clustering during the study period is investigated formally.

Patient characteristics

Ages at diagnosis ranged from 8 to 19 years, with a median age of 15 years (Table 1). There were 8 black boys, 7 white boys, 6 black girls, and 5 white girls (Table 1).

These tumors arose in all portions of the large bowel (Fig. 1). Specifically there were 5 primary tumors of the cecum, 3 of the ascending colon, 2 of the hepatic

Correa, P. and Haenszel, W. (eds.), Epidemiology of Cancer of the Digestive Tract.
© *1982 Martinus Nijhoff Publishers. The Hague/Boston/London. ISBN-13:978-94-009-7504-0*

Table 1. Characteristics of 26 adolescents with colorectal carcinoma.

Patient	Age years	Race/sex	Primary site	Histology	Stage at diagnosis (Duke's)	Documented metastases
1	10.7	BB	Hepatic flexure	M	C	Mesenteric nodes
2	11.8	BB	Cecum	M	D	Peritoneum, retroperitoneal nodes, sigmoid
3	15.4	BG	Rectum	M	B	Perirectal fat
4	16.4	BB	Cecum	M	D	Peritoneum, pelvis
5	15.5	BG	Sigmoid	M	D	Peritoneum, retroperitoneal nodes, ovaries, liver
6	13.0	BG	Descending	M	D	Peritoneum, retroperitoneal and mesenteric nodes, abdominal wall, uterus
7	14.2	BG	Splenic flexure	M	D	Peritoneum, retroperitoneal nodes, liver, mediastinum, cervical nodes, liver, adrenals, pancreas, kidneys, bladder, lungs, heart, skin, bone marrow (A)
8	15.4	WG	Transverse	M	C	Peritoneum, retroperitoneal nodes, ovaries, uterus, abdominal wall (A)
9	16.7	BG	Splenic flexure	M	D	Peritoneum, retroperitoneal nodes, ovaries
10	8.8	WG	Cecum	M	D	Peritoneum, retroperitoneal nodes
11	15.1	BB	Descending	M	D	Peritoneum, retroperitoneal and mediastinal nodes, liver, spleen, adrenals, pancreas, gallbladder, urinary bladder, thyroid, lungs, brain meninges, bones and bone marrow (A)
12	18.9	BB	Splenic flexure	M	B	Peritoneum, retroperitoneal nodes, pancreas, abdominal wall
13	16.5	WG	Ascending	M	C	Peritoneum, mesenteric nodes
14	17.0	BB	Hepatic flexure	M	C	Peritoneum, pancreas, spleen, abdominal wall, lungs

Outcome	Resident of State	Residence population characteristic	Known exposure to environmental hazards	Other
DOD 9 mo.	AL	Rural	?	
DOD 13 mo.	TN*	Rural	?	
NED 10 yrs.+	AR*	Rural	?	
DOD 7 mo.	MS*	Rural	?	
DOD 8 mo.	MS*	Rural	Agricultural sprays for crops	
DOD 40 mo.	LA	Urban	None	Single juvenile polyp 12 cm from anus found at routine examination following multiple surgical resections
DOD 5 mo.	MS*	Rural	Agricultural sprays for crops	Sibling died of neuroblastoma at age 14 yrs.
DOD 36 mo.	MS*	Rural	?	Cholinesterase deficiency
DOC 10 days	MS*	Rural	Agricultural sprays for crops	
DOD 10 mo.	WI	Rural	Farm sprays for animals	
DOD 9 mo.	MS*	Rural	Agricultural sprays for crops	
DOD 17 mo.	TN*	Rural	Farm sprays	
DOD 6 mo.	IN	Urban	None	
DOD 26 mo.	TN*	Rural	Farm sprays	

130

Table 1. Continued.

Patient	Age years	Race/sex	Primary Site	Histology	Stage at diagnosis (Duke's)	Documented metastases
15	15.3	WB	Rectum	M	D	Perirectal area, perito-neum, bladder, prostate, sacrum, axillary and inguinal nodes
16	18.8	WB	Rectum	M	D	Peritoneum retroperi-toneal nodes, perirectal area, abdominal wall, bone marrow
17	19.2	WB	Cecum	M	D	Peritoneum, retroperi-toneal nodes, liver, pleura
18	17.7	WB	Descending	M	D	Peritoneum
19	13.2	WB	Sigmoid	Non-M	D	Peritoneum, retroperi-toneal nodes, liver
20	15.5	BB	Ascending	M	D	Peritoneum, mesenteric nodes, pelvis
21	15.6	WG	Ascending	M	D	Peritoneum, retroperi-toneal nodes, liver, kidney, lungs, heart, brain (A)
22	13.8	WG	Transverse	Non-M	B	Serosa, pericolic fat
23	19.8	BG	Sigmoid	Non-M	D	Peritoneum, retroperi-toneal nodes, ovaries, liver, chest wall
24	18.6	WB	Rectosigmoid	M	D	Peritoneum, mesenteric amd retroperitoneal nodes, liver
25	14.9	BB	Sigmoid	M	C	Peritoneum mesenteric nodes, pelvis
26	18.2	WB	Cecum	Non-M	D	Peritoneum, mesenteric nodes

BB = Black boy   AL = Alabama   MS = Mississippi
BG = Black girl   TN = Tennessee   WI = Wisconsin
WB = White boy   AR = Arkansas   IN = Indiana
WG = White girl   LA = Louisiana   TX = Texas
M = Mucinous   MO = Missouri
Non-M = Non-mucinous

Outcome	Resident of State	Residence population characteristic	Known exposure to environmental hazards	Other
DOD 11 mo.	AR*	Rural	Agricultural sprays for crops	Single juvenile polyp removed at time of initial biopsy of rectal tumor
DOD 5 mo.	TN*	Rural	Agricultural sprays for crops	
DOD 9 mo.	AR*	Rural	Agricultural sprays for crops	
DOD 6 mo.	AL	Rural	Agricultural sprays for crops	
DOD 5 mo.	MO	Urban	Agricultural sprays for crops	Congenital rubella syndrome with deafness; juvenile polyposis coli diagnosed at 4 yrs.
LWD 25 mo.	AR*	Rural	Agricultural sprays for crops	
DOD 6 mo.	MS*	Urban	Agricultural sprays for crops	Benign carcinoid found in appendix removed at time of initial laparotomy
NED 16 mo.	AR*	Rural	Agricultural sprays for crops	
DOD 6 mo.	MS*	Rural	Agricultural sprays for crops	
LWD 5 mo.	TN*	Urban	Agricultural sprays for crops	
LWD 9 mo.	MS	Urban	Pesticides for mosquitoes	Single juvenile polyp detected in mucous fistula 6 months after primary diagnosis
LWD 3 mo.	TX	Urban	None	

DOD = Died of disease
NED = No evident disease
DOC = Died of complication
A = Autopsy
LWD = Living with disease
* = Residence within 75 miles of Mississippi River

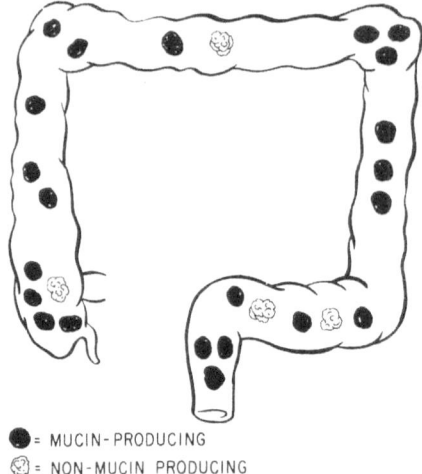

= MUCIN-PRODUCING
= NON-MUCIN PRODUCING

Figure 1. Primary sites of colorectal carcinoma in 26 adolescents.

flexure, 2 in the mid-transverse colon, 3 of the splenic flexure, 3 in the descending colon, 4 in the sigmoid, 1 in the rectosigmoid and 3 in the rectum.

The frequency of various symptoms and signs in these 26 patients is outlined in Table 2. Abdominal pain was the most frequently encountered symptom; only one patient with primary tumor in the transverse colon failed to complain of abdominal discomfort. For most patients, the abdominal pain or discomfort was vague and caused a delay in seeking medical attention. Other common symptoms were related to bowel dysfunction. Bowel obstruction was demonstrated for 6 subjects. Six of the nine patients with tumors in the rectum or sigmoid had rectal bleeding. Duration of symptoms ranged from 4 days to 12 months, with a median duration of $2\frac{1}{2}$ months.

Most patients had extensive tumors at the time of diagnosis (Table 1). Three patients had Duke's stage B tumors, 5 stage C, and 18 had stage D tumors with widespread intra abdominal metastatic tumor or other distant metastatic involvement.

The histology of the primary and metastatic tumors was that of poorly differentiated mucin-producing carcinoma in 22 subjects (Table 1). Four subjects had well-differentiated non-mucin producing carcinomas; these lesions were located in the cecum, transverse colon and sigmoid.

Results of treatment

Treatment methods included surgery, chemotherapy and radiation therapy (9).

Table 2. Presenting signs, symptoms of 26 adolescents with colorectal carcinoma.

Abdominal pain	25
Nausea, vomiting	15
Weight loss	15
Constipation	10
Diarrhea	9
Anorexia	8
Anemia	7
Obstruction	6
Distension	5
Rectal bleeding	5
Palpable abd. mass	4
Cervical lymphadenopathy	1

For many subjects, surgery was limited by the extensive nature of the tumor at the time of diagnosis. Similar chemotherapy, consisting of a combination of 5-fluorouracil, methyl-CCNU and vincristine was administered to 20 of the subjects admitted since 1974. Several patients have additionally received treatment with investigational agents. Radiation therapy was delivered to 2 primary tumors of the rectum or rectosigmoid.

As of Octover 1980, 2 of the 26 patients are surviving continuously free of disease at 16 and 130 months from diagnosis (Table 1). Four patients are living with disease at 2, 4, 10 and 25 months from diagnosis. Twenty patients died of tumor 10 days to 38 months (median 9 months) from diagnosis (Fig. 2). The overall median survival is estimated to be 9 months.

Those patients who remain continuously free of tumor had stage B tumor at diagnosis. Patient 3 received pre-operative irradiation prior to definitive surgery, followed by post-operative 5-fluorouracil therapy. Patient 22 continues to receive adjuvant 5-FU, methyl-CCNU and vincristine. For 11 patients who received these 3 agents for treatment of measurable primary or metastatic tumor, partial responses were observed in 3 patients as measured by physical examination or diagnostic imaging techniques. For 8 patients who received these agents in an adjuvant situation, recurrence of tumor was detected between 5 and 23 months (median 14 months). Two patients admitted since 1974 received no chemotherapy; one patient died early from complications of tumor, and the other patient refused additional treatment following surgical resection of tumor.

General epidemiology

Standard questionnaires, specifically designed for the subjects of this study, were utilized to assess various aspects of the epidemiologic features of the latter 22 of these subjects admitted since 1973. These earlier studies were undertaken with

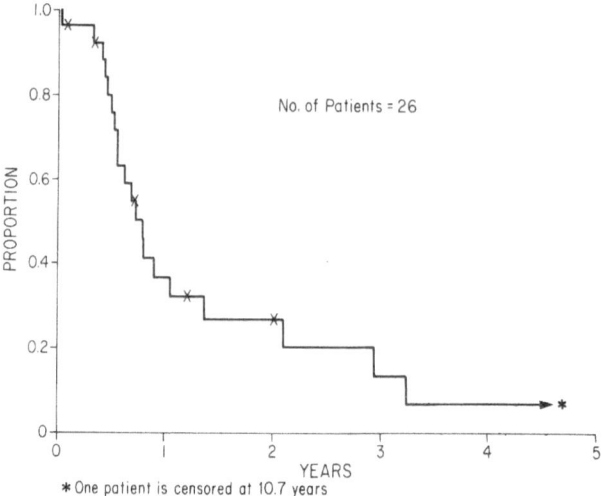

Figure 2. Survival time from diagnosis, 26 adolescents with colorectal carcinoma.

the cooperation of the Cancer Branch, Chronic Disease Division of the Center for Disease Control; some of the results of these surveys have been published in part (1), or are to be reported shortly (9).

For the latter 22 subjects, specific inquiries were made regarding exposure to various chemicals. These questions were more relevant after the determination that 3 white boys admitted to 1976 had been intimately involved in the spraying operations for cotton and soybean production. Seventeen of these 22 subjects had histories of exposure to chemicals used in farm operations for crops-14 or livestock-3 (Table 3). One additional patient, who resided in an urban area, had repeated exposure to pesticides used for mosquito control.

Only one (patient 19) of the 26 patients in this series (Table 1) had multiple juvenile polyps; this diagnosis had been made at the age of 4 years, but he had not been re-examined between the ages 7 and 13 years, the time of diagnosis of carcinoma of the sigmoid colon. This patient, with congenital rubella syndrome, had central deafness without congenital heart disease or cataracts.

Three other patients had single juvenile polyps. For patient 15, an anal polyp was found at the time of diagnosis of rectal carcinoma. The polyps of patients 6 and 25 were found 6 and 24 months after the diagnosis of carcinoma.

Some isolated findings of interest are: patient 21 had a benign carcinoid found in the appendix which was resected at the time of the initial laparotomy; patient 8 had cholinesterase deficiency detected at the time of laparotomy; her maternal uncle had a similar deficiency; a 14-year-old male sibling of patient 17 had died of generalized neuroblastoma 6 years before her diagnosis of carcinoma of the splenic flexure.

Table 3. History of exposure to chemicals.

	Documented Exposure	None	Unknown
Rural	14	0	1
Urban	4	3	0

Detailed pedigrees were constructed for each of the 22 subjects referred since 1973. In no family was there any evidence of consanguinity or a family cancer syndrome.

Dietary histories additionally were obtained from most of recently referred patients. To date, no specific influences could be associated with the development of tumors within our patients, as has been implied for adults with this neoplasm (10–14). Such influences would be difficult to detect with this number of patients in any case.

Incidence and disease clustering

When an apparently large number of cases of a disease are referred to a single institution, it is natural to ask whether or not there is (or was) an epidemic of the disease during this time period. This question is difficult to answer for any chronic disease and requires special approaches when the institution is not a geographical or population-based referral center.

There previously have been reports of high incidence of colorectal carcinoma involving our referral area (15, 16). Specifically, the lower Mississippi River valley area has been demonstrated to be such an area; however, a younger than expected median age at death from colorectal carcinoma has not been reported within this geographic area.

We consider two questions in this section: (1) Has there been an unusually high incidence of colorectal cancer in children in this area during the past 15 years? (2) Is there any evidence of time or space clustering of disease during this time period?

Both questions need to be made more precise, both with respect to time and geographical region and with respect to terminology. The time period covered for this analysis is January 1, 1966 through July 31, 1980. The geographical region considered is part of three states (Tennessee, Arkansas and Mississippi) from which the hospital receives most of its referrals. All counties within these three states and located within 75 miles of the Mississippi River constitute the area of interest (Fig. 3). This region was chosen because of the historic referral pattern to this institution. Also, we will restrict attention to children

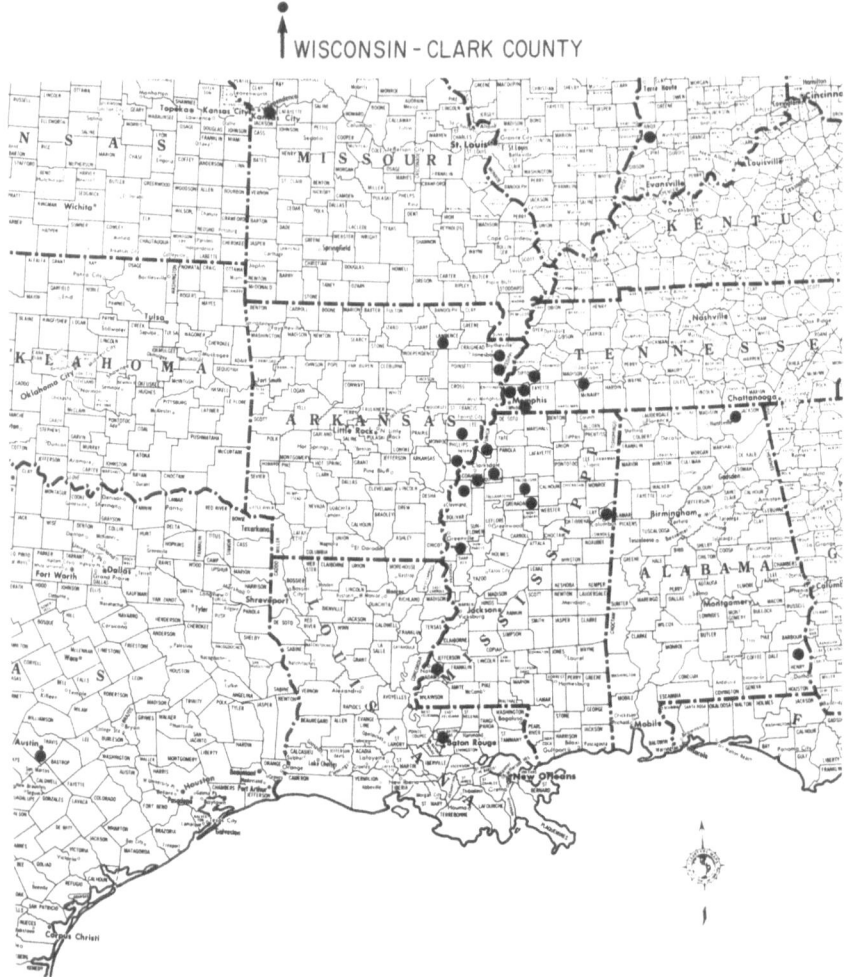

↑ WISCONSIN - CLARK COUNTY

Figure 3. Place of residence at time of referral, 26 adolescents with colorectal carcinoma.

between the ages of 10 and 19 (inclusive) because of the extreme rarity of the disease under 10 years of age. In this section, 'children' will refer to persons in this age range. Patients meeting these criteria are indicated by an asterisk in Table 1.

First, we are interested in testing whether the average annual incidence (for the study period) of colorectal cancer in children living in the study region is significantly larger than that reported in the Third National Cancer Survey, which is taken as our standard of comparison (8).

To calculate incidence rates, we need to know the number of newly-diagnosed cases occurring in the study region during the study period. In our case, this is impossible since all cases from this region are not referred to this institution.

Table 4. Number of children within 75 miles of Mississippi River, Tennessee, Arkansas and Mississippi.

	Cases referred to SJCRH	All cases[a]	Expected cases, TNCS
Tennessee	5	7.5	7.3
Arkansas	5	6.4	5.2
Mississippi	8	11.2	7.1
	18	25.1	19.6
Annual incidence rate per 10^6 children:	2.136	2.978	2.278

[a] See Appendix 1

However, by the methods given in Appendix 1, we can perhaps be close enough to determine whether or not the observed incidence rate is unusual.

There were 18 patients meeting the above criteria and referred to this institution: 8 from Mississippi and 5 each from Arkansas and Tennessee (see Table 4). The total estimated number of cases in the area including those that were not referred to this institution is also given in Table 4. This number was calculated from death certificate information and estimated survival probabilities as indicated in Appendix 1. Finally, the expected number of cases based on the Third National Cancer Study is given (8).

The average annual incidence rate for the region was 2.14 per 1,000,000 children if only cases referred to this institution and 2.98 if the estimated additional cases are added. Neither of these rates are even close to being significantly different from the incidence rate of 2.28 derived from the Third National Cancer Survey (8). Thus, there is absolutely no evidence that the overall incidence rate for colorectal carcinoma in children in the study area during the past 15 years is unusually high or low.

However, since an unusual pattern of occurrences can exist even if the overall incidence rate is unremarkable, it is still of interest to test for time or space clustering within the study period and study region. For this analysis we consider only those 18 cases referred to this institution.

There are three different types of clustering considered here: time, space and time-space as discussed in Appendix 2. The first two are clusterings of the cases with respect to time of diagnosis or residence at diagnosis considered individually. Time space clustering of the cases is clustering in which cases occurring close together in time also tend to occur close together in space.

In order to obtain some idea of time clustering, the study period of January, 1966 through July, 1980 was arbitrarily broken into 7 consecutive time intervals of 25 months each. This breakdown was chosen so that the expected incidence in

138

Table 5. Time clustering. States

Time interval	TN	AR	MS	Total
January 66 – January 68	1	0	0	1
February 68 – February 70	0	1	0	1
March 70 – March 72	0	0	0	0
April 72 – April 74	0	0	1	1
May 74 – May 76	2	0	5	7
June 76 – June 78	1	2	0	3
July 78 – July 80	1	2	2	5
	5	5	8	18
$X^2 =$	4.80	7.60	18.25	15.44
$P =$	0.57	0.27	< 0.01	0.02

each time interval would be sufficient for a reasonable test of randomness. Assuming that the population structure has not changed appreciably during the year under study, the number of cases occurring in each time interval should follow a Poisson distribution. In fact, the size of the population of children in this study area has not changed dramatically during this time period, with a net gain of only approximately 7,000 children under 20 years of age from January, 1966 to July, 1980 (the population estimate in July, 1980 was 1,149,000) (17).

As indicated in Table 5, a standard Poisson heterogeneity test (18) indicates that, overall, there is significant evidence of disease clustering in time ($X^2 = 15.44$, 6 *df*, $P = 0.02$). This conclusion is largely due to 7 of the 18 cases occurring during the period from May, 1974 through May, 1976. In fact, 6 of these cases were diagnosed between October, 1974 and October, 1975. Also, when the three states are examined separately, it appears that the only state with any evidence of time clustering is Mississippi, with 5 of the total 8 cases from Mississippi diagnosed during this period ($X^2 = 18.25$, 6 *df*, $P < 0.01$.

Other tests statistics could be used for time clustering, such as the maximum number of cases diagnosed in any time interval (19, 20), but there would seem to be little gain in information by the use of these techniques here.

With respect to geographic clustering (often referred to as space clustering), the study region was divided into six areas. This was accomplished by dividing the counties in each of the three states into two categories: 'river' counties and 'non-river' counties. River counties are those counties with a boundary in the Mississippi River. Non-river counties are those within the 75 mile restriction but not directly on the river. These region were chosen partly for convenience and partly because of the intrinsic interest in the Mississippi River valley itself.

The results are given in Table 6. Overall, there is a statistically significant difference among the regions with respect to the observed rate ($X^2 = 14.89$, 5 *df*,

Table 6. Space clustering.

		No. cases	Average population	γ^a
River counties:	TN	4	289	0.95
	AR	4	72	3.80
	MS	5	119	2.88
	River total:	13	480	1.86
Non-river counties:	TN	1	128	0.54
	AR	1	222	0.31
	MS	3	285	0.72
	Non-river total:	5	635	0.54
	Total:	18	1,115	1.11

Significance tests
Overall: $X^2 = 14.89, 5\ df, P = 0.01$
States: $X^2 = 0.79, 2\ df, P = 0.67$
River vs non-river: $X^2 = 6.23, 1\ df, P = 0.01$
[a] γ = Average annual incidence rate per 10^6 children; all children under 20 years of age ($\gamma = 1.13$ in TNCS).

$P = 0.01$), indicating that space clustering is present. Here, contingency table analysis is used rather than a Poisson heterogeneity test since the average population varies widely from region to region. There is no difference among the 3 states but a significant difference between the river and non-river regions ($X^2 = 6.23, 2\ df, P = 0.01$). The river region had an incidence rate more than 3 times the non-river region, a finding somewhat muted by the low incidence rate, compared to the Third National Cancer Survey (8), in the non-river region.

To investigate space time clustering, the procedure of Knox (21) will be used for simplicity. Other procedures, such as those developed by Mantel (22), may be more generally applicable but the method of Knox seems adequate in this setting. Specifically, we define close in time (i.e., time of diagnosis) as less than 1 year apart and 'close in space' (i.e., residence at diagnosis) as less than 50 miles. Each pair of cases is classified in this way. Of the 153 possible pairs of 18 patients, 8 were close in time and space (Table 7), quite close to the expected 7.1 pairs under the hypothesis of randomness. Thus, there is no evidence that cases occurring close in space tend to occur close in time.

Discussion

From the study of these subjects with colorectal carcinoma, certain differences between adolescents and adults with this tumor have been identified (1). The

140

Table 7. Space time clustering.

		Within 1 year		
		Yes	No	Total
Within 50 miles	Yes	8	24	32
	No	26	95	121
	Total	34	119	153

$Z = 0.33$
$P = 0.74$

primary sites for our subjects were located throughout the large bowel and the colon. For adults, approximately 60% of primary colorectal carcinomas are located within 40 cm of the anus, in the descending colon, sigmoid and rectum. Among adults there is evidence of increasing disease located in the more proximal segments of the bowel (23–25). At the present time it is unknown whether younger adults between 20 and 40 years of age have a greater incidence of proximal as opposed to distal large bowel primary sites (26–30).

The histopathologic picture for 22 of our 26 subjects was that of poorly differentiated, mucin-producing carcinoma, a histologic variant of colorectal carcinoma which has been estimated to occur in 15% of adults with this primary type of bowel cancer (31). Previous reports have indicated that this is the most common histologic variety of large bowel cancer to appear in children and adolescents with this disease (1, 3–5).

Before diagnosis, the signs and symptoms experienced by adolescents consists of vague intermittent abdominal pain, nausea and vomiting and minor change in bowel habits; intestinal obstruction is uncommon in adolescents with this tumor. Most adolescents experience a delay in the diagnosis of their tumors, primarily due to lack of suspicion of this type of cancer occurring in persons of this age group.

The extent of tumor within our subjects differed remarkably from the findings of adults (32, 33). Eighteen of the 26 patients had evidence of metastatic disease involving sites distant from the primary tumor site, with intraperitoneal, hepatic, pelvic or other non-visceral involvement. Tumor confined to the bowel was rare in our subjects, in contradistinction to adults with colorectal carcinoma.

The extent of disease at the time of diagnosis reflected on the outcome for our patients, with long-term disease free survival of only one patient (33, 34). The failure of chemotherapy to produce complete or partial responses in most patients was common to patients with measurable tumor activity and the lack of success was reflected in the development of recurrent tumor by subjects who received multiple agent chemotherapy in an adjuvant situation. Information is not available regarding chemotherapy response of adult patients with the mucinous histologic subtype for comparison with adults with the non-mucinous varieties of colorectal tumors (31).

The response of our patients to chemotherapy as well as their survival time has differed from that reported for adults with similar stages of disease; responses were encountered only rarely among patients treated for measurable disease (35). The median survival time of 9 months is in marked contrast to that of adult subjects with Duke's stage B, C or D colorectal carcinoma (33, 34).

Only 1 of these 26 adolescents with colorectal carcinoma was considered to be a person at extremely high risk for the development of this tumor (36–38). This was the patient with multiple polyposis of the colon first diagnosed at the age of 4 years. The 3 patients who had either the concurrent or later diagnosis of single juvenile polyps had no indications of polyposis prior to the development of colorectal carcinoma. Additionally, none of the subjects gave a history of previous radiation therapy for genitourinary tract cancer, previous history of ulcerative colitis or prior bowel cancer and none of the subjects had a family history of colorectal carcinoma. None of the subjects had Gardner's syndrome, Turcot's syndrome, or the Peutz-Jegher syndrome.

It may be conjectured that 2 populations of patients are included within this group of 26 subjects, the majority of which represent those with the unique histology found in adolescents and the minority being representative of the rare case of sporadic bowel cancer which appears in younger adults. The ages of our subjects with the non-mucinous variety of colorectal carcinoma were 13 years 1 month, 13 years 9 months, 18 years 2 months, and 19 years 10 months.

Colorectal carcinoma represents the most frequently encountered 'adult-type' cancer which has been referred to this institution. Seventy-eight of 1611 patients with malignant solid tumors, or 4.9%, treated at our hospital have had these carcinomas, which are more commonly encountered in adults than in children (39). The second most common carcinoma at our institution has been lympho-epithelioma; 22 subjects with this tumor have been treated at this hospital since 1962. Other 'adult-type' cancers referred to our center have included hepatocellular carcinoma, thyroid, adrenal, renal, and pancreatic carcinomas, and melanoma.

Implications have been made regarding the possible etiology of colorectal carcinoma within these patients. This history of exposure to pesticides and herbicides used in agricultural spraying operations or for other non-agricultural farm uses indicated the frequency of chemical exposure among our subjects from rural areas (9). The additional history of exposure by subjects from urban backgrounds contributed to the conclusions regarding the causal association of these events with the later development of colorectal carcinoma. Although serum pesticide levels were elevated for several of 10 subjects from Tennessee, Arkansas and Mississippi studied for DDT, dieldrin and heptachlor residues, studies have not yet been completed on herbicide levels in the serum of these subjects. The obtained history of exposure to herbicides was elicited more frequently than that of exposure to pesticides.

The interpretation of the incidence and disease clustering data is rather uncertain both because of ascertainment difficulties and because clustering may be an artifact of referral patterns. It appears that the overall incidence during the past 15 years in the region studied is quite close to that which would have been expected but that those cases are not randomly distributed in time and space. More cases were found in counties adjacent to the Mississippi River than in nearby counties not adjacent to the river. An exceptionally large number of cases were diagnosed in 1974 and 1975. However, there appeared to be little evidence for space-time clustering. That is, there is little evidence that cases occurring close in time tended to also occur close in space.

The clustering along the river is interesting but the clustering in 1974 and 1975 is inexplicable in light of our current knowledge. Changes in referral patterns may partly explain this latter finding but it seems it is unlikely that such an abrupt change would have occurred in those years only. It may, of course, simply be a chance occurrence. On balance, it seems that evidence is not strong enough to conclude that any strikingly unusual incidence or pattern of colorectal cancer in children has ocurred in this area during the past 15 years. However, there is sufficient evidence to warrant further monitoring of the area for cancer as well as other health problems.

Acknowledgments

The authors express their gratitude to Dr Matthew Zack of the Chronic Disease Division, Center for Disease Control, Atlanta, Georgia, for death certificate information regarding Arkansas and Mississippi, to Ms Audrey Collins of the Department of Health and Human Resources, Office of Health Services and Environmental Quality, Public Health Statistics, for death certificate information from the State of Louisiana, and to the Tennessee State Center for Health Statistics for similar information. The contributions of Mr David Facklam, Epidemiology Program Coordinator, Mrs Lee C. Liu and Mrs Laurel Drake, Computer Programming, St. Jude Children's Research Hospital, are gratefully acknowledged.

This work was supported by Childhood Cancer Program Project Grant CA-23099, Cancer Research Support (CORE) Grant CA-21765, and by ALSAC.

References

1. Pratt CB, Rivera G, Shanks E, et al.: Colorectal carcinoma in adolescents: implications regarding etiology. Cancer 40(5) (Suppl):2464–2472, 1977.
2. Johnson JW, Judd ES, Dahlin DC: Malignant neoplasms of the colon and rectum in young persons. Arch Surg 79:365–372, 1959.
3. Middlekamp JN, Haffner H: Carcinoma of the colon in children. Pediatrics 32(4):558–571, 1963.
4. Sessions RT, Riddell DH, Kaplan HJ, Foster JH: Carcinoma of the colon in the first two decades of life. Ann Surg 162(2):279–284, 1965.
5. Pissiotis CA, Gulessarian HP, Condon RE: Colorectal carcinoma in the first twenty-five years of life. J Surg Oncol 6(1):87–91, 1971.
6. Chabalko JJ, Fraumeni JF Jr: Colorectal cancer in children – Epidemiologic aspects. Dis Colon Rectum 18(1):1–3, 1975.
7. Enker WE, Paloyan E, Kirsner JB: Carcinoma of the colon in the adolescent. A report of survival and review of the literature. Am J Surg 133(6):737–741, 1977.
8. Third National Cancer Survey: Incidence data (Table 19B). Average annual age-specific incidence rates per 100,000 population, by primary site, males plus females, all races, all areas combined, 1969–1971. Bethesda, MD, NCI Monograph No 41, 1975, p 102.
9. Caldwell GC, Cannon SB, Pratt CB, Arthur RD: Serum pesticide levels in childhood colorectal carcinoma patients. Cancer (in press).
10. Sherlock P, Lipkin M, Winawer SJ: Predisposing factors in carcinoma of the colon. Adv Intern Med 20:121–150, 1975.
11. Reddy BS, Weisburger JH, Wynder EL: Effect of dietary fat level and dimethylhydrazine on fecal acid and neutral sterol excretion and colon carcinogenesis in rats. J Natl Cancer Inst 52(2):507–511, 1974.
12. Graham S, Haenszel W, Bock FG, Ryon JL: Need to pursue new leads in the epidemiology of colorectal cancer. J Natl Cancer Inst 63(4):79–81, 1979.
13. Hill MJ: Carcinogenesis of gastrointestinal cancer. Front Gastrointest Res 4(1):1–16, 1979.
14. Colorectal Cancer. Epidemiology: incidence, diet and metabolic factors. In: Weisburger JH, et al. (eds): Colorectal Cancer. International Union Against Cancer. Geneva: UICC, 1975, pp 4–33.
15. Blot WJ, Fraumeni JF, Stone BJ, McKay FW: Geographic patterns of large bowel cancer in the United States. J Natl Cancer Inst 57(6):1225–1231, 1976.
16. Jansson B, Seibert B, Speer JF: Gastrointestinal cancer: Its geographic distribution and correlation to breast cancer. Cancer 36(6)(Suppl):2373–2384, 1975.
17. Current Population Reports, 'Federal-State Cooperative Program for Population Estimates', Series P-25 and P-26, 1960–1980.
18. Armitage P: Statistical Methods in Medical Research. Oxford: Blackwell Scientific Publications, 1971, pp 214–216.
19. Ederer F, Myers M, Mantel N: 'A statistical problem in space and time: Do leukemia cases come in clusters?' Biometrics 20(3):626–638, 1964.
20. Mantel N, Kryscio RJ, Myers M: Tables and formulas for extended use of the Ederer-Myers-Mantel disease-clustering procedure. Am J Epidem 104(5):576–584, 1976.
21. Knox G: The detection of space-time interactions. Appl Statistics 13(1):25–2, 1964.
22. Mantel N: The detection of disease clustering and a generalized regression approach. Cancer Res 27(2):209–220, 1967.
23. Snyder DN, Heston JF, Meigs JW, Flannery JT: Changes in site distribution of colorectal carcinoma n Connecticut, 1940–1973. Am J Diag Dis 22(9):791–797, 1977.
24. Rhodes JB, Holmes FF, Clark GM: Changing distribution of primary cancers in the large bowel. JAMA 238(15):1641–1643, 1977.
25. Abrams JS, Reines HD: Increasing incidence of right-sided lesions in colorectal carcinoma. Am J Surg 137(4):522–526, 1979.
26. Correa P, Haenszel W: The epidemiology of large-bowel cancer. Adv Cancer Res 26:1–141, 1978.

144

27. Berg JW, Haenszel W, Devesa SS: Epidemiology of gastrointestinal cancer. Proc Natl Cancer Conf 7:459–464, 1973.
28. Wynder EL: The epidemiology of large bowel cancer. Cancer Res 35(11)(Pt 2):3388–3394, 1975.
29. Miller AB: Epidemiology and colorectal cancer. Am J Surg 21(3):209–210, 1978.
30. Lyon JL, Sorenson AW: Colon cancer in a low-risk population. Am J Clin Nutr 31(10 Suppl): 5227–5230, 1978.
31. Symonds DA, Vickery AL Jr: Mucinous carcinoma of the colon and rectum. Cancer 37(4): 1891–1900, 1976.
32. Hoth DF, Petrucci PE: Natural history and staging of colon cancer. Sem Oncol 3(4):331–336, 1976.
33. Evans JT, Vana J, Aronoff BL, et al.: Management and survival of carcinoma of the colon: Results of a national survey by the American College of Surgeons. Ann Surg 188(6):716–720, 1978.
34. Silverman DT, Murray JL, Smart CR, et al.: Estimated median survival times of patients with colorectal cancer based on experience with 9,745 patients. Amer J Surg 133(3):289–297, 1977.
35. Moertel CG, Schutt AJ, Hahn RG, Reitemeier RJ: Therapy of advanced colorectal cancer with a combination of 5-fluorouracil, methyl-1, 3-cis(2-chloroethyl)-1-nitrosourea, and vincristine. J Natl Cancer Inst 54(1):69–71, 1975.
36. Fraumeni JF Jr, Mulvihill JJ: Who is at risk of colorectal cancer? In: Schottenfeld D (ed): Cancer Epidemiology and Prevention. Springfield, IL: Charles C. Thomas, 1975, pp 404–415.
37. Stemper TJ, Kent TH, Summers RW: Juvenile polyposis and gastrointestinal carcinoma: A study of a kindred. Ann Int Med 83(5):639–646, 1975.
38. Lynch HT, Giurgis H, Swartz M, et al.: Genetics and colon cancer. Arch Surg 106(5):669–675, 1973.
39. Pratt CB, Murphy SB, Green AA, et al.: Carcinomas in children. Proc Am Assoc Cancer Res and ASCO 20:155, 1979.
40. Klauber MR: Space-time clustering tests for more than two samples. Biometrics 31(3):719–726, 1975.
41. Siemiatycki J: Mantel's space-time clustering statistic: computing higher moments and a comparison of various data transforms. J Statist Comput Simul 7(1):13–31, 1978.

Appendix 1

Use of death certificate information

In an attempt to identify cases of colorectal cancer occurring in the study area not referred to SJCRH, death certificates were obtained from the states of Tennessee, Arkansas and Mississippi. All patients dying in one of the countries of the study region from January 1, 1966 to the present under 25 years of age at death with colorectal carcinoma listed as a cause of death were identified. From these lists it was possible to identify those patients referred to SJCRH by matching on date of death, age at death, race and sex.

For the remaining cases identified by death certificate but not referred to SJCRH, it was ordinarily not possible to know with certainty (from death certificate information only) whether the patient met the requirements for inclusion into this study: (i) under 20 years of age at diagnosis; (ii) residing in the study area at diagnosis; (iii) diagnosed no earlier than January 1, 1966. Thus, in order to estimate the expected number of cases as used in Table 4 of the text, the following approach was taken:

(1) Assume the patient was residing in the study area at diagnosis. This is probably a reasonable assumption given the overall migration pattern for this area but, in any case, it is a necessary one.

(2) For *each* case, the probability that the patient was both under 20 at diagnosis and diagnosed no earlier than January 1, 1966 was calculated conditional on the observed age and date of death and the survival pattern as observed for the 26 patients referred to this institution.

Details are omitted but, qualitatively, this implies that the older patients are not very likely to have been under 20 at diagnosis due to the small probability of survival for more than one or two years after diagnosis. Also, in a few cases, the probability is exactly zero (e.g., a patient age 23 at death in 1967 could not possibly have been diagnosed after January 1, 1966 at an age less than 20). On the other hand, a patient age 18 at death in 1976 is almost certain to meet the requirements.

Based on these probabilities an 'expected' number of additional cases not referred to SJCRH, can be calculated. This number is added to the number of cases seen at SJCRH and reported as 'all cases' in Table 4. This explains the non-integer number of cases. Overall, an estimated 7.1 cases were diagnosed during this period but not referred to SJCRH. This number can be inflated by approximately 10% if desired to account for patients who do not appear in the death certificate information because they are cured of their disease. However, this was not done in this paper and, in any case, would not affect the conclusions reached here.

Appendix 2

Disease clustering

There is a fairly extrusive literature on statistical techniques useful in detecting disease clustering (19, 20, 22, 40, 41).

Clustering can be in space, in time, or in both, so-called space time clustering. 'Space' refers to primary geographic residence at diagnosis and 'time' refers to date of diagnosis. Clustering means that the cases tend to be closer together (in the metric used) than would be expected from a random distribution of cases. Space time clustering means that cases close together in space also tend to be close together in time, a type of statistical interaction.

It is important to note the limitations of this type of analysis. Many factors can lead to clustering which have no relevance to the disease itself. For example, a shift in referral patterns or population characteristics over time can lead to a clustering of disease even if the incidence has remained constant over time.

In this paper we use very simple techniques to test for clustering:

(1) For time clustering, we arbitrarily consider seven 25-month time intervals. This number was chosen because it breaks the total time period of 175 months into an integer number of months and because the expected number of cases in a given interval is not too small (approximately 2.6). A Poisson heterogeneity test is used to test for clustering since the population structure within these time periods has been reasonably constant.

(2) For space clustering, the study region is broken into two categories: river counties and non-river counties. River counties are those bordering on the Mississippi River. Non-river counties are those counties within 75 miles of the river but not directly bordering it. Considering the three states involved yields six distinct geographic regions. To test for clustering, an ordinary X^2 test for the homogeneity of incidence rates is used. This is necessary since the population varies widely from region to region.

(3) For space-time clustering, we use for simplicity the method of Knox (21) rather than the more general tests of Mantel (22). For each pair of patients, 'close' in time is taken as within 1 year and 'close' in space as within 50 miles. Then the observed number of patients close in *both* space and time is compared to that expected under the hypothesis of randomness.

6. Epidemiology of Gastrointestinal Lymphomas

CLARK W. HEATH, Jr

Introduction

The gastrointestinal tract and its system of lymphatic drainage are commonly involved in cases of human lymphoma. Over half of all autopsied lymphoma cases examined by Rosenberg et al. (1) showed such abdominal involvement. In less than 5 percent of cases, however, did the disease appear clinically to have originated in gastrointestinal or gastrointestinal lymphoid tissue. Primary gastrointestinal lymphoma is generally, therefore, a rare disease. Although direct measurements of lymphoma incidence exist only by histologic type and not by organ system (overall rates being in the range of 50 to 100 cases per million population per year in most countries (2)), incidence of primary gastrointestinal lymphomas can be estimated at about 2 to 5 cases per million per year.

Since gastrointestinal lymphomas are relatively rare, their epidemiology has not been intensively studied. What little epidemiologic data do exist, however, present problems in interpretation. Case ascertainment is difficult because of the relative inaccessibility of gastrointestinal and abdominal tissues for clinical diagnostic study. Different series of cases are therefore hard to compare, both because of potential variability in intensity of case detection and because of difference in case classification. Classification problems are of 2 kinds: (1) definition of tissue site (whether to classify, for example, an ileocecal tumor as originating in large or small intestine; at what site to classify multicentric or diffuse tumors; how to classify tumors within bowel wall as opposed to tissues in adjacent nodal tissue); and (2) histopathologic classification (varying systems of cell-type classification and differences in thoroughness or expertise in microscopic diagnosis). These fundamental difficulties should be borne in mind as one considers the data reviewed in this chapter.

General etiologic considerations

There appear to be no strong reasons to suppose that the causes of gastrointestinal lymphomas differ greatly from those of lymphomas generally. Although the etiology of lymphoma is no more precisely known than for most

Correa, P. and Haenszel, W. (eds.), Epidemiology of Cancer of the Digestive Tract.
© *1982 Martinus Nijhoff Publishers. The Hague/Boston/London. ISBN-13:978-94-009-7504-0*

other forms of cancer, it seems reasonable that the same spectrum of interacting risk factors are involved: oncogenic chemicals, ionizing radiation, oncogenic viruses or infectious agents, genetic constitution, and immunologic capacity. Limited amounts of data suggest possible roles for chemicals, radiation, and familial patterns in lymphoma etiology (3). Most work has focused, however, on the possible influence of immunologic factors and infectious agents, partly because reticuloendothelial tissues serve immunologic functions and provide tissue defenses against infection. Epidemiologic, virologic, and immunologic studies of Hodgkin's disease and Burkitt's lymphoma have provided most of the evidence in this regard. Geographic, age, and social class patterns in Hodgkin's disease occurrence are indirectly compatible with polio-like viral disease (4). For Burkitt's lymphoma, however, more direct virologic evidence, in addition to descriptive epidemiologic features, strongly suggest an etiologic relationship between Epstein-Barr herpesvirus infection, host immunologic factors, and the development of that particular form of childhood lymphoma (5).

For some forms of gastrointestinal lymphoma, epidemiologic patterns and some laboratory observations strongly suggest immunologic reasons for tumor development. Although direct links with gastrointestinal infections have not been made, the repeated exposure of gastrointestinal tissue to various infectious agents, particularly in certain socio-economic settings, and the important physiologic role of gastrointestinal lymphoid tissue in protecting the body from intestinal entry of infectious agents make disturbed immunologic function and immune tissue structure attractive hypotheses for explaining the particular development of lymphoid tumors in such tissues.

The selective review provided here of the epidemiology of gastrointestinal lymphomas includes malignancies arising both in the gastrointestinal wall itself and in related lymphoid tissue (mesenteric nodes). The practical difficulty of discriminating clearly between these 2 groups of tumors, especially when diagnosis is made after tumor spread has occurred, is self evident and has led to wide use of the term 'abdominal lymphoma' to encompass not only gastrointestinal and gastrointestinal lymphoid tumors but also lymphomas arising in other abdominal organs. As far as possible, however, this review will avoid such generalizations and will focus on tumors of gastrointestinal and gastrointestinal lymphoid origin.

Patterns of case occurrence

In most western developed countries, distributions of gastrointestinal lymphomas seem relatively uniform by age, sex, and tissue site. Where data are available in less developed parts of the world, however, or for less developed populations in developed countries (Israel and South Africa, for example), recognizable patterns of age, sex, and tissue site differences are apparent.

Geographic differences

Table 1 summarizes lymphoma frequencies in different countries by specific gastrointestinal location (1,6–18). The data are drawn primarily from clinical series of cases seen at individual hospitals or groups of hospitals. In some instances, however, cases closely approximate total case occurrence in a country (Israel (10)) or in a region of a country (Fars Province, Iran (9)). Data are most plentiful from the United States (14–19) where quite uniformly about 50 to 60% of cases occur in the stomach with 25 to 30% in the small intestine (primarily ileum) and 10 to 15% in the large intestine. Although numbers of reported cases are small in most other countries, patterns outside the United States vary from predominance of stomach tumors in India (8), to relatively greater frequencies for colon tumors in Hong Kong Chinese (7) and in Uganda (13), and to striking frequencies of small intestinal lymphomas in Iran (9), South Africa (12), Lebanon (11) and Israel (10). For Iran, in fact, about one quarter of all lymphomas appear to arise in the gastrointestinal tract, of which about 80% primarily involve the small intestine. The case series from Great Britain (6) is difficult to interpret in terms of the national origin of cases since it includes a substantial number of small intestinal cases referred from other parts of the world. Cases arising in the esophagus are extremely rare in all case series.

Distribution by age, sex, ethnic origin, and organ site

Among cases in the United States, age and sex patterns are similar for different gastrointestinal tissue sites, except that, as elsewhere, cases arising in the stomach are rarely seen in children and young adults (19, 20). Male cases outnumber female in varying degrees, and diagnoses are made most often in persons over age 50. Cases affecting the large intestine show a 2-fold male predominance (21, 22) and seem most frequent in the cecal region (21, 22). Data from the multi-hospital case series of Freeman et al. (17) illustrate these patterns.

Elsewhere in the world, striking differences are apparent. Where small intestinal lymphomas are more frequent, younger age groups are involved together with a more equal distribution of cases between the sexes (10–12). Whereas small intestinal lymphoma in the United States more often affects ileum than jejunum (23–25), the reverse appears true in countries where small intestinal lymphoma is more common (9, 26). In Israel and South Africa, where cases are seen from diverse ethnic groups, small intestinal cases show decided ethnic predilections, in Israel both for Jews of non-Ashkenazi or eastern origin and for Arabs (10, 27),

Table 1. Frequency of gastrointestinal lymphoma by country and gastrointestinal site (1, 6–18).

Country	Investigator	Year of case diagnosis	Total cases	Esophagus		Stomach		Small intestine		Large intestine	
				No.	%	No.	%	No.	%	No.	%
England	Henry et al. (6)	to 1977	125	–	–	51	40.8	53	42.4	21	16.8
Hong Kong	Ho et al. (7)	1964–74	46[a]	–	–	18	39.1	16	34.8	12	26.1
India	Desai et al. (8)	1941–60	21	–	–	15	71.4	3	14.3	3	14.3
Iran	Barekat et al. (9)	1962–69	80	1	0.8	11	13.8	64	80.0	5	6.3
Israel	Modan et al. (10)	1960–64	119[b]			46	38.7	56	47.1	16	13.4
Lebanon	Gedeon (11)	1946–68	32	–	–	11	34.4	14	43.8	7	21.9
South Africa	Kahn et al. (12)	1952–69	57	–	–	19	33.3	34	59.6	4	7.0
Uganda	Owor (13)	1964–75	40	–	–	10	25.0	9	22.5	21	52.5
USA	Allen et al. (14)	1913–53	7?	1	1.3	44	55.7	25	31.6	9	11.4
	Rosenberg et al. (1)	1930–61	58	–	–	31	53.4	19	32.8	8	13.8
	Loehr et al. (15)	1932–69	100	–	–	63	63.0	25	25.0	12	12.0
	Naqui et al. (16)	1935–65	190	–	–	116	61.1	56	29.5	18	9.5
	Freeman et al. (17)	1950–64	541	3	0.6	346	64.0	110	20.3	82	15.2
	Lewin et al. (18)	1968–75	111	–	–	48	43.2	37	33.3	26[c]	23.4

[a] Chinese only.
[b] Excludes 47 cases for which a primary gastrointestinal site could not be determined.
[c] Includes 13 cases classified as 'ileocecal'.

Table 2. Age, sex, and histologic patterns by gastrointestinal site among cases of gastrointestinal lymphoma in the United States (adapted from Freeman et al (17)

	Stomach	Small intestine	Large intestine
Total number of cases	346	110	82
Percent male	57	62	50
Percent age 0–19	0	11	9
20–49	17	16	16
50+	83	73	75
Percent lymphosarcoma	41	45	37
Reticulum cell sarcoma	48	40	46
Other histologic types	11	15	17

and in South Africa for persons of mulatto background (12).

Distribution by cell type

Differing schemes of cell-type classification make it hard to compare cell-type patterns over time and between different series of cases. On the whole, it appears that both histiocytic (reticulum cell sarcoma) and lymphocytic (lymphosarcoma) forms of lymphoma can occur at all gastrointestinal sites, with histiocytic forms somewhat more frequent in stomach and large intestine than in small intestine (Table 2). Hodgkin's disease is variably mentioned as a diagnosis, as is Burkitt's lymphoma. Recent British histopathologic studies (6) have suggested, however, that plasmacytic forms of lymphoma are much more common among gastro-intestinal cases than previously reported, particularly in cases arising in ileocecal tissue. In that particular series of cases, plasmacytomas were diagnosed in 39% of 125 cases, 29% in stomach (15 of 51 cases), 43% in small intestine (23 of 53 cases) and 52% in large intestine (11 of 21 cases). No cases of Hodgkin s disease were diagnosed. As described below, lymphoplasmacytic infiltration is commonly found in those forms of small intestinal lymphoma associated with malabsorption and so-called alpha chain disease. As a reflection of the prevalence of such cases in Middle Eastern countries, among 145 small intestinal lymphomas diagnosed in Baghdad, Iraq, 89 (61%) were classified as lympho-plasmacytic (26).

Relation to coeliac disease and idiopathic steatorrhea

The association of sprue-like illness or steatorrhea with lymphoma of intestines or mesenteric nodes was first described in 1936 by Golden (28) and in 1937 by Fairley and Mackie (29). Since that time, the clinical association of small intestinal lymphoma with adult coeliac disease and idiopathic steatorrhea has been repeatedly confirmed, both in Europe (30–35) and in North America (36–39). While for some time it was postulated that malabsorption in such cases was the result and not the precursor of lymphoma, a study of patients with adult coeliac disease in England eventually showed conclusively that intestinal malabsorption preceded and predisposed to intestinal or mesenteric lymphoma (30). Among 202 patients with adult coeliac disease in that study, 14 developed lymphoma, all but one involving gastrointestinal tract (10 cases) or mesenteric nodes (3 cases), total expected lymphoma incidence being 0.115 case. Duration of intestinal symptoms before diagnosis of lymphoma averaged 21.2 years. By the end of 1975, further follow-up of this case series showed the occurrence of 4 additional cases of reticulum cell sarcoma, all involving small intestine (33). Treatment of malabsorption symptoms by means of gluten-free diet appeared not to prevent the eventual appearance of lymphoma.

Cases of intestinal or mesenteric lymphoma following coeliac disease or idiopathic steatorrhea appear mostly to affect older or middle-aged persons, males slightly more often than females. Jejunal tumors seem somewhat more frequent than at other intestinal sites, in keeping with the fact that the fundamental pathologic lesion of coeliac disease consists of jejunal villous atrophy and crypt hyperplasia. Among lymphomas in such cases, histiocytic or reticulum cell tumors seem more usual than small cell lymphomas, with underlying mucosal and submucosal plasmacytic infiltration being a regular feature (34).

Relation to dermatitis herpetiformis

A further clinical association has been observed between the occurrence of gastrointestinal lymphoma and the presence of dermatitis herpetiformis, a skin disorder often accompanying adult coeliac disease. This association was first recorded from Sweden in 1970 in a 44-year-old male patient with a jejunal reticuloenthelial tumor, a long-standing history of diarrhea, and dermatitis herpetiformis first diagnosed 18 years earlier (40). Subsequent case reports from Scandinavia, Ireland, and Canada have confirmed this association, firmly establishing a syndrome of intestinal lymphoma, malabsorption, and skin disease (41–44) (Table 3).

Immunoproliferative small intestinal disease

The most striking epidemiologic findings with respect to gastrointestinal lymphomas have concerned certain small intestinal tumors occurring in young persons primarily from under-priviledged backgrounds in Mediterranean and

Table 3. Published cases of gastrointestinal lymphoma associated with dermatitis herpetiformis (DH).

Author, year of publication, country	Age at time of lymphoma diagnosis	Sex	Clinical Features
Gjone at al., 1970 (40) (Norway)	44	M	Reticuloendothelial tumor of jejunum; malabsorption for 23 years and DH for 18 years.
Andersson et al., 1971 (41) (Sweden)	60	F	Lymphoreticulosarcoma of transverse colon and splenic flexure; malabsorption for 26 years and DH for 44 years.
Connon et al., 1975 (42) (Ireland)	52	M	Reticulum cell sarcoma of jejunum; malabsorption for 3 years (?) and DH for 10 years.
Tonder et al., 1976 (43) (Norway)	59	F	Reticulosarcoma of distal ileum; malabsorption (coeliac disease) for 25 years and DH for 5 months.
Freeman et al., 1977 (44) (Canada)	60	M	Histiocytic lymphoma of stomach with jejunal villous atrophy; DH for 20 years.
	42	M	Histiocytic lymphoma of jejunum and proximal ileum with atrophy of intestinal mucosa; DH for 6 months.
	62	M	Diffuse undifferentiated lymphoma of jejunum and proximal ileum following 'benign ulcerative non-granulomatous jejunitis'; DH for 5 years.

southwest Asian countries and associated with intestinal malabsorption, lymphoplasmacytic infiltration of small intestine (primarily jejunum), and the frequent presence in serum of an abnormal 1gA immunoprotein consisting of heavy chain immunoglobulin fragments (alpha chains) (45). Since the condition was first described from countries near the Mediterranean Sea, it was initially called 'Mediterranean lymphoma.' When the 1gA abnormality was subsequently identified, the term 'alpha chain disease' was introduced. As understanding of the disease grew, however, and it became apparent that alpha chain fragments were not always present and that the condition could exist entirely as lymphoplasmacytic infiltration of intestine without overt malignancy, the more general term 'immunoproliferative small intestinal disease' (IPSID) came into use.

The first reports of this condition came from Israel (46, 47), describing a total of 22 patients (12 male, 10 female, age range 16–42 years with mean age at diagnosis 23.7 years). The most striking finding was the entirely Middle Eastern origin of cases (9 Arabs, 1 Circassian, and 12 Jews, all of non-Ashkenazi background [India, Iran, Iraq, Libya, Syria, Tunisia, and Yemen]). The cases differed from those seen in association with sprue or coeliac disease both in their ethnic/geographic origins and in their strikingly young age distribution.

In 1968, French investigators described the presence of alpha chain fragments in serum from a young Syrian Arab woman with abdominal lymphoma, malabsorption, and diffuse small intestinal lymphoplasmacytic infiltration (48), with further immunologic studies reported soon after in three additional patients, 2 Kabyles from Algeria and a Eurasian of French/Cambodian extraction (49). Although subsequent work by many groups of investigators have confirmed the frequent occurrence of alpha chain fragments in such lymphoma patients, it is recognized that this immunologic protein marker can occasionally occur in other clinical settings. In particular, two cases of infiltrative lung disease have been described, one in a 4-year-old Dutch girl (50), the other in a 76-year-old British man (51), in which alpha chain fragments were a feature. That this protein marker can also be seen in lymphomas distinct from the IPSID syndrome is suggested by the recent finding of alpha heavy chains in a 39-year-old man from the United States with multiple polypoid lymphocytic lymphomas affecting colon and rectum, lymphoma of peripheral nodes, and terminal acute lymphoid leukemia (52).

The histopathology of IPSID lymphomas in Middle Eastern patients and the nature of the associated lymphoplasmacytic intestinal infiltration has suggested a spectrum of related malignant and premalignant upper intestinal lesions arising in a setting of chronic immunologic deficiency or disturbance (53). The clonal unity of IPSID lymphoma cells and the cells infiltrating intestinal mucosa has subsequently been suggested by cellular studies of alpha chain fragment production (54).

The initial impression that IPSID was exclusively found in Middle Eastern and Mediterranean countries was proven wrong by reports of cases among mulatto residents of South Africa (55–57). The observation that such cases primarily affect that particular segment of the South African population, despite the presence of large white and black populations, suggest the potential importance of socio-economic factors in development of the disease. While the nature of such factors is unclear, they perhaps involve patterns of diet and intestinal infection in lower socio-economic populations undergoing transitional adjustment to western living patterns.

At present, case reports in the literature suggest that IPSID may occur to varying degrees in developing populations in many parts of the world. In addition to South Africa and to the Middle Eastern nations already mentioned, cases have been described from Mexico (58), Italy (59), Pakistan (60), Bangladesh (60), Greece (61), Colombia (62), and Nigeria (63). Although the disease has been recognized for too short a time to allow full understanding of its geographic distribution and incidence trends over time, it may be significant that cases in Israel seem now to be appearing less frequently than 10 years ago, the mean annual incidence in Israel having fallen from 4.8 cases per million in 1960–67 to 3.6 in 1968–75 (64). Conceivably, this trend (if confirmed in future studies) may be the result of improvements in socio-economic conditions among developing populations, supporting the hypothesis that such improvements are accompanied by changes in living and dietary habits which in turn may lessen the prevalence of intense and continuous gastrointestinal infections in infancy and early life, the possible etiologic stimuli for later IPSID development.

Possible association with ulcerative colitis

The idea that ulcerative colitis may predispose to the development of lymphoma in the large intestine, as it does for adenocarcinoma, has been suggested by published reports of cases in which the two diseases have been found to coexist (65–67). In two series of colonic lymphoma cases (21, 22), 3 of 50 cases and 2 of 27 cases respectively were said to be associated with ulcerative colitis. While the hypothesis seems reasonable that a disease like ulcerative colitis, involving possible autoimmune abnormalities, might lead to eventual lymphoid neoplasia, such cases are clearly infrequent. This fact, together with the uncertainties involved in distinguishing between lymphoma and colitis in the same patients and knowing for certain that one illness precedes the other (68), makes any conclusion about such an etiologic relationship uncertain at present.

Familial gastrointestinal lymphoma

The relative infrequency with which multiple cases of gastrointestinal lymphoma are reported in families makes it seem unlikely that heritable factors play any direct major role in the etiology of such diseases. Three reports describe multiple case families, 2 from the Middle East (69, 70) and 1 from the United States (71) (Table 4). In only one family was parental consanguinity reported (69). Pre-adolescent children were involved in two families, young adults in the third. In the family reported from Iran (70), the two affected sibs had upper intestinal lymphoma. Studies of non-familial cases elsewhere in the Middle East (72) have suggested the occurrence of immunoglobulin abnormalities in close family relatives. Such observations at least raise the hypothesis that genetic and/or familial/environmental factors may produce immunologic changes as potential precursors to tumor development. Similar immunologic abnormalities were sought but not found among members of the remarkable multiple case family reported from the United States (71).

Table 4. Familial gastrointestinal lymphoma.

Author, year of publication, country	Relatives affected	Age, sex, year of diagnosis and case descriptions
Pevsner et al., 1973 (69) (Israel)	2 brothers, Arab family; parents are first cousins	4 M, 1966, Burkitt's-like lymphoma of mesenteric nodes 4–1/2 M, 1972, poorly differentiated lymphoma of distal ileum and abdominal nodes
Banihashermi et al., 1973 (70) (Iran)	Sister and brother diagnosed 6 months apart	22 F, lymphosarcoma of upper small intestine 28 M, reticulum cell sarcoma of jejunum and mesenteric nodes
Maurer et al., 1976 (71) (United States)	3 brothers and their nephew	3 M, 1962, malignant retroperitoneal lymphoma involving colon, kidney, liver 5 M, 1965, poorly differentiated lympho-cytic lymphoma of cecum, colon, ab-dominal nodes, and viscera 7 M, 1967, mixed cell lymphoma involving abdominal nodes and mid-ileum 2 M (nephew), 1969, mixed cell lymphoma involving mesenteric nodes and distal ileum

Summary

The rarity of primary gastrointestinal lymphomas, together with difficulties in case diagnosis, have made it impractical to conduct extensive epidemiologic studies in this particular area of oncogenesis. Existing epidemiologic information, as a result, is primarily descriptive and is usually not population-based. One, therefore, can make only limited comparisons regarding lymphoma frequency by age, sex, organ site, histologic type, geographic patterns, and perhaps time trends. Analytic epidemiologic studies, whereby the strength of potential etiologic associations can be tested between case occurrence and the presence of particular risk factors, have been essentially limited to British follow-up studies regarding cancer risk among patients with coeliac disease (30, 33).

Nevertheless, existing descriptive data, coupled with immunologic studies, suggest etiologic patterns which make biologic sense with respect to gastro-intestinal tumors and to lymphomas in particular. Of greatest value are ob-servations (1) regarding IPSID and (2) regarding the clinical complex of coeliac disease/dermatitis herpetiformis/lymphoma. Taken together, findings in these two areas support the notion that immunologic dysfunction of small intestinal lymphoid tissue can eventually predispose to lymphoma production, either in intestinal mucosa itself or in mesenteric nodes. The mechanism by which on-cogenesis occurs and the sequence of events leading to local tissue immune dysfunction are not clear and represent two prime areas for future biologic research. The epidemiologic background against which IPSID occurs – poverty and frequent gastrointestinal infections in early life – suggests that intense and unremitting local infection may trigger the eventual chain of events leading to pathologic immune dysfunction and lymphoma. Specific mechanisms for tumorigenesis, however, may involve interaction with ubiquitous viral material possessing oncogenic potential, perhaps in the mode postulated for Burkitt's lymphoma in relation to herpesvirus infections.

References

1. Rosenberg SA, Diamond HD, Jaslowitz B, Craver LF: Lymphosarcoma: a review of 1269 cases. Medicine 40:31–84, 1961.
2. Doll R, Muir C, Waterhouse J: Cancer incidence in five continents. International Union Against Cancer, Vol 3, 1975.
3. Aisenberg AC: Malignant Lymphoma. New Engl J Med 288:883–941, 1973.
4. Gutensohn N, Cole P: Epidemiology of Hodgkin's disease. Sem Oncol 7:92–102, 1980.
5. De-The G: The epidemiology of Burkitt's lymphoma: evidence for a causal association with Epstein-Barr virus. Epid Rev 1:32–54, 1979.
6 Henry K, Farrer-Brown G: Primary lymphomas of the gastrointestinal tract. I: Plasma cell tumors. Histopath 1:53–76, 1977.
7. Ho F, Gibson B: Gastrointestinal lymphomas in Hong Kong Chinese. Israel J Med Sci 15: 382–385, 1979.
8. Desai PB, Meher-Homji DR, Paymaster JC: Malignant lymphoma: A clinical study of 800 Indian patients. Cancer 18:25–33, 1965.
9. Barekat AA, Saidi F, Dutz W: Cancer survey of South Iran with special reference to gastrointestinal neoplasms. Int J Cancer 7:353–363, 1971.
10. Modan B, Shani M, Goldman B, Modan M: Incidence of nodal and extranodal malignant lymphoma in Israel: An epidemiological study. Brit J Haemat 16:53–59, 1969.
11. Gideon EM: Primary malignant lymphoma of the digestive tract. Leb Med J 23:1–10, 1970
12. Kahn LB, Selzer G, Kaschula RDC: Primary gastrointestinal lymphoma – a clinicopathologic study of fifty-seven cases. Amer J Dig Dis 17:219–232, 1972.
13. Owor R: Malignant lymphoma of the gastrointestinal tract in Uganda – a report of 40 cases. East Afr Med J 54:666–669, 1977.
14. Allen AW, Donaldson G, Sniffen RC, Goodale F Jr: Primary malignant lymphoma of the gastrointestinal tract. Ann Surg 140:428–438, 1954.
15. Loehr WJ, Mujahed Z, Zahn FD, et al.: Primary lymphoma of the gastrointestinal tract: A review of 100 cases. Ann Surg 170:232–238, 1969.
16. Naqui MS, Burrows L, Kark AE: Lymphoma of the gastrointestinal tract: prognostic guides based on 162 cases. Ann Surg 170:221–231, 1969.
17. Freeman C, Berg JW, Cutler SJ: Occurrence and prognosis of extranodal lymphomas. Cancer 29:252–260, 1972.
18. Lewin KJ, Ranchod M, Dorfmann RF: Lymphoma of the gastrointestinal tract. A study of 117 cases presenting with gastrointestinal disease. Cancer 42:693–707, 1978.
19. Taylor ES: Primary lymphosarcoma of the stomach. Ann Surg 110:200–221, 1939.
20. Friedman AI: Primary lymphosarcoma of the stomach. Amer J Med 26:783–796, 1959.
21. Wychulis AR, Beahrs OH, Woolner LB: Malignant lymphoma of the colon. A study of 69 cases. Arch Surg 93:215–225, 1966.
22. Glick DD, Soule EH: Primary malignant lymphoma of colon or appendix. Arch Surg 92: 144–151, 1966.
23. Marcuse PM, Stout AP: Primary lymphosarcoma of the small intestine. Analysis of 13 cases and review of the literature. Cancer 3:459–474, 1950.

24. Fy YS, Perzin KH Lymphosarcoma of the small intestine. A clinicopathologic study Cancer 29:645–659 1972.
25. Faulkner JW, Dockerty MB: Lymphosarcoma of the small intestine. Surg Gyn Obst 95:76–84, 1952.
26 Al-Saleem T, Zardawi IM: Primary lymphomas of the small intestine in Iraq: a pathological study of 145 cases. Histopath 3:89–106, 1979.
27. Shani M, Modan B, Goldman B, et al.: Primary gastrointestinal lymphoma. Israel J Med Sci 5:1173–1177, 1969.
28. Golden R: The small intestine and diarrhea. Amer J Roentgenol 36:892–901, 1936.
29. Fairley NH, Mackie FP: The clinical and biochemical syndrome in lymphadenoma and allied diseases involving the mesenteric lymph glands. Brit Med J 1:375–380, 1937.
30. Harris OD, Cooke WT, Thompson H, Waterhouse JAH: Malignancy in adult coeliac disease and idiopathic steatorrhea. Amer J Med 42:899–912, 1967.
31. Austad WI, Cornes JS, Gough KR, et al.: Steatorrhea and malignant lymphoma. The relationship of malignant tumors of lymphoid tissue and coeliac disease. Am J Dig Dis 12:475–490, 1967.
32. Brunt PW, Svicus W, MacLean N: Neoplasia and coeliae syndrome in adults: Lancet 1:180–184, 1969.
33. Holmes GKT, Stokes PL, Sorahan TM, et al.: Coeliac disease, gluten-free diet, and malignancy. Gut 17:612–619, 1976.
34. Isaacson P, Wright DH: Intestinal lymphoma associated with malabsorption. Lancet 1:67–70, 1978.
35. Brandt L, Hagender B, Norden A, Stenstam M: Lymphoma of the small intestine in adult coeliac disease. Acta Med Scand 204:467–470; 1978.
36. Sleisinger MH, Almy TP, Barr DP: The sprue syndrome secondary to lymphoma of the small bowel. Amer J Med 15:666–674, 1953.
37. Benson GD, Kowlessar OD, Sleisinger MH: Adult coeliac disease with emphasis upon response to gluten-free diet. Medicine 43:1–40, 1964.
38. Kent TH: Malabsorption syndrome with malignant lymphoma. Arch Path 78:97–103, 1964.
39. Spence WJE, Ritchie S: Lymphomas of small bowel and their relationship to idiopathic steatorrhea. Canad J Surg 12.207–209, 1969.
40. Gjone E, Nordoy A: Dermatitis herpetiformis, steatorrhea, and malignancy. Brit Med J 1:610, 1970.
41. Andersson H, Dotevall G, Mobacken H: Malignant mesenteric lymphoma in a patient with dermatitis herpetiformis, hypochlorhydria, and small-bowel abnormalities. Scand J Gastroent 6:397–399, 1971.
42. Connon JJ, McFarland J, Kelly A, et al.: Acute abdominal complications of coeliac disease. Scand J Gastroent 10:843–846, 1975.
43. Tonder M, Sorlie D, Kearny MS: Adult coeliac disease. A case with ulceration, dermatitis herpetiformis, and reticulosarcoma. Scand J Gastroent 11:107–111, 1976.
44. Freeman HJ, Weinstein WM, Schmitka TK, et al.: Primary abdominal lymphoma. Presenting manifestation of celiac sprue or complicating dermatitis herpetiformis. Am J Med 63:585–594, 1977.
45. World Health Organization: Alpha-chain disease and related small-intestinal lymphoma: a memorandum. Bull WHO 54:615–624, 1976.
46. Ramot B, Shanin N, Bubis JJ: Malabsorption in lymphoma of small intestine. A study of 13 cases. Israel J Med Sci 1:221–226, 1965.
47. Eidelman S, Parkins RA, Rubin CE: Abdominal lymphoma presenting as malabsorption: A clinico-pathologic study of nine cases in Israel and a review of the literature. Medicine 45:111–137, 1966.
48. Seligman M, Danon F, Hurez D, et al.: Alpha-chain disease: a new immunoglobulin abnormality. Science 162:1396–1397, 1968.
49. Seligman M, Mihaesco E, Hurez D, et al.: Immunochemical studies in four cases of alpha chain disease. J Clin Investig 48:2374–2389, 1969.
50. Stoop JW, Ballieux RE, Hijmans W, Zegers BJM: Alpha-chain disease with involvement of the respiratory tract in a Dutch child. Clin Exp Immunol 9:625–635, 1971.

51. Florin-Christensen A, Doniach D, Newcomb PB: Alpha-chain disease with pulmonary manifestations. Brit Med J 1:413–415, 1974.
52. Cohen HJ, Gonzalvo A, Krook J, et al.: New presentation of alpha heavy chain disease: North American polypoid gastrointestinal lymphoma. Clinical and cellular studies. Cancer 41:1161–1169, 1978.
53. Rappaport H, Ramot B, Hulu N, Park JK: The pathology of so-called Mediterranean abdominal lymphoma with malabsorption. Cancer 29:1502–1511, 1972.
54. Ramot B, Levanon M, Hahn Y, et al.: The mutual clonal origin of the lymphoplasmacytic and lymphoma cell in alpha-heavy chain disease. Clin Exp Immunol 27:440–445, 1977.
55. Novis BH, Bank S, Marks IN, et al.: Abdominal lymphoma presenting with malabsorption. Quart J Med 40:521–540, 1971.
56. Levin KJ, Kahn LB, Novis BH: Primary intestinal lymphoma of 'western' and 'Mediterranean' type, alpha chain disease and massive plasma cell infiltration. A comparative study of 37 cases. Cancer 38:2511–2528, 1976.
57. Novis BH: Primary intestinal lymphoma in South Africa. Israel J Med Sci 15:386–389, 1979.
58. Jinich H, Rojas E, Webb JA, Kelser JR Jr: Lymphoma presenting as malabsorption. Gastroenterology 54:421–425, 1968.
59. Bonomo L, Dammacco F, Marano R, Bonomo GM: Abdominal lymphoma and alpha chain disease. Report of three cases. Amer J Med 52:73–85, 1972.
60. Doe WF, Henry K, Hobbs JR et al.: Five cases of alpha chain disease. Gut 13:947–957, 1972.
61. Manousos ON, Economidon JC, Georgiadou DE, et al.: Alpha chain disease with clinical, immunological, and histological recovery. Brit Med J 2:409–412, 1974.
62. Pittman FE, Tripathy K, Isobe T, et al.: IgA heavy chain disease. A case detected in the western hemisphere. Amer J Med 58:424–430, 1975.
63. Whicher JT, Ajdukiewicz A, Davies JD: Two cases of alpha chain disease from Nigeria. J Clin Path 30:678–681, 1977.
64. Selzer G, Sacks M, Sherman G, Naggan L: Primary malignant lymphoma of the small intestine in Israel. Israel J Med Sci 15:390–396, 1979.
65. Corres JS, Smith JC, Southwood WFW: Lymphosarcoma in chronic ulcerative colitis with report of two cases. Brit J Surg 49:50–53, 1961.
66. Sataline LR, Mobley EM, Kirkham W: Ulcerative colitis complicated by colonic lymphoma. Gastroenterology 44:342–347, 1963.
67. Nugent FW, Zuberi S, Bulan MB, Legg MA: Colonic lymphoma in ulcerative colitis: report of four cases. Lahey Clin Fdn Bull 21:104–111, 1972.
68. Friedman HB, Silver GM, Brown CH: Lymphoma of the colon simulating ulcerative colitis. Amer J Dig Dis 13:910–917, 1968.
69. Pevsner S, Leef F: Childhood abdominal lymphoma in two brothers. Israel J Med Sci 9:914–917, 1973.
70. Banihashemi A, Nasr K, Hedayatee H, Mortazavee H: Familial lymphoma including a report of familial primary upper small intestinal lymphoma. Blut 26:363–368, 1973.
71. Maurer HS, Gotoff SP, Allen L, Bolan J: Malignant lymphoma of the small intestine in multiple family members. Association with an immunologic deficiency. Cancer 37:2224–2231, 1976.
72. Alsabti EAK: Paraproteinemia in normal family members of eight cases with primary intestinal lymphomas in Iraq. Oncology 35:68–72, 1978.

7. Epidemiology of Primary Liver Cancer

NUBIA MUÑOZ and ALLEN LINSELL

Introduction

This chapter is concerned mainly with the epidemiology and etiology of hepato-cellular carcinoma (HCC)*, the most frequent of the liver malignancies. In early epidemiological studies this cancer was not always distinguished from other primary liver cancers, such as those derived from intrahepatic biliary cells. However, detailed histological studies, culminating in the acceptance of classifi-cations of liver tumors proposed by international bodies such as the World Health Organisation (1) and, more recently, the introduction of a serological test, the alpha-fetoprotein (AFP) estimation, which is found in high levels in patients with HCC and some testicular tumors, but almost never in patients with intrahepatic biliary cells cancer, have done much to refine the definition of HCC.

As the liver is so frequently the site of secondary cancers, one would expect clinical diagnosis of primary liver cancer (PLC) to be difficult. However, in those areas of the world – some developing countries – where PLC is frequent and tumors of the colon much less so, clinical diagnosis is confirmed in a large proportion of cases by biopsy or autopsy (2). Even in Europe and North America the cancer often follows long-standing liver disease and clinical diagnosis fre-quently proves to be accurate, and with the introduction of the AFP estimation we now have a new diagnostic tool.

As will be seen later, HCC is exceptionally frequent in some developing countries with large populations, and so globally it is probably among the most common cancers affecting man. Search for etiological clues in the environment are mostly carried out in the developing world rather than in the industrialized countries where the potential exists for hazards from many chemicals which produce HCC in animals, but where on the other hand HCC in man is in-frequent.

Abbreviations: HCC - hepatocellular carcinoma; AFP - alpha-fetoprotein; PLC - primary liver cancer; RNA - ribonucleic acid; EBV - Epstein-Barr virus; CMV - cytomegalovirus; HBV - hepatitis B virus; HBsAg - hepatitis B surface antigen; anti-HBs - antibody to surface antigen; anti-HBc - antibody to core antigen; RR - relative risk; HBcAg - hepatitis B core antigen; DNA - Deoxyribonuc-leic acid; WHV - woodchuck hepatitis virus; ppb - part per billion; UV - ultraviolet; ISG - immune serum globulin; HBIG - hepatitis B immunoglobulin.

Correa, P. and Haenszel, W. (eds.), Epidemiology of Cancer of the Digestive Tract.
© *1982 Martinus Nijhoff Publishers. The Hague/Boston/London.ISBN-13:978-94-009-7504-0*

The original studies on HCC in the tropics attempted to associate the frequent nutritional disorders of children, often with severe liver damage, with this cancer. It is now known that the profound changes produced in the liver by Kwashiorkor, for example, may, if treatment is adequate, be repaired with no apparent structural damage (3).

Recent studies on hepatitis provide evidence, however, that infection in early life may indeed be related to an elevated risk of liver cancer, and investigations over the last two decades of the possible role of the mycotoxins have gone a long way to substantiate the anecdotal reports of the early 1960s that fungal contamination of food might be an etiological factor. Evidence from the virological and chemical studies will be presented and the importance of seizing the opportunity to investigate a cancer, which may serve as a model of the role of a virus and a chemical in the etiology of a cancer, will be stressed.

Geographical distribution

Hepatocellular carcinoma (HCC) is one of the most common malignant tumors in sub-Saharan Africa and in South-East Asia. It is also relatively frequent in some European countries, such as Switzerland, Spain, France and Greece. This geographical distribution is illustrated by three different kinds of data.

Relative frequencies

These data must be interpreted with caution as they are subject to many biases which are exaggerated by using exclusively histologically proven cases, but they are the only data available from some areas of the world. Table 1 shows the relative frequencies of primary liver cancer (PLC) without a precise separation by cell type in autopsy and biopsy series. High relative frequencies have been reported for Hong Kong (4), Thailand (5), Uganda (6), Kenya (6), Tanzania (6), and Malawi (7). Intermediate rates for France (8) and Sudan (9) and low rates for India (10), Pakistan (11), Mexico (12), Peru (13), Denmark (14) and the USA (15).

Mortality rates

Although these rates are a good indicator of incidence considering the very poor survival of HCC, they also have serious limitations, particularly as a considerable proportion of cases are registered in national records as liver cancer of unspecified origin. The proportion of these cases of unspecified origin to the total

Table 1. Relative frequencies of PLC in autopsy and biopsy series.

		Autopsies		
Country	Period	Total no. of autopsies	PLC No.	%
Hong Kong (4)	1964–1966	1,480	100	6.8
Thailand (5)	1954–1970	12,265	297	2.4
France (8)	1959–1966	2,540	42	1.7
Peru – Lima (13)	1966	558	6	1.0
Mexico (12)	1953–1966	6,558	37	0.6
USA – Boston (15)	1917–1968	14,000	84	0.6
India, Bombay (10)	1947–1968	12,616	45	0.3
Denmark (14)	1938–1959	14,881	50	0.3
Pakistan, Decca (11)	1960–1965	5,450	11	0.2

		Biopsies		
Country	Period	Total no. of biopsies	PLC No.	%
Uganda (6)	1954–1960	2,926	199	6.8
Kenya (6)	1957–1961	2,747	143	5.2
Malawi (7)	1964–1966	648	27	4.1
Tanzania (6)	1957–1961	2,940	88	3.0
Sudan (9)	1954–1961	2,234	36	1.6

mortality from liver cancer in 28 countries has been studied and it ranges from 1% to 100% (16). It is more than 90% in Mauritius, Japan and Greece; it varies from 65% to 75% in France, Italy and Germany and it is less than 20% in the remainder of Europe, Israel and New Zealand (16). Table 2 shows the combined age-adjusted death rates (primary liver cancer plus unspecified liver cancer) for 28 countries. High rates were reported for Hong Kong, Greece, Japan, Latin and Eastern European countries and low rates in the USA, Australia, New Zealand and Scandinavian countries.

Within country variation in mortality rates for HCC has also been reported in China. A three years' mortality survey (1975–78) has recently been completed in the People's Republic of China, covering a population of 840 million people (17). The geographical distribution of 15 malignant tumors by province and county, has been summarized in an Atlas of Cancer Mortality for the People's Republic of China (18). In males, liver cancer is the third most common cancer after gastric and esophageal cancers. Very high mortality rates are observed in the north-east province of Jilin, in the east-coastal areas of the provinces Jiangsu, Zhejiang, Fujian and Guangdong and in the south-east in Guangxi province

Table 2. Age-adjusted combined death rates[a] per 100000 population, 1971.

High rates >7 × 100000 males				Intermediate rates 3.7 × 100000 males				Low rates <3 × 100000 males			
Country	Males	Females	Sex ratio	Country	Males	Females	Sex ratio	Country	Males	Females	Sex ratio
Hong Kong	38.9	8.6	4.5	Czechoslovakia	6.2	4.4	1.4	New Zealand	2.6	0.9	2.9
Greece	16.8	8.9	1.9	Belgium	5.7	3.7	1.5	Sweden	2.5	1.5	1.7
Japan	12.5	6.2	2.0	Austria	5.6	2.8	2.0	UK, Scotland	2.5	0.9	2.8
Italy	10.7	7.7	1.4	FR of Germany	5.1	3.5	1.5	Ireland	2.5	1.9	1.3
Spain	10.4	9.2	1.1	Switzerland	4.4	1.5	2.9	Mauritius	2.4	1.5	1.6
Bulgaria	10.4	6.6	1.6	Thailand	4.1	1.4	2.9	Norway	2.0	0.9	2.2
Poland	7.7	8.9	0.9	Israel	3.7	3.8	1.0	USA	1.4	0.6	2.3
Yugoslavia	7.5	4.9	1.5	Denmark	3.2	2.2	1.5	Australia	1.4	0.7	2.0
France	7.1	3.7	1.9	Finland	3.1	2.0	1.6	UK, England and Wales	0.9	0.4	2.2
Hungary	7.0	5.2	1.3								

[a]Rates adjusted to the world standard population. Combined rates include deaths from primary and unsuspected liver cancer (16).

Incidence data

Data from cancer registries contained in Volumes I, II, and III of 'Cancer incidence in five continents' (19–21) and other publications (22–23) provide a more accurate, but also more selective, picture of the frequency of HCC in contrast to data derived from mortality statistics. Table 3 shows selected areas classified arbitrarily in three groups: high incidence (age-adjusted incidence rate higher than 20 per 100,000 males), intermediate and low incidence (less than 5 per 100,000 males). High rates are seen in populations in South and West Africa and among Chinese populations in Singapore and in the USA; intermediate rates in Malay and Indian populations of Singapore, Nigeria, Recife, Brazil, Switzerland, Spain, Poland, Maori populations of New Zealand, American Indian in New Mexico, Jamaica and Cuba; low rates are observed in other populations in the USA, Latin America, Europe, white populations in South Africa and in Israel and India. Urban/rural differences in the incidence of HCC have been reported from Norway and Poland, the rates being 2–3 times higher in the urban than in the rural areas.

Time trends

Data from the three volumes of 'Cancer incidence in five continents' have been analyzed for 37 populations in 18 countries over an average period of eight years. In 17 (46%) of the 37 populations a statistically significant median increase of 3.7 per year for males and of 6.7 for females in 10 populations was observed. This increase was clearly identifiable in Kracow - Poland, Bombay - India, Alberta - Canada, and in the Jewish population of Israel. In the other populations a decrease was observed but it was statistically significant in only one population, Latins from El Paso (USA) (24).

The most obvious explanation for the observed increase in HCC is an improvement in diagnostic procedures and changes in registration practices. However, this will not explain why the increase in HCC is greater in certain populations having similar diagnostic and registration services. Another reason for the observed increase may be the better survival of cirrhotic patients which will increase the chances of neoplastic transformation of cirrhotic livers (24).

In countries with a very high risk for HCC, not included in the study by Saracci and Repetto (24), such as South Africa and Mozambique, it would appear that the rates are falling. Over half a million African patients were admitted between 1948 and 1964 to the Baragwanath Hospital, Johannesburg. The liver cancer incidence rates for this population for 1958–1962 were half the rates recorded for 1953–1955 (25). This trend is confirmed by studies on mine workers from Mozambique working in South Africa. A drop in the crude incidence rates for

Table 3. Age-adjusted incidence rates of liver cancer.[a]

High incidence >20 × 100000 males	M	F	Sex ratio	Intermediate incidence 5–20 × 100000 males	M	F	Sex ratio	Low incidence <5 × 100000 males	M	F	Sex ratio
Mozambique (19)	99.3	31.7	3.1	Singapore, Malay	14.6	6.8	2.1	Romania, Timis	4.6	5.0	0.9
Rhodesia, Bulawayo	64.6	25.4	2.5	Singapore, Indian	11.4	6.9	1.7	USA, Bay Area: black	4.2	1.7	2.5
Singapore, Chinese	34.2	8.0	4.3	Brazil, Recife	10.7	10.3	1.0	Japan, Okayama	4.1	2.9	1.4
South Africa, Natal. African	28.4	6.9	4.1	Nigeria	10.4	3.9	2.7	Puerto Rico	3.3	2.4	1.4
Senegal, Dakar (19)	24.5	10.0	2.5	South Africa, Natal: Indian	9.5	3.8	2.5	USA, New Mexico: Spanish	3.0	2.4	1.3
USA, Bay Area Chinese	21.1	4.5	4.7	Switzerland, Geneva	9.4	1.4	6.7	USA, Bay Area: white	2.8	1.4	2.0
				Poland, Warsaw City	8.5	5.8	1.5	Israel	2.5	1.4	1.8
				Spain, Zaragosa	7.3	6.2	1.3	Colombia, Cali	2.4	2.5	1.0
				New Zealand, Maori	7.7	3.6	2.1	Canada, British Columbia	2.1	1.1	1.9
				France; Côte d'Or (22)	7.6	1.4	5.4	USA, Connecticut	2.0	0.7	2.9
				USA, New Mexico: American Indian	5.8	0.6	9.7	India, Bombay	1.4	0.6	2.3
				Jamaica	5.2	1.0	5.2	South Africa, Cape Province: white	1.2	0.6	2.0
				Cuba	5.1	5.0	1.0	UK, Birmingham	1.0	0.5	2.0

[a] Adjusted to world standard population. From: Cancer incidence in five continents, Vols I, II and III (19–21).

HCC was found from 1964 (crude rate: 25.4 per 100,000) to 1971 (crude rate: 18.3 per 100,000) (26). In Mozambique it has been suggested that although the hospital incidence rates of the Imhambane rural district of 16 per 100,000 per year, was undoubtedly an under-estimate, there was evidence of a decrease in HCC (27). The reason for this decline is unknown but it has been suggested that it may be related to an improvement in living conditions, specifically in diet (26).

Sex and age distribution

In general, males are more prone to develop HCC than females. Male/female ratios higher than 4.0 are observed in Hong Kong (Table 2), Chinese in Singapore and in the USA, in South Africa, Switzerland, France, Jamaica and American Indians (Table 3). In these countries the male predominance is most marked in the younger age groups. In most populations the sex ratio varies from 1.5 to 4.0. Sex ratios near 1.0 or below 1.0 are observed in some Latin populations such as: Spain, Italy (Table 2), Recife – Brazil, Cuba and Cali – Colombia (Table 3), and other populations such as: Israel, Poland, Hungary, Ireland and Czechoslovakia (Table 2). The higher frequency of HCC in males than in females in most populations might be explained by a higher susceptibility, genetic or acquired, or by a higher exposure to the environmental factors responsible for HCC. Several studies have shown that femaler rats are more resistant to both toxic and carcinogenic effects of aflatoxin and this tendency is observed even at lower doses of aflatoxin (28). In most populations there is a higher prevalence of HBsAg carriers among males than among females and this difference was most striking in the younger age groups (29).

In all populations, independently of the risk, the incidence rates increase progressively with age with a tendency to level off in the older age groups. In the high incidence areas, such as Rhodesia, there is a shift towards the younger age groups. In these high-risk populations the tumor is seen not infrequently under 40 years of age, but it does not occur at this age in populations with low or intermediate rates (Fig. 1). Thus, in Mozambique, the male incidence in the 25–34 years age group was approximately 500 times that of the equivalent white population of the United States or the United Kingdom, but in the 65+ age group it was 15 times that observed in the US or UK (21).

Age of exposure to suspected risk factors might explain the higher differential in risk observed in the younger age groups between high-incidence and low-incidence populations.

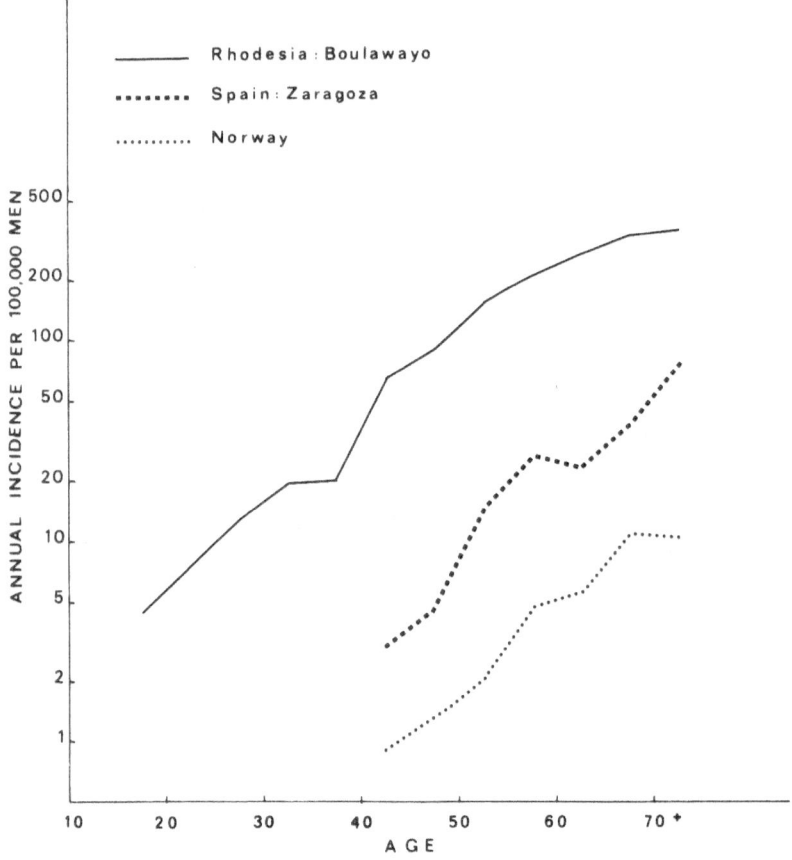

Figure 1. Age distribution of hepatocellular carcinoma in populations with high-, intermediate- and low-risk.

Hepatocellular carcinoma

As shown in Table 3, Chinese populations who have migrated to low-risk countries such as Singapore and the USA retain their high risk for HCC. However, a decrease in risk in the second generation is suggested by studies in Singapore showing that the risk for HCC is 75% higher among China-born Chinese than among Singapore-born Chinese (30). This suggests that exposure during early life to the suspected risk factors is one of the determinants of the risk for HCC later in life. On the other hand, Europeans who migrate from low-incidence areas to high-incidence areas, such as some African countries, retain their low rates, and it has been suggested that this is due to the fact that these migrants maintain the life style of their home countries (31).

Associated conditions

Viral hepatitis

The general term viral hepatitis refers to infections caused by hepatitis virus type A, type B and a more recently identified infection referred to as 'non-A:non-B' hepatitis. Recent data suggest that there are at least two types of non-A:non-B hepatitis virus; one with long incubation period and long duration caused by a virus immunologically and morphologically similar to hepatitis B virus and another with short incubation and short duration, associated with RNA particles which are being characterized, and which appear to be similar to hepatitis A virus (32–33). Chronic liver disease can develop after acute type B hepatitis and even more frequently after non-A:non-B hepatitis. Although tests for hepatitis A virus have been available for some years, it has not yet been shown that hepatitis A infection can progress to chronic liver disease (34). Other viruses producing hepatitis in humans, such as EBV and CMV, have not been associated with chronic liver disease. The association between hepatitis B virus (HBV) and HCC will be discussed below under risk factors.

Cirrhosis and hepatocellular carcinoma

An association between cirrhosis and HCC has long been recognized, but it has not been clearly understood. No correlation has been observed between the mortality from cirrhosis and the mortality from HCC in different geographical areas. The highest death rates for cirrhosis are observed in Chile, Mexico, Portugal, France, Puerto Rico, Italy, Ireland and Austria, which have low rates for HCC, and lower death rates for cirrhosis are reported in Thailand, Hong Kong,

Greece and Switzerland, which have high rates for HCC. This information is derived from material available at the WHO Data Bank. Cirrhosis is a dynamic condition of varied etiologies and with different malignant potential, which may explain why no agreement has been reached concerning a morphological classification and why no correlation has been observed between death rates for cirrhosis as a whole and HCC. The simple morphological classification of macronodular and micronodular is useful to explain the association of cirrhosis with liver cancer. The macronodular type is more frequent in Africa and South East Asia, high incidence areas for HCC, and the micronodular type is prevalent in the low-risk areas of Europe and the USA. The macronodular type appears to be more often associated with hepatitis B virus and it seems to be more prone to evolve to HCC. It has been estimated that 40% of the cirrhoses in Africa and South East Asia terminate in HCC and that 60% to 80% of HCC arise in cirrhotic livers. A widely held view is that the association between HBV and HCC is stronger among patients with cirrhosis than among those without cirrhosis (35), but this has not always been noted (36). However, a considerable proportion of HCC arising in non-cirrhotic livers occurs in asymptomatic HBsAg carriers with mild or no hepatic lesions (37). On the other hand, the micronodular type is prevalent in the low-risk areas for HCC, i.e., Europe and the USA, and it is often of alcoholic etiology. Only 5% to 10% of these cirrhoses appear to terminate in HCC, but as high as 80% to 90% of the HCC in these areas arise in cirrhotic livers (31, 38–42). In reformed alcoholics, however, liver cancer appears more frequently and is superimposed on a cirrhosis which has developed macronodular changes.

Experimental data indicate that in general, low doses of hepatocarcinogens induce HCC without concomitant cirrhosis of the liver while high doses induce both cirrhosis and HCC (43). However, as will be discussed below, aflatoxins have been shown to have carcinogenic activity in many species of animals but only in a few species do they induce both cirrhosis and HCC (44).

Risk factors

Viral infections – hepatitis B virus

An association between hepatitis B virus (HBV) infection and HCC has been observed in several sero-epidemiological case control studies (36, 45–50). These have recently been reviewed (51–52). In the earlier sero-epidemiological studies, before the identification of the core antigen and antibody, the presence of hepatitis B surface antigen (HBsAg) was used as the only marker of chronic active HBV infection. These studies show that individuals who are carriers of

Table 4. Prevalence of HBsAg among HCC patients and controls.

Country	No. of patients		Presence of HBsAg		
	HCC	Control	HCC %	Control %	Relative risk
Senegal (36)	165	328	61.2	11.3	12.4
South Africa (45)	158	200	59.5	9.0	14.9
Kenya (46)	42	450	54.8	4.7	24.7
Japan (46)	215	10738	36.7	2.7	20.6
Singapore: (47) Chinese	117	150	51.0	8.0	12.1

HBsAg are at a higher risk of developing HCC than appropriate controls. Some of these studies, in which sensitive methods (radioimmunoassay or immune adherence hemagglutination assay) have been used, are summarized in Table 4. In the study in Senegal, two groups of sex- and age-matched hospital controls were used: one non-cancer control and one other cancer control which included patients with cancer other than HCC (36). Only the non-cancer control is included in Table 4. The control groups for the studies in South Africa, Kenya, Japan and Singapore were blood donors, or apparently healthy subjects, not matched by sex or age to the cases (45–47). It is of interest to note that the antigenaemia rates among the control groups correlate quite well with the HCC risk in these populations. Japan with the lowest rates has the lowest antigenaemia rate; Senegal, South Africa and Chinese in Singapore, with high incidence rates for HCC, also have high rates of antigenaemia and Kenya has intermediate rates both for HCC and HBsAg. The prevalence of past or present HBV infection, as evidenced by the presence of HBsAg or anti-HBs was higher among the HCC cases than among the controls in all populations and ranged from 42% in Japan to 79% in Senegal. However, the main difference between cases and controls is seen in the prevalence of antigenaemia with relative risks ranging from 12 in the Chinese in Singapore to 25 in Kenya. Since patients with only anti-HBs have been found to have a similar risk for HCC as those lacking all markers (49), these two groups of patients should be grouped together in a referent basal category with a relative risk equal to 1. As it was not possible to do this from the published data, the relative risks given in Table 4 are underestimates of the true relative risks.

More recent case-control studies include an additional marker, the antibodies to the core antigen indicating active HBV infection. Active HBV infection was defined as the presence of HBsAg (with or without other markers) or anti-HBc (without anti-HBs). Studies which have used radioimmunoassay are summarized in Table 5 (48–50). The controls for the South African and Greek studies

Table 5. Prevalence of present or past HBV infection and of active HBV infection among HCC patients and controls.

Country	Number of patient		Present or past HBV infection[a]		Active HBV infection[b]		
	HCC	Control	HCC %	Control %	HCC %	Control %	RR
South Africa (48)	74	104	96.0	62.3	80.0	21.1	14.7
Greece (49)	80	160	80.0	58.7	48.8	10.0	10.4
Zambia (50)	19	40	100.0	62.5	68.4	12.5	15.2
Uganda (50)	47	50	93.6	76.0	72.3	8.0	30.1
USA (50)	27	200	74.1	5.0	40.7	1.0	68.1

[a]Positive for one or more HBV markers.
[b]Positive for HBsAg (with or without anti-HBs) or for anti-HBc (without anti-HBs).

were hospital controls matched for sex and age to the HCC patients, but the controls for Zambia were healthy villagers, and for Uganda were patients with Kaposi's sarcoma or melanoma, while for the USA they were blood donors. None of these groups were matched for sex and age to the HCC cases. Again a higher prevalence of past or present HBV infection was observed among HCC patients than among controls. It ranges from 74% in the HCC cases from the USA to 100% among the HCC cases from Zambia, and from 5% in the controls of the USA to 76% among the Ugandan controls. A good correlation between the prevalence of active HBV infection in the control populations and the HCC risk is evident. The prevalence of active HBV infection is at most 1% in US blood donors and 0.1 to 0.3% in the general population and HCC risk is very low. In South African blacks the prevalence of active HBV infection was 21% and their HCC risk is very high. Striking differences in the prevalence of active HBV infection between cases and controls were also observed in all populations. The relative risks ranged from 10.4 in Greece to 68.1 in the USA. The relative risks for South Africa, Zambia, Uganda and the USA were estimated from published data which, once more, rendered impossible the correction for the similar risk for HCC associated with the presence of only anti-HBs and the absence of all markers.

Since the higher the relative risk the stronger the association between a risk factor and the disease in question, and since strong associations are usually causal, these RR over 10 indicate that the association between HBV and HCC may indeed be considered causal. The higher RR observed in the USA indicate that in populations where the prevalence of the HBsAg carrier state is very low, the association of HBV with HCC is stronger. However, as HCC is quite rare in the USA, the absolute number of HCC associated with HBV is much less than in high-risk countries where the HBV may account for most HCC, although the RR is smaller.

Very few risk factors associated with human cancer have given relative risks of this magnitude (heavy smoking and lung cancer RR $\simeq 20$; diethylstilboestrol and adenocarcinoma of the vagina and cervix RR $\simeq 100$). That this association besides being strong is also specific, is suggested by the lack of association of HBV with other cancers (36) and with metastatic liver cancer (49).

That the association does not reflect HBV infection of patients who already had HCC is suggested by the results of follow-up studies which have revealed the sequential development from acute and chronic hepatitis with persistent anti-genaemia to cirrhosis and HCC (53–54) and by seroepidemiological studies showing that the peak of antigenaemia in most populations occurs in childhood or young adulthood (55–56). That active HBV infection precedes the develop-ment of HCC is also suggested by the high rate of perinatal HBV transmission from asymptomatic carrier mothers to their babies in high-risk populations for HCC in the Far East (57–58) and by a case-control study of 28 HCC patients and their families and 28 control patients and their families, where the antigenaemia prevalence rate in the mothers of HCC patients was 71% compared with 14% in the mothers of control patients (59). These data suggest that maternal trans-mission of HBV during the perinatal period is a crucial factor in the development of HCC.

Additional data supporting this conclusion have recently been reported from the UK. The transmission rate of HBsAg from 297 carrier mothers to their babies was high among Chinese (64%), intermediate among Afro-Caribbean (30%) and low among Asian (8%) and European (0) (60).

However, the strongest evidence indicating that the HBV infection precedes the development of HCC comes from ongoing cohort studies. Preliminary re-sults from studies of this type in Taiwan and Japan indicate that the RR among carriers may be as high as 50 (61–62).

Studies on the localization of the different antigens of HBV in fixed liver tissue complement well the seroepidemiological studies discussed above. Recently methodology has been developed which makes possible the determination and localization of the different HBV antigens not only in electron microscopical and frozen sections of fresh liver tissue, but also in fixed liver tissue by immuno-specific (fluorescence and peroxidase) and other empirical stains (Shikata's orcein stain) (63). It has been shown that while HBsAg can be reliably localized by immuno-peroxidase and immunofluorescence techniques, Shikata's orcein stain is also specific for this antigen and offers great advantages for large-scale retrospective studies (64). Since the distribution of HBsAg in the liver tissue is focal, the sensitivity of these techniques greatly depends on the amount of tissue studied (64–65). Correlation studies between HBV antigens in serum and liver tissue have shown that in 50 to 85% of HBsAg seropositive subjects the HBsAg

174

Table 6. Proportion of orcein positive liver diseases in populations with high-, intermediate- and low-risk for HCC.

Risk for HCC	Cirrhosis											Miscellaneous		Total
	HCC		Alcohol		Non-alcohol		Non specif.		Total					
	No.	%	No.	%	No.	%	No.	%	No.	%		No.	%	No.
High	91	71.4	5	0	17	58.8	17	52.9	39	48.7		42	4.8	172
Intermediate	69	79.7	7	0	8	62.5	66	66.6	81	60.5		71	2.8	221
Low	117	30.8	141	2.8	37	21.6	46	21.7	224	9.8		170	0.6	511
Total	277	56.3	153	2.6	62	37.1	129	48.8	344	26.2		283	1.8	904

can be demonstrated in liver tissue (66–67) and that patients with HBsAg or anti-HBc in the serum have also HBsAg or HBcAg in the liver tissue in 93% of the cases (67).

To extend the observations derived from seroepidemiological studies a collaborative study was carried out on 904 postmortem liver specimens from patients with HCC, cirrhosis and other liver diseases from high, intermediate and low incidence areas for HCC. The HBsAg in liver tissue was determined by Shikata's orcein stain. The results are summarized in Table 6. A high prevalence of HBsAg in the liver tissue of patients with HCC and non-alcoholic cirrhosis was observed in all geographical areas, but it was higher in the high and intermediate risk group than in the low-risk countries for HCC. On the contrary, very low prevalence rates of the antigen were observed in liver tissue of patients with alcoholic cirrhosis and miscellaneous liver diseases (68). These findings are in agreement with previous reports from the USA (40,67).

The above epidemiological evidence strongly suggests that HBV is causally associated with HCC. The experimental evidence, on the other hand, is incomplete. The study of the role of HBV in cell transformation has been hampered by the lack of an in vitro system for propagation of the virus. However, indirect experimental evidence suggests that HBV may indeed play a role in the neoplastic transformation of liver cells. HBV markers such as HBsAg or non-integrated viral DNA sequences have been detected in tumor tissue and in a cell line derived from an HCC of a Mozambican male (69–70). The ability of this cell line to grow rapidly in tissue culture as well as in soft agar (71) and to induce HBsAg positive tumors in nude mice (72) indicates a malignant phenotype. The recent cloning of HBV-DNA in Escherichia Coli (73) has greatly facilitated the molecular hybridization studies. Using this cloned HBV-DNA as a probe, several groups have now reported the presence of integrated HBV-DNA in the cellular genome of both human HCC tissue and of the cell line derived from a HCC of a Mozambican male (74–76). Integration of HBV in a malignant cell does not imply that the virus is the oncogenic agent. However, viral transformation is usually associated with the integration of viral sequences into host chromosomal DNA.

The ultimate experimental evidence of oncogenicity of HBV will be the induction of HCC in experimental animals. However, this is difficult to achieve because the chimpanzee is the only reliable model for in vivo studies of HBV. Although this animal model has been of great value in studies on the infectivity, transmission and in vivo replication of HBV and especially to test the efficacy and safety of HBV vaccines (77) it is not very practical to study the oncogenic potential of this virus. In this context, the recent report of a virus similar to human HBV associated with chronic hepatitis and HCC in woodchucks (78) is of great interest. These two viruses, human HBV and the woodchuck hepatitis virus (WHV) have properties which distinguish them from any known class of DNA viruses: infection with either virus results in the accumulation in the blood of

176

large amounts of excess surface antigen in the form of spherical and tubular particles of 20nm in diameter, and complete virions have a small, circular double-stranded DNA with a portion of partially single-stranded DNA polymerase. The endogenous DNA polymerase reaction uses the DNA as template, and both viruses are associated with chronic hepatitis and HCC (79). Two antigenic systems recently identified in the WHV (79) increase the potential value of this animal model for studying the mechanisms of induction of HCC by both WHV and HBV.

In summary, the evidence of a causal association between HBV and HCC is compelling, but since it may not be the only virus, the possibility should not be overlooked that the type of non-A, non-B hepatitis virus associated with chronic hepatitis may also play a part in the development of HCC. When serological markers for this virus become available this possibility could be seriously explored.

Chemicals as risk factors

Naturally occurring liver chemical carcinogens. The naturally occurring substances for which there is sufficient laboratory evidence of carcinogenicity to justify an investigation of the possibility that they cause human cancer are listed below:

Mycotoxins
  Aflatoxins
  Cyclochlorotine
  Luteoskyrin
  Sterigmatocystin
Pyrrolizidine alkaloids
  Isatidine
  Lasiocarpine
  Monocrotaline
  Retrorsine
Cycasin
Safrole
Tannic acid

The first, the aflatoxins, are justly as well as alphabetically at the top of the list, as they are probably at the moment the most investigated group of chemical liver carcinogens as reviewed below. Cyclochlorotine and luteoskyrin are metabolites of *Penicillium icelandicum*, which is frequently associated with contamination of rice and grain in Japan and Africa. Although there is laboratory evidence of carcinogenicity of the fungus and indeed of the purified mycotoxins in mice and rats, there is no direct evidence of the mycotoxins occurring in human food. Sterigmatocystin is a metabolite of a number of fungi that have been detected on cereals and other crops in South Africa. It is similar in some chemical features to the aflatoxins and, if it were found frequently as a food contaminant, would represent a toxic and possibly carcinogenic hazard to humans (80). The doses of sterigmatocystin required to produce tumors in rats, however, are much higher than those of the aflatoxins, and a survey of foodstuffs in southern Africa failed to indicate that sterigmatocystin was a health hazard. These three mycotoxins appear, therefore, to have the common feature that whereas the parent fungi are detected on foodstuffs, the isolate or pure derivatives on which the experimental evidence of carcinogenicity is based are not so found. There is at this time no evidence linking ingestion of these chemicals to human disease.

Over 100 pyrrolizidine alkaloids have been characterized, of which about 30 are hepatotoxic. There is still disagreement about the carcinogenicity of some of these compounds, but the four listed above are credited with malignant properties. Acute poisoning from the drinking of herbal teas and medicines in Jamaica has been associated with the alkaloids. It is noted, however, that the frequency of HCC is not significantly higher in Jamaicans than, for example, in black Americans in the United States. Investigation of the medicinal but possibly toxic effects of these traditional medicines, which are widely used in many populous parts of the world, is a much neglected field of research. Epidemics of vascular occlusive disease of the liver, which has been associated with the pyrrolizidine alkaloids, have been reported recently from India and Afghanistan (81–82) and it is probable that outbreaks of this kind are much more frequent than we suppose.

Cycasin occurs in the cycads, which are hardy plants able to survive drought conditions in tropical countries, and their seeds and roots are used as food in such emergencies. The toxic properties of the cycads are recognized by those living in the tropics and detoxification by sun drying and water extraction is practised. The active principle of cycasin, methylazoxymethanol, has chemical similarities to dimethylnitrosamine, and it produces liver tumors in a number of laboratory animals. The global use of cycads is obviously limited and there is no evidence that there is an increased frequency of liver cancer in areas where their ingestion is common (83).

Safrole occurs in many essential oils and was used until recently as a flavoring agent. This use is no longer permitted in the United States. Safrole compounds are carcinogenic not only for the liver, but also for the esophagus (84–85). However, there are no case reports or epidemiology evidence linking the safroles to human disease.

Tannic acid and the tannins are powerful hepatotoxic agents that produce liver tumors when subcutaneously injected (86). Tannic acid has a number of industrial uses and is used medicinally. Total sales for this purpose in the United

Table 7. Frequency of tumors in different animal species after exposure to aflatoxin.

Species	Dose	Duration of observation	Tumor frequency
Duck	30 μg/kg in diet	14 months	8 in 11 – 72%
Trout	8 μg/kg in diet	1 year	27 in 65 – 40%
Tree shrew	24 – 66 mg total	3 years	9 in 12 – 75%
Marmoset	5.0 mg total	2 years	2 in 3 – 65%
Monkeys	100 – 800 mg total	over 2 years	3 in 42 – 7%
Rats	100 μg/kg in diet	54 – 88 weeks	28 in 28 – 100%
Mice	150 mg/kg in diet	80 weeks	0 in 60 – 0%

States amount to 10,000 kg annually. In addition to its natural occurrence in tea or coffee, it is used as a flavoring agent and in brewing and winemaking. It is estimated that the annual consumption in the United States is about 50,000 kg (87), but there are again no case reports or other evidence linking these products to human cancer.

Aflatoxin. The dramatic discovery of the mycotoxins elaborated by the *Aspergillus flavus* fungi was related to fatal epidemics in poultry from toxic doses. There are four major members of the group, aflatoxin B_1 being the most potent. An epidemic of acute aflatoxicosis in man was reported in India in 1975, where over 100 people were said to have died (88). Following the discovery of liver tumors in trout accidentally fed aflatoxin-contaminated food, the carcinogenicity of aflatoxin was sought in a wide variety of laboratory animals. It was found that aflatoxin is a powerful carcinogen, producing tumors, mostly in the liver, in many animal species. There is a great variation in the susceptibility of many animals to aflatoxin (Table 7), although it is difficult to correlate the parameters of the different experiments (89).

The rat has been the most commonly used experimental animal and the dose response in a particularly susceptible strain is shown in Table 8 (90). At a dose of

Table 8. Dose-response to aflatoxin B_1 in male fisher rats.

Dietary levels ppb	Duration weeks	Liver cancer frequency
0	74 – 109	0/18
1	78 – 105	2/22 – 10%
5	65 – 93	1/22
15	69 – 96	4/22
50	71 – 97	20/25
100	54 – 88	28/28

1 part per billion (ppb) aflatoxin B_1, approximately 10% of the animals had cancer. The response is dose related to 100 ppb with cancer in all animals surviving 18 months. Tumors have been reported in rats a year after a single dose of aflatoxin and subsequent normal feeds (91).

From Table 7 it will be noted that the mouse is resistant to doses many times greater than those which produced tumors in rats. However, infant hybrid mice develop tumors when given repeated injections in the perinatal period (92).

Several studies have shown that female rats are more resistant to both toxic and carcinogenic effects (28) and this tendency is observed even at lower doses of aflatoxin. Other factors which could influence the response in man have been examined in animal experiments. The evidence of the influence of protein malnutrition, so important in those areas of the world where liver cancer is common, is contradictory. The effects of sunlight, again, would be of interest when considering the applicability of these results to man, as liver cancer is more frequent in the tropics. Rats UV irradiated after low doses of aflatoxin show a decrease of tumor frequency and it is suggested that endogenous photo-sensitized riboflavin may complex with aflatoxin and inhibit the production of the ultimate carcinogenic agent (93). A protective role against the carcinogenicity of aflatoxin has been demonstrated in rats with sodium phenobarbital, and it has been suggested that induction of liver microsomal enzymes that metabolize the aflatoxin to non-carcinogenic products may be responsible (94).

The animal evidence, therefore, indicates that aflatoxin is a very potent carcinogen in many species, including monkeys (95). The tumors are more readily produced in males and in the young. A dose-response relationship has been demonstrated.

It was recognized at an early stage of the investigations in man that the aflatoxins, although available worldwide, would be found most frequently in hot, humid climatic conditions. It was precisely from countries with such a climate that higher frequencies of liver cancer had been reported. Investigations soon demonstrated that samples of cereals and nuts from markets and home stores in tropical countries had impressive levels of contamination. However, such high levels were not detected when food ready for ingestion was examined. Housewife selection of cereals and other simple cooking methods play an important role in protection against these hazards. Long-term studies of plate samples of food ready for ingestion were therefore undertaken, assuming that an assessment of current exposure would be relevant to current cancer rates. This is perhaps a bold assumption but it is known that diet, storage and cooking habits had not changed markedly over the years in rural Africa and Asia, where most food is grown on small individual farms. The choice of populations for these studies was dictated by the possibility of measuring cancer frequencies, not an easy task in countries with a minimal infrastructure of health services predominantly concerned with infectious and tropical diseases. The recognition of a

180

Table 9. Summary of available data on aflatoxin ingestion levels and primary liver cancer incidence in adults.

Country	Area	Aflatoxin Estimated average daily intake in adults: ng/kg body weight/day[a]	Liver cancer No. of cases	Incidence per 10[5] of total population/year
Kenya	High altitude	3.5	4	1.2
Thailand	Songkhla	5.0	2	2.0
Swaziland	High veld	5.1	11	2.2
Kenya	Middle altitude	5.9	33	2.5
Swaziland	Mid-veld	8.9	29	3.8
Kenya	Low altitude	10.0	49	4.0
Swaziland	Lebombo	15.4	4	4.3
Thailand	Ratburi	45.0	6	6.0
Swaziland	Low veld	43.1	42	9.2
Mozambique	Inhambane	222.4	460	13.0[b]

[a]Excludes any aflatoxin present in native beers.
[b]Revised incidence estimate taken from van Rensburg (1974).

biological marker for hepatocellular cancer, AFP, enabled a more accurate diagnosis to be made under these conditions than had previously been possible. The results of studies to assess the level of contamination and cancer frequency, both in Africa and Asia are shown in Table 9 (96). It may be unwise to use these statistics in any sophisticated analysis without recognizing the numerous biases which might be present in such field studies. This is particularly pertinent when considering the registration of cancer cases in rural Africa and Asia. In the Kenya study the area of low frequency was that with the less well-developed medical services, and as the number of cancer cases was small, the detection of every case was vital. To check this, a study similar in design was carried out in Swaziland, where the ratio of hospitals to liver cancer frequency was reversed, and where one could be more confident of case detection (97). It would appear, however, that what evidence we have in man does indicate a good correlation which has special significance considering the fact that those epidemiological studies were set up to test a specific hypothesis derived from experimental studies.

One of the great difficulties in the transfer of the experimental evidence to the human situation is the disparity of levels of exposure, and it will have been noted that the human studies record exposures of nanogram amount of aflatoxin. However, it has been suggested by Shank (98) that the exposures of man and rats may be of the same order of magnitude and we must recognize the undoubted potency of aflatoxin, at least in some animals.

To summarize the evidence of the carcinogenicity for man, it can be said that aflatoxin-contaminated food is freely available in those countries where the tumor is frequent. It is known that man ingests this food and that in Africa and Asia a parallelism has been demonstrated between the levels of aflatoxin in food ready for ingestion and liver cancer rates. The practical difficulties of extending these correlation studies to analytical studies measuring individual exposure make us dependent on the assessment of intervention by improvement of harvest and storage practices. The assessment of such trials is not only difficult, but demands a very long-term study. However, possibilities of assessing individual exposure are being explored. A case-control study on HCC assessing individual exposure to aflatoxin by questionnaire and by actual determinations of aflatoxin in urine is under way in the Philippines (99). A more specific marker of exposure is being sought by the characterization of aflatoxin adducts.

Synthetic liver carcinogens. Selected synthetic compounds whose carcinogenicity has been evaluated are listed below:

Nitrosamines and nitrosamides
Chlorinated hydrocarbons
   Organochlorines
   Polychlorinated biphenyls
   Carbon tetrachloride
   Chloroform

The experiments on the carcinogenicity of the nitrosamines date back 20 years and it is now clear that humans could be exposed either to nitrosamines as such in food or, and, perhaps more importantly, to those produced in vivo after the ingestion of nitrites and nitrosatable compounds. In experimental animals the nitroso compounds can cause a wide range of cancers and they are remarkably tumor specific. The detection of food contaminated by nitroso compounds may not represent a major problem, although there are considerable unresolved analytical questions, but the possibility of their in vivo formation from nitrites and amines, amides, etc., is much more difficult to estimate. Nitrites are available directly as food additives, but can also be formed by the reduction of nitrates found in drinking water by a large number of microorganisms. The formation of nitrites from nitrates by intestinal bacteria and the subsequent production of nitroso compounds has also been suggested, so the number of potentially nitrosatable substances in food is considerable. However, epidemiological evidence relating them to human disease is still scanty, and many advances in analytical methodology are required before the field problems can be tackled effectively.

Many of the organochlorine pesticides are very stable and persist in the environment. Human exposure is mainly dietary, but domestic and public use of the pesticides undoubtedly adds to the risks. There is much information on the carcinogenicity of these compounds in experimental animals, mostly mice, but its interpretation has led to controversy (100). However, the ability of these chemicals to produce tumors in mice has been considered sufficient evidence of carcinogenicity to warrant changes in national regulations governing the use of pesticides. In contrast to the wealth of information on the effects of the organochlorines in animals, there is still little evidence directly relating them to human disease. The same can be said for the polychlorinated biphenyls, which have been used for forty years and which are known to be widely disseminated in the environment. However, action has been taken to minimize production in many countries. In the United States their use is restricted to close-system electrical applications, and their production has been prohibited in Japan.

The solvents carbon tetrachloride and chloroform may be available in trace amounts to humans by a number of routes, including drinking water supplies. There are no long-term studies on exposure in humans, and occasional cases of liver tumors following acute intoxication by carbon tetrachloride are of doubtful significance.

Alcoholism

The proportion of alcoholics who develop chronic liver disease is unknown, but it is probably low. Usually, chronic liver disease occurs in those who have been drinking excessively for many years.

Alcohol is probably the most important factor in the causation of chronic liver disease in most European countries, in the Americas and in Australia. The special susceptibility of the liver to alcohol is probably due to the fact that it is the only organ metabolizing it. Fatty change is readily induced and is a common finding, but does not itself lead to chronic liver disease. The most significant lesion is chronic alcohol hepatitis, characterized by neutrophil polymorph inflammatory reaction especially around liver cells containing Mallory's hyaline, fibrosis of portal tracts and centrilobular areas, and fatty changes (41). Alcoholic hepatitis is likely to terminate in cirrhosis, especially when drinking continues. Alcoholic cirrhosis is usually fatty and micronodular, but a macronodular pattern is commonly seen in reformed alcoholics. This macronodular pattern is associated with an increased risk for HCC, but in a small minority HCC arises in alcoholics without cirrhosis (41). It is unlikely that alcohol per se is carcinogenic, but it may facilitate or promote the action of specific carcinogens.

Smoking

A significant association between smoking and HCC negative for HBsAg has recently been reported in Greece (101). This association was not substantially

Table 10. Relationship between HCC and HBV, aflatoxin and alcoholism.

	Africa and South-East Asia	Europe and North America
Incidence of HCC	high	low[a]
Age-group affected	young to middle	middle to old
Type of cirrhosis	often macronodular	often micronodular
Aetiology of cirrhosis	often HBV	often alcoholic
% cirrhosis evolving to HCC	40 – 50%	5 – 10%
Exposure to aflatoxin	high	very low
% HCC associated with HBV	60 – 80%	30 – 50%

[a]Except Greece, Switzerland and Spain which have intermediate rates.

affected after controlling for alcohol intake. Similar epidemiological studies are needed to confirm or disprove that report.

Conclusion

The three risk factors discussed in detail above, HBV, aflatoxin and alcohol, probably account for most liver cancers around the world. The relative contributions of these three factors in high- and low-risk areas for liver cancer are summarized in Table 10. It can be concluded that in the high-risk areas, in Africa and South East Asia, HBV and aflatoxin probably account for most of the HCC. On the other hand, in Europe and in North America alcohol and smoking may be equally or even more important than HBV in the etiology of HCC, and aflatoxin is irrelevant. There have been long-standing speculations that this was indeed so (39), but the identification of the hepatitis A, B, and non-A, non-B viruses and the availability of HBV markers have enabled us to confirm this. The possible role of a non-A, non-B hepatitis virus in the etiology of HCC may be clarified as serological markers for this virus are being identified.

Relation between HBV and aflatoxin and HCC

The evidence discussed above indicates an association between HBV, aflatoxin and HCC. The next step will be to investigate whether they act together to induce HCC or whether they act independently. That aflatoxin may not have an appreciable carcinogenic role in man, was suggested by Prince in 1978 (102). He estimates the risk of developing HCC among HBsAg carriers in Senegal, Mozambique and the United States and obtains a risk of approximately 1 case of HCC among 250 male carriers per year and this figure is similar for the three countries. As aflatoxin exposure is much higher in the high-risk countries for HCC, namely, Mozambique and Senegal, than in the United States, which has a low risk for HCC, he concludes that aflatoxin does not play an important role in the development of human HCC. Lutwick, expanding Prince's argument concludes that aflatoxin does not act as a primary carcinogen but as an immunosuppresive agent causing an increase in HBV carriers (103). A further expansion of their argument is shown in Table 11 which summarizes the absolute risk of developing HCC among HBsAg carriers in four high-risk populations: Chinese in Singapore, blacks in South-Africa – Senegal, Greece and two low-risk populations, namely whites in the USA and Japan. Table 11 shows that the absolute risk of developing HCC among carriers parallels the HCC risk in all of these populations.

These correlations should be interpreted with caution as the prevalence rates of HBsAg carriers in both HCC patients and controls have been obtained from selected samples and therefore do not represent the true prevalence of carriers among the total number of HCC patients and among the general populations of each geographical setting for which the incidence rates have been obtained. However, if we compare the absolute risk of developing HCC among carriers of South Africa and Senegal where aflatoxin exposure is high, with the absolute risk of developing HCC among carriers in Japan and the USA where aflatoxin exposure is low, we see that this absolute risk is twice as high in Senegal and South Africa than in Japan and the USA, while the difference in HCC incidence between the two sets of populations is 6–10-fold. These data indicate that there might be a slight interaction between HBV and aflatoxin but this by no means excludes the possibility that aflatoxin also acts as a liver carcinogen independently of HBV, and that it may account for a considerable proportion of HCC in high risk countries for HCC, such as Mozambique, South Africa and Senegal.

If we make the following assumptions, the incidence of HCC non-associated with HBV in high and low-risk countries for HCC would be estimated:

– the proportion of HCC associated with HBV (proportion positive for HBsAg) is about 60% in high-risk countries and about 30% in low-risk countries for HCC;

– the proportion of HBsAg carriers in the male population of high-risk countries for HCC is around 10% and in the low-risk countries it is not higher than 1%.

Therefore, the proportion of HCC non-associated with HBV is about 40% in the high-risk countries and about 70% in the low-risk countries and the proportion of non-HBsAg carriers among the male population of high-risk countries is about 90% and 99% in the low-risk countries.

The incidence of HCC non-associated with HBV among male non-carriers will be:

Table 11. Absolute risk of developing HCC among male hepatitis carriers.

	Singapore (Chinese)	South Africa (blacks)	Senegal	Greece	Japan (Okayama)	USA Houston (whites)
Incidence of HCC per 100 000 per year	34.2[a] (21)	28.4 (21)	24.5 (19)	23.3 (128)	4.1 (21)	2.5 (21)
Proportion of HCC positive for HBsAg	51% (47)	60% (45)	61% (36)	50% (49)	37% (46)	30% (50)
Incidence of HCC positive for HBsAg/100 000/yr	17.3	17.0	15.3	11.5	1.5	0.75
Proportion of carriers among the general population	8% (47)	11% (45)	11% (36)	7.5% (49)	2.1 (56)	0.9 (56)
Number of HCC developing among male carriers per year	17 in 8 000 or 1 in 460	17 in 11 000 or 1 in 647	15 in 11 000 or 1 in 733	11.5 in 7 500 or 1 in 652	1.5 in 2 100 or 1 in 1 400	0.75 in 900 or 1 in 1 200

[a]Numbers in parentheses indicate references.

(a)	High-risk countries	
	TOTAL HCC incidence:	$30 \times 100,000$
	non-HBV associated HCC:	40% of 30 = 12
		12/90 000 or 13.3 $\times$ 100 000
(b)	Low-risk countries	
	TOTAL HCC incidence:	$4 \times 100,000$
	non-HBV associated HCC:	70% of 4 = 2.8
		2.8/99 000 or 2.8 $\times$ 100 000

Therefore, the incidence of non-HBV associated HCC is five times higher in the high-risk populations where the exposure to aflatoxin is high than in the low-risk populations where exposure to aflatoxin is negligible. In the low-risk countries, alcoholism will probably account for most of the non-HBV associated HCC. The non-A, non-B hepatitis type associated with chronic liver diseases may also account for some of the HCC non-associated with HBV in both high- and low-risk countries.

Other risk factors

Parasites

There is little evidence to suggest that parasites such as schistosoma may play a direct role in the development of HCC, but an association between intra-hepatic bile duct carcinoma and infestations with *clonorchis sinensis* (104) or with *opistorchis viverrini* (105) is suggested. *Clonorchis sinensis* is one of the commonest species of distoma found mainly in Thailand. It dwells in the lumen of bile ducts where it induces mucus cell hyperplasia, metaplasia and adenomatous proliferation (4).

Thorotrast

Thorotrast is an aqueous, colloidal solution containing approximately 25% of thorium dioxide (ThO_2). Thorium is a radioactive element decaying so slowly that from a practical standpoint it can be considered as remaining in the body indefinitely, mainly in the liver. It has been used extensively from 1930–1960 as a multipurpose contrast medium, particularly for arteriography. In experimental animals it induces sarcomas mainly at the site of injection (106). In humans approximately 120 liver tumors have been reported in patients many years after the administration of thorotrast; 33% of these tumors were classified as hemangiosarcomas, 32% as cholangiocarcinomas, 20% as HCC and 15% as bile duct carcinoma or combinations of these histological types (107). More tumors associated with thorotrast are likely to be reported as there are still many carriers of this substance.

Sex hormones

Androgens. Several case reports of HCC developing in patients with aplastic anemia after long-term treatment with androgenic-anabolic steroids have been published (108–109). However, doubt has been raised regarding the malignant nature of these tumors, as some of them regress after discontinuation of therapy (110). Moreover, these findings are difficult to interpret, because liver conditions such as hemosiderosis and post transfusion hepatitis, which are also associated with HCC have frequently been described in patients with aplastic anemia.

Oral contraceptives. Over 170 cases of liver cell adenomas have been reported in young women using oral contraceptives for long periods of time (111). The association between liver cell adenomas and oral contraceptives suspected from these case reports has been confirmed in two case-control studies (112–113). A few cases of HCC have also been reported in oral contraceptive users, but the exposure period was in general short and in some cases less than one year (114–116). However, no controlled studies have been reported.

Vinyl chloride

Vinyl chloride monomer has been shown to be carcinogenic for several animal species, producing tumors at several sites, including angiosarcomas of the liver (117). An increased risk for angiosarcomas of the liver and tumors of the brain, lung and lymphohematopoietic system, has been reported in subjects occasionally exposed to vinyl chloride in several countries (117).

Hemochromatosis

The relationship between HCC and idiopathic hemochromatosis, or iron accumulation, probably due to a genetically determined metabolic error, and secondary hemosiderosis, usually found in alcoholic cirrhosis and following multiple transfusions, is unclear. In some high-risk populations for HCC, such as the South African Bantu, hemochromatosis is commonly seen. However, this popu-

188

lation is also highly exposed to aflatoxin, HBV and alcoholic beverages with a high content of iron (118). Moreover, in other African populations with a high risk for HCC, hemochromatosis is rarely seen (41).

Future perspectives

Although the future of treatment of liver cancer cannot be considered promising, there may be very real prospects for the primary prevention of this cancer, which affects so many in large, heavily populated countries of the Far East and Africa. It is felt that the emphasis should fall on primary prevention rather than on early detection, as screening would have to be at very frequent intervals in very large populations (119–120). These estimates are based on the extremely rapid growth of the tumor. Studies in China and South Africa would indicate that screening would be required at least every six months, but the effectiveness of screening in reducing HCC mortality is unlikely.

The evidence associating three major risk factors with HCC has been discussed. This evidence is quite strong for HBV, less strong for aflatoxin and weak for alcohol. The object of primary prevention should be directed to decrease exposure to these hazards.

Alcoholism is a worldwide problem, control of which is the subject of much effort in many countries. Undoubtedly the important sequelae of alcoholism are cirrhoses and other cancers such as esophageal and laryngeal, but if its possible role in the etiology of HCC is confirmed, its control would also reduce HCC mortality.

The importance of reducing the contamination of food by mycotoxins such as aflatoxin is obvious, as apart from their potential as carcinogens they are also acute toxic hazards. Such contamination is primarily a problem for developing countries where agriculture is based mainly on small subsistence farms. The measures that will reduce contamination of foodstuffs by the aflatoxins, improved methods of harvesting and storage, will also reduce food losses from insect and rodent damage and therefore should have a general appeal for agricultural administrations. However, it is difficult to assess the success of such intervention on liver cancer, as this will require almost experimental conditions and most certainly a long observation period.

It is suggested that the prevention of hepatitis B could be the most successful form of primary prevention for HCC. Three ways of prevention of HBV infection are currently being explored.

(1) Passive immunization, which has been used for pre- and post-exposure prophylaxis. Both conventional immune serum globulin (ISG) and hepatitis B immunoglobulin (HBIG) have been utilized in pre-exposure prophylaxis in mentally retarded children in institutions, US troops going to HBV endemic

areas and in hemodialysis units. Both ISG and HBIG were found to be effective provided they were used at regular 3–4 month intervals during the period of exposure (121). This involves the problems of cost and the risk of induction of sensitization to human serum protein alloantigens. It has been suggested that HBIG may be more effective than ISG for post-exposure prophylaxis in infants born to HBsAg carrier mothers and after percutaneous exposure and has also been proved quite effective in protecting individuals sexually exposed to acute HB cases. The timing of the initial dose of globulin appears to be of critical importance as it has to be administered as soon as possible after exposure (122).

(2) Antiviral compounds such as interferon and adenine arabinoside have been utilized in patients with chronic hepatitis (123) but the response to treatment is so variable that considerable work is needed before its use can be assessed.

(3) Vaccines. As the HBV cannot be propagated in vitro, several vaccines have been prepared from HBsAg purified from the plasma of chronic carriers of the antigen. They have been proved to be safe, antigenic and capable of stimulating protection against infection with HBV, when tested in chimpanzees. These vaccines provide protection not only when they are administered before but also after exposure to the virus (124–125). However, because these vaccines are not very antigenic and because there is concern about the possibility of eliciting adverse reactions, other approaches to vaccine development are being considered. A vaccine prepared by extraction and purification of certain polypeptides from HBsAg is being evaluated for safety and efficacy in chimpanzees (126). The recent cloning of HBV-DNA in *Escherichia Coli* may provide an alternative and a simpler way of producing an ideal vaccine.

The human population groups in which this vaccine will be of immediate use will be the high-risk populations for HBV infection such as staff of hemodyalisis units and of similar hospital environments, staff and residents of homes for the mentally retarded, spouses of HBsAg carriers and male homosexuals, those travelling to areas of high HBV endemicity and those who have had a recent exposure such as a needlestick. The results of a controlled randomized double-blind trial to evaluate the efficacy of an HB vaccine (Merck vaccine) in 1,083 homosexual men from the United States have been recently reported. A 92% reduction of hepatitis B or subclinical infection among vaccines was observed (127). The first target of vaccine campaigns to prevent HCC will probably be newborn HBV-negative babies born to positive mothers, after appropriate prophylaxis with immunoglobulin. The most logical extension of a vaccine campaign would be to HBV-negative children, especially females, in high-risk populations such as those in the Far East and in Africa.

In summary, the prospects are bright for the prevention of HBV infection through a safe and efficient HB vaccine which may ultimately affect not only the incidence of acute HB and the pool of chronic carriers, but may also reduce the morbidity and mortality from chronic active hepatitis, cirrhosis and HCC.

190

References

1. Gibson JB, Sobin LH, et al.: Histological Typing of Tumours of the Liver, Biliary Tract and Pancreas. International Histological Classification of Tumours No. 20. Geneva: World Health Organisation, 1978.
2. Davies JNP: Primary Liver Carcinoma in Uganda. Acta Un Int Cancer 17:787–797, 1961.
3. Cook GC, Hutt MSR: The Liver after Kwashiorkor. Brit Med J 3:454–457, 1967.
4. Gibson JB: Parasites, Liver Disease and Liver Cancer. In: Liver Cancer, pp 42–50. IARC Scientific Publication, No 1, 1971.
5. Stitnimankarn T: Primary hepatic carcinoma in Thailand. Gann Monograph on Cancer Research 18:123–127, 1976.
6. Linsell CA: Cancer in Kenya. In: Clifford P, Linsell CA, Timms GL (eds): Cancer in Africa. East African Medical Journal and East African Publishing House, Kenya, 7–12, 1968.
7. Borgstein JAA: Notes on the Incidence of Cancer in Malawi. In: Clifford P, Linsell CA, Timms GL (eds): Cancer in Africa. East African Medical Journal and East African Publishing House, Kenya, 31–36, 1968.
8. Péquignot H, Etienne JP, Delavierre P, Petite JP: Cancers primitifs du foie sur cirrhose. Augmentation de fréquence et observation chez des cirrhotiques connus et suivis. Presse Méd 75:2595–2600, 1967.
9. Daoud EH, El Hassan AM, Zak F, Zakova N: Aspects of malignant disease in Sudan. In: Clifford P, Linsell CA, Timms GL (eds): Cancer in Africa. East African Medical Journal and East African Publishing House, Kenya, 43–50, 1968.
10. Patwardhan JR, Kshirsagar VH, Gadgil RK: Primary Carcinoma of the Liver in Bombay. Indian J Cancer 7:113–118, 1970.
11. Islam AKN: Primary Carcinoma of the Liver. E Pak Med J 13:92–96, 1969.
12. Lopez-Corella E, Ridaura-Sanz C, Albares-Saavedra J: Primary Carcinoma of the Liver in Mexican Adults. Cancer 22:678–685, 1968.
13. Vega Rizo-Patron L: Fatal Hepatitis, Cirrhosis and Hepatoma Incidence in Lima, Peru. Int Path (Wash) 9:12–17, 1968.
14. Glennert J: Primary carcinoma of the liver. A post-mortem study of 104 cases. Acta path microbiol, Scand 53:50–60, 1961.
15. Purtilo DT, Gottlieb LS: Cirrhosis and Hepatoma occurring at Boston City Hospital (1917–1968). Cancer 32:458–462, 1973.
16. Aoki K: Cancer of the Liver, International Mortality Trends. World Health Statistics Report 31:28–50, 1978.
17. Li FP, Shiang EL: Cancer Mortality in China. J Natl Cancer Inst 65:217–221, 1980.
18. Cancer Control Office, Ministry of Health: Atlas of Cancer Mortality for the People's Republic of China (in press).
19. Doll R, Payne P, Waterhouse J (eds): Cancer incidence in five continents, Vol. I, A Technical Report. Berlin, Heidelberg, New York: Springer-Verlag, 1966.
20. Doll R, Muir C, Waterhouse J (eds): Cancer incidence in five continents, Vol. II, Berlin, Heidelberg, New York: Springer-Verlag, 1970.
21. Waterhouse JAH, Muir CS, Correa P, Powell J (eds): Cancer incidence in five continents, Vol. III. Lyon, France: International Agency for Research on Cancer, 1976.
22. Quenum C, Tuyns A, Leblanc L, Sankale M: Essai de détermination de l'incidence du cancer primitif du foie dans la région du Cap-vert. Médecine d'Afrique Noire 20(1):27–35, 1973.
23. Faivre J, Milan C, Bugnon P et al.: Primary liver cancer in côte d'Or (Burgundy). Results of Three Years' Systematic Registration in a Well-defined French Population. Biomédecine 31:150–152, 1979.
24. Saracci R, Repetto F: Time Trends of Primary Liver Cancer: Indication of Increased Incidence in Selected Cancer Registry Populations. J Natl Cancer Inst 65:241–247, 1980.
25. Robertson MA, Harington JS, Bradshaw E: The cancer pattern in Africans at Baragwanath Hospital, Johannesburg. Br J Cancer 25:377–384, 1971.
26. Harington HS, McGlashan ND, Bradshaw E, et al.: A Spatial and Temporal Analysis of Four Cancers in African Gold Miners from Southern Africa. Br J Cancer 31:665–678, 1975.

27. Van Rensburg SJ, Van Der Watt JJ, Purchase IFH, et al.: Primary Liver Cancer Rate and Aflatoxin Intake in a High Cancer Area. S A Med J 48:2508a–2508d, 1974.
28. Newberne PM, Wogan GN: Sequential Morphologic Changes in Aflatoxin B_1 Carcinogenesis in the Rat. Cancer Res 28:770–781, 1968.
29. Blumberg BS, Sutnick AI, London WT, Melartin L: Sex Distribution of Australia Antigen. Arch Inter med 130:227–231, 1972.
30. Shanmugaratnam K, Tye CY: Liver Cancer Differentials in Immigrant and Local-born Chinese in Singapore. J Chron Dis 23:443–448, 1970.
31. Hutt MSR: Epidemiology of Human Primary Liver Cancer. In: Liver Cancer. IARC Scientific Publication, No 1, 21–29, 1971.
32. Tateda A, Kikuchi K, Numazaki Y, Shirachi R, Ishida N: Non-B Hepatitis in Japanese Recipients of Blood Transfusions: Clinical and Serologic Studies after the Introduction of Laboratory Screening of Donor Blood for Hepatitis B Surface Antigen. J Infect Dis 139:511–518, 1979.
33. Sohier R, Trepo C: Hepatitis non-A non-B. Etat actuel des connaissances. Revue d'épidémiologie et de santé publique 28(3):000–000 (in press).
34. Mathiesen LR, Hardt F, Dietrichson O, et al.: The Role of Acute Hepatitis Type A, B, and non-A, non-B in the development of chronic active liver disease. Scand J Gastroenterol 15:49–54, 1980.
35. Anon. More on the Aflatoxin-Hepatoma Story. Brit Med J ii:647–648, 1975.
36. Prince AM, Szmuness W, Michon J, et al.: A Case/Control Study of the Association between Primary Liver Cancer and Hepatitis B Infection in Senegal. Intl J Cancer 16:376–383, 1975.
37. Mazzur S, Szmuness W: Summary of Workshop A-5: Chronic Carriers of HBsAg. In: Vyas GN, Cohen SN, Schmid R (eds): Viral Hepatitis, pp 661–663. Philadelphia: Franklin Institute Press, 1978.
38. Linsell CA, Higginson J: The Geographic Pathology of Liver Cell Cancer. In: Cameron HM, Linsell CA, Warwick GP (eds): Liver Cell Cancer, pp 1–16. Amsterdam, New York, Oxford: Elsevier Scientific Publishing Company, 1976.
39. Higginson J: The Epidemiology of Primary Carcinoma of the Liver. In: Pack GT, Islami AH (eds): Recent Results in Cancer Research, No 26 – Tumours of the Liver, p 38. New York: Springer Verlag, 1970.
40. Peters RL: Pathology of Hepatocellular Carcinoma. In: Okuda K, Peters RL (eds): Hepatocellular Carcinoma, pp 107–168. Wiley Series on Diseases of the Liver. New York, London, Sydney, Toronto: John Wiley and Sons, 1976.
41. Anthony PP: The Background of Liver Cell Cancer. In: Cameron HM, Linsell CA, Warwick GP (eds): Liver Cell Cancer, pp 93–120. Amsterdam, New York, Oxford: Elsevier Scientific Publishing Company, 1976.
42. Shikata T: Primary Liver Carcinoma and Liver Cirrhosis. In: Okuda K, Peters RL (eds): Hepatocellular Carcinoma, pp 53–71. Wiley Series on Diseases of the Liver. New York, London, Sydney, Toronto: John Wiley and Sons, 1976.
43. Farber E: The Pathology of Experimental Liver Cancer. In: Cameron HM, Linsell CA, Warwick GP (eds): Liver Cell Cancer, pp 243–277. Amsterdam, New York, Oxford: Elsevier Scientific Publishing Company, 1976.
44. Wogan GN: The Induction of Liver Cell Cancer by Chemicals. In: Cameron HM, Linsell CA, Warwick GP (eds): Liver Cell Cancer, pp 121–152. Amsterdam, New York, Oxford: Elsevier Scientific Publishing Company, 1976.
45. MacNab GM, Urbanowicz JM, Geddes EW, Kew MC: Hepatitis-B Surface Antigen and Antibody in Bantu Patients with Primary Hepatocellular Cancer. Br J Cancer 33:544–548, 1976.
46. Nishioka K, Levin AG, Simons MJ: Hepatitis B Antigen, Antigen Subtypes and Hepatitis B Antibody in Normal Subjects and Patients with Liver Disease. Bull WHO 52:293–300, 1975.
47. Simons MJ, Yu M, Shanmugaratnam K: Immunodeficiency to Hepatitis B Virus Infection and Genetic Susceptibility to Development of Hepatocellular Carcinoma. Ann N Y Acad Sci 259:181–195, 1975.
48. Kew MC, Desmyter J, Bradbourne AF, MacNab GM: Hepatitis B Virus Infection in Southern African Blacks with Hepatocellular Cancer. J Natl Cancer Inst 62:517–520, 1979.

49. Trichopoulos D, Gerety RJ, Sparros L, Tabor E, Xirouchaki E, Muñoz N, Linsell CA: Hepatitis B and Primary Hepatocellular Carcinoma in a European Population. Lancet ii:1217–1219, 1978.

50. Tabor E, Gerety RJ, Voegel CL, et al.: Hepatitis B Virus Infection and Primary Hepatocellular Carcinoma. J Natl Cancer Inst 58:1197–1200, 1977.

51. Blumberg BS: Australian Antigen and the Biology of Hepatitis B. Science 197:7–25, 1977.

52. Szmuness W: Hepatocellular Carcinoma and the Hepatitis B Virus: Evidence for a Causal Association. Progr Med Virol 24:40–69, 1978.

53. Dudley FJ, Scheuer PJ, Sherlock S: Natural History of Hepatitis-Associated Antigen-Positive Chronic Liver Disease. Lancet ii:1388–1394, 1972.

54. Kubo Y, Okuda K, Musha H, Nakashima T: Detection of Hepatocellular Carcinoma during a Clinical Follow-up of Chronic Liver Disease. Gastroenterol 74:578–582, 1978.

55. Szmuness W, Prince AM, Diebolt G, et al.: The Epidemiology of Hepatitis B Infections in Africa: Results of a Pilot Survey in the Republic of Senegal. Am J Epidemiol 98:104–110, 1973.

56. Sobeslavsky O: Global Aspects of Hepatitis B Infection. In: Japan Medical Research Foundation (eds): Hepatitis Viruses, pp 111–124, Tokyo, Japan: University of Tokyo Press, 1978.

57. Schweitzer IL: Vertical Transmission of the Hepatitis B Surface Antigen. In: Natural Academy of Sciences (eds): Proc Symposium on Viral Hepatitis. Amer J Med Sciences, CBS, 287, 1975.

58. Beasley RP, Trepo C, Stevens CE, Szmuness W: The Antigen and Vertical Transmission of Hepatitis B Surface Antigen. Amer J Epidemiol 105:94–98, 1976.

59. Larouze B, London WT, Saimot G, et al.: Host Responses to Hepatitis B Infection in Patients with Primary Hepatic Carcinoma and their Families. Lancet ii:534–538, 1976.

60. Derso A, Boxall EH, Tarlow MJ, Flowett TH; Transmission of HBsAg from Mother to Infant in Four Ethnic Groups. Brit Med J 1:949–952, 1978.

61. London WT: Observations on Hepatoma. In: Vyas GN, Cohen SN, Schmid R (eds): Viral Hepatitis, pp 455–458. Philadelphia: Franklin Institute Press, 1978.

62. Beasley RP: Open Discussion. In: Vyas GN, Cohen SN, Schmid R (eds): Viral Hepatitis, pp 460–461. Philadelphia: Franklin Institute Press, 1978.

63. Shikata T, Uzawa T, Yoshiwara N, Akatsuka T, Yamazaki S: Staining Methods of Australian Antigen in Paraffin Section – Detection of Cytoplasmic Inclusion Bodies. Jap J Exp Med 44:25–36, 1974.

64. Nayak NC, Sachdeva R: Localization of Hepatitis B Surface Antigen in Conventional Paraffin Sections of the Liver. Am J Path 81:479–490, 1975.

65. Nayak NC, Dhar A, Sachdeva R, et al.: Association of Human Hepatocellular Carcinoma and Cirrhosis with Hepatitis B Virus Surface and Core Antigens in the Liver. Intl J Cancer 20:643–654, 1977.

66. Cohen C, Berson SD, Geddes EW: Hepatitis B Antigen in Black Patients with Hepatocellular Carcinoma. Cancer 41:245–249, 1978.

67. Omata M, Afroudakis A, Liew CT, Ashcavai M, Peters RL: Comparison of Serum Hepatitis B Surface Antigen (HBcAg) and Serum Anticore with Tissue HBsAg and Hepatitis B Core Antigen (HBsAg). Gastroenter 75:1003–1009, 1979.

68. Muñoz N, Nayak NC, Quenum C, Mandard AM, Cuello C, Papharalambus: Hepatitis B Virus Antigen in Liver Tissue of Patients with Hepatocellular Carcinoma, Cirrhosis and Miscellanoues Liver Diseases from High-, Intermediate- and Low-Risk Areas for Hepatocellular Carcinoma (in preparation).

69. Thung SN, Gerber MA, Sarno E, Popper H: Distribution of Five Antigens in Hepatocellular Carcinoma. Lab Invest 41:101–105, 1979.

70. Summers J, O'Connell A, Maupas P, et al.: Hepatitis B Virus DNA in Primary Hepatocellular Carcinoma Tissue. J Med Virol 2:207–214, 1978.

71. Alexander J, MacNab G, Sanders R: Perspectives Virol 10:103–120, 1978.

72. Desmyter J, Ray MB, Bradburne AF, Alexander JJ: Human HBsAg-positive Hepatoma in Nude Athymic Mice. In: Vyas GN, Cohen SN, Schmid R (eds): Viral Hepatitis, pp 459–463. Philadelphia: Franklin Institute Press, 1978.

73. Burrell CJ, Mackay P, Greenaway PJ, et al.: Expression in *Escherichia coli* of Hepatitis B Virus DNA Sequences Cloned in Plasmid pBR322. Nature 279:43–47, 1979.

74. Chakraborty PR, Ruiz-Opazo N, Shouval D, Shafritz DA: Identification of Integrated Hepatitis B Virus DNA and Expression of Viral DNA in an HBsAg-producing Human Hepatocellular Carcinoma Cell Line. Nature 286:531–533, 1980.
75. Brechot C, Pourcel C, Louise A, Rain B, Tiollais P: Presence of Integrated Hepatitis B Virus DNA Sequences in Cellular DNA of Human Hepatocellular Carcinoma. Nature 286:533–535, 1980.
76. Edman JC, Gray P, Valenzuela P, Rall LB, Rutter WJ: Integration of Hepatitis B Virus Sequences and their Expression in a Human Hepatoma Cell. Nature 286:535–538, 1980.
77. Barker LF, Maynard JE, Purcell RH, Hoofnagle JH, Berquist KR, London WT, et al.: Viral Hepatitis Type B in Experimental Animals. Am J Med Sci 270:189–195, 1975.
78. Summers J, Smolec JM, Snyder R: A Virus Similar to Human Hepatitis B Virus Associated with Hepatitis and Hepatoma in Woodchucks. Proc Natl Acad Sci USA 75:4533–4537, 1978.
79. Werner BG, Smolec JM, Snyder R, Summers J: Serological Relationship of Woodchuck Hepatitis B Virus. J Virol 32:314–322, 1979.
80. Stoloff L: Occurrence of Mycotoxins in Foods and Feeds. In: Rodricks JV (ed): Mycotoxins and Other Fungal Related Food Problems, pp 23–50, Washington, DC: American Chemical Society, 1976.
81. Tandon BN, Tandon RK, Tandon HD, Narndranathan M, Joshi YK: An Epidemic of Veno-Occlusive Disease of Liver in Central India. Lancet ii:271–272, 1976.
82. Mohabbat O, Srivastava RN, Shafiq Younos M, Gholam Ghaos Sediq Merzad AA, Aram GN: An Outbreak of Hepatic Veno-occlusive Disease in North-western Afghanistan, Lancet ii:269–271, 1976.
83. Hirono I, Kachi H, Kato T: A Survey of Acute Toxicity of Cycads and Mortality Rate from Cancer in the Miyako Islands, Okinawa. Acta Pathol Jpn 20:327–337, 1970.
84. Long EL, Jenner PM: Esophageal Tumours Produced in Rats by the Feeding of Dihydrosafrole. Fed Proc 22:275, 1963.
85. Long EL, Nelson AA, Fitzhugh OG, Hansen WH: Liver Tumours Produced in Rats by Feeding Safrole. Arch Pathol 75:595–604, 1963.
86. Korpássy B, Mosonyi M: The carcinogenic activity of tannic acid. Liver tumours induced in rats by prolonged subcutaneous administration of tannic acid solutions. Brit J Cancer 4:411–420, 1950.
87. International Agency for Research on Cancer: Some Naturally Occurring Substances. Monogr 10, Lyon, 1976.
88. Krishnamachari KAVR, Bhat RV, Nagarajan V, Tilak, TBG: Hepatitis Due to Aflatoxicosis – an Outbreak in Western India. Lancet i:1061–1063, 1975.
89. Wogan GN: Mycotoxins and Other Naturally Occurring Carcinogens. In: Kraybill HF, Mehlman MA (eds): Environmental Cancer. Advances in Modern Toxicology, Vol. 3, pp 263–290. New York: John Wiley and Sons, 1977.
90. Wogan GN, PaglialungaS, Newberne PM: Carcinogenic Effects of Low Dietary Levels of Aflatoxin B_1 in Rats. Food Cosmet Toxicol 12:681–685, 1974.
91. Carnaghan RBA: Hepatic Tumours and Other Chronic Liver Changes in Rats Following a Single Oral Administration of Aflatoxin. Br J Cancer 21:811–814, 1967.
92. Vesselinovitch SD, Mihailovich N, Wogan GN, Lombard LS, Rao KVN: Aflatoxin B_1, a Hepatocarcinogen in the Infant Mouse. Cancer Res 32:2289–2291, 1972.
93. Joseph-Bravo PI, Findley M, Newberne PM: Some Interactions of Light, Riboflavin and Aflatoxin B_1 in vivo and in vitro. J Toxicol Environ Health 1:353–376, 1976.
94. Swenson DH, Lin JK, Miller EC, Miller JA: Aflatoxin B_1-2,3-axide as a Probably Intermediate in the Covalent Binding of Aflatoxins B_1 and B_2 to Rat Liver DNA and Ribosomal RNA in vivo. Cancer Res 37:172–181, 1977.
95. Adamson RC, Correa P, Sieber S, McIntire RK, Dalgard D: Carcinogenicity of Aflatoxin B, in Rhesus Monkeys: Two Additional cases of Primary Liver Cancer. J Natl Cancer Inst 57:67–78, 1976.
96. Linsell CA, Beers FG: Field Studies on Liver Cell Cancer. In: Hiatt HH, Watson JD, Winsten JA (eds): Origins of Human Cancer, pp 549–556. Cold Spring Harbor, NY: Cold Spring Harbor Laboratory, 1977.

194

97. Peers FG, Gilman GA, Linsell CA: Dietary Aflatoxins and Human Liver Cancer. A Study in Swaziland. Int J Cancer 17:167–176, 1976.
98. Shank RC: Epidemiology of Aflatoxin Carcinogenesis. In: Kraybill HF, Mehlman MA (eds): Environmental Cancer. Advances in Modern Toxicology, Vol. 3, pp 291–318. New York: John Wiley and Sons, 1977.
99. Personal Communication with Bulato-Jayme J.
100. International Agency for Research on Cancer: Some Organochlorine Pesticides. Monogr 5. Lyon: IARC, 1974.
101. Trichopoulos D, MacNahon B, Sparros L, Merikas G: Smoking and Hepatitis B-Negative Primary Hepatocellular Carcinoma. J Natl Cancer Inst 65:111–114, 1980.
102. Prince AM: Open Discussion. In: Vyas GN, Cohen S, Schmid R (eds): Viral Hepatitis, p 460. Philadelphia, 1978.
103. Lutwick L: Relation between Aflatoxin, Hepatitis-B Virus and Hepatocellular Carcinoma. The Lancet, 755–757, 1979.
104. Hou PC: The Relationship between Primary Carcinoma of the Liver and Infestation with *Clonorchis Sinensis*. J Path Bact 72:239–246, 1956.
105. Bhamarapravati N, Virranuvatti V: Liver Diseases in Thailand. An Analysis of Liver Biopsies. Am J Gastroenterol 45:267–275, 1966.
106. Selbie FR: Tumours in Rats and Mice following the Injection of Thorotrast. Br J Exp Pathol 29:100, 1938.
107. Battifora HA: Thorotrast and Tumours of the Liver. In: Okuda K, Peters RL (eds): Hepatocellular Carcinoma, pp 83–93, 1976.
108. Johnson FL, Feagler JR, Lerner KG, Majerus PW, Siegel M, Hartmann JR, Thomas CD: Association of Androgenic-Anabolic Steroid Therapy with Development of Hepatocellular Carcinoma. Lancet ii:1273–1276, 1972.
109. Shapiro P, Ikeda RM, Ruebner BH, Connors MH, Halsted CC, Abildgaard CF: Multiple Hepatic Tumors and Peliosis Hepatitis in Fancon's Anemia Treated with Androgens. Am J Dis Child 131:1104–1106, 1977.
110. Farrell GC, Joshua DE, Uren RF, Baird PJ, Perkins KW, Kronenberg H: Androgen-induced Hepatoma. Lancet i:430–432, 1975.
111. Letoublon C, Champetier J, Benbassa A, Durand A, Laborde Y, Pasquier D: Benign Liver Tumours and Oral Contraceptives (Fr.) Lyon Chir 74:121–124, 1978.
112. Edmondson HA, Henderson B, Benton B: Liver-cell Adenomas Associated with the Use of Oral Contraceptives. New Engl J Med 294:470–472, 1976.
113. Rooks JB, Ory HW, Ishak KG, Strauss LT, Greenspan JR, Tyler GW Jr: The Association between Oral Contraception and Hepatocellular Adenoma – a Preliminary Report. Int J Gynaecol Obstet 15:143–144, 1977.
114. Thalassionis NC, Lymberatos C, Hadjioannou J, Gardikas C: Liver-cell Carcinoma after Long-term Oestrogen-like Drugs. Lancet i:270, 1974.
115. Glassberg AB, Rosenbaum EH: Oral Contraceptives and Malignant Hepatoma. Lancet i:479, 1976.
116. Menzies-Gow N: Hepatocellular Carcinoma Associated with Oral Contraceptives. Br J Surg 65:316–317, 1978.
117. IARC Monographs on the Evaluation of the Carcinogenic Risk of Chemicals to Humans. Vol 19:377–437, 1979.
118. Higginson J, Grobbelaar BG, Walker ARP: Hepatic Fibrosis and Cirrhosis in Man in Relation to Malnutrition. Am J Pathol 33:29–53, 1957.
119. Leblanc L, Tuyns AJ, Masseyeff R: Screening for Primary Liver Cancer. Digestion 8:8–14, 1973.
120. Personal Communication with Li HK, Lei LM, Fang KS, Kang HS, from the Unit of Biochemical and Immunological Diagnosis, Shanghai Cancer Institute.
121. Prince AM, Szmuness W, Mann MK, et al.: Hepatitis B Immune Globulin: Final Report of a Controlled Multicenter Trial of Efficacy in Prevention of Dialysis-Associated Hepatitis. J Infect Dis 137:131–144, 1978.
122. Grady GF: Viral Hepatitis: Passive Prophylaxis with Globulins – State of the Art in 1978. In:

Vyas GN, Cohen SN, Schmid R (eds): Viral Hepatitis, pp 467–476. Philadelphia: Franklin Institute Press, 1978.

123. Merigan TC, Robinson WS: Antiviral Therapy in HBV Infection. In: Vyas GN, Cohen SN, Schmid R (eds): Viral Hepatitis, pp 575–579. Philadelphia: Franklin Institute Press, 1978.

124. Purcell RH, Gerin JL: Hepatitis B Vaccines: A Status Report. In: Vyas GN, Cohen SN, Schmid R (eds): Viral Hepatitis, pp 491–505. Philadelphia: Franklin Institute Press, 1978.

125. Hilleman MR, Bertland AU, Buynak EB, et al.: Clinical and Laboratory Studies of HBsAg Vaccine. In: Vyas GN, Cohen SN, Schmid R (eds): Viral Hepatitis, pp 525–537. Philadelphia: Franklin Institute Press, 1978.

126. Hollinger FB, Dreesman GR, Sanchez Y, et al.: Experimental Hepatitis B Polypeptide Vaccine in Chimpanzees. In: Vyas GN, Cohen SN, Schmid R (eds): Viral Hepatitis, pp 557–567. Philadelphia: Franklin Institute Press, 1978.

127. Szmuness W, Stevens CE, Harley EJ, et al.: Demonstration of Efficacy in a Controlled Clinical Trial in a High-Risk Population in the United States. New Engl J Med 303:833–841, 1980.

128. Trichopoulos D, Violaki M, Sparros L, Xirouchaki E: Epidemiology of Hepatitis B and Primary Hepatic Carcinoma. The Lancet:1038–1039, 1975.

8. Ethnogeographic Patterns in Gallbladder Cancer

ERIC J. DEVOR*

Introduction

In the past few years a great deal of information has been compiled regarding interpopulation variation in carcinoma of the gallbladder. The primary purpose of the present paper is to review this information. A secondary purpose is to consider the form and pattern of interpopulation variation in the light of recent work on gallbladder cancer in the tri ethnic population of New Mexico. Finally, a series of conclusions will be drawn about the meaning of such variation as it pertains to a possible causal mechanism for the disease.

The terms pattern and coherence, frequently used in this paper, describe interpopulational variation. Patterns in and of themselves do not, however, have any explanatory power. It is only when two or more patterns are compared that potential causal explanations may begin to appear. This naturally leads to the concept of coherence which is used here to mean the overall congruence of two or more patterns. High coherence may not necessarily mean that patterns are related through the same causal mechanism. It is, of course, obvious that the more patterns that are found to be coherent with the original causal pattern, the more likely it is that they share some common causal features or explanation.

In assessing the possible causal pathways influencing the population patterning of gallbladder cancer one must pay strict attention to the dichotomy between environmental factors (primarily cultural and dietary practices) and host factors (primarily age, sex, race, and preexistent disease).

An instructive example of this dichotomy may be seen in the relationship between the prevalence of diabetes and the genetic population structure of certain southwestern American Indian tribes. Workman (1) has shown that the patterning of intertribal genetic differentiation, as measured by red cell antigens, and that of hyperglycemia, as measured by two hour plasma glucose levels, among the Pima, Papago, and Zuni display low coherence.

Pima and Papago, members of the Piman linguistic subfamily of the Uto-Aztecan group, share a recent common origin on the basis of archaeological, ethno-historical and genetic evidence (2). Zuni, by contrast, are an amalgam of

* This work was completed while the author was a Visiting Professor at the University of Kansas.

Correa, P. and Haenszel, W. (eds.), Epidemiology of Cancer of the Digestive Tract.
© *1982 Martinus Nijhoff Publishers. The Hague/Boston/London. ISBN-13:978-94-009-7504-0*

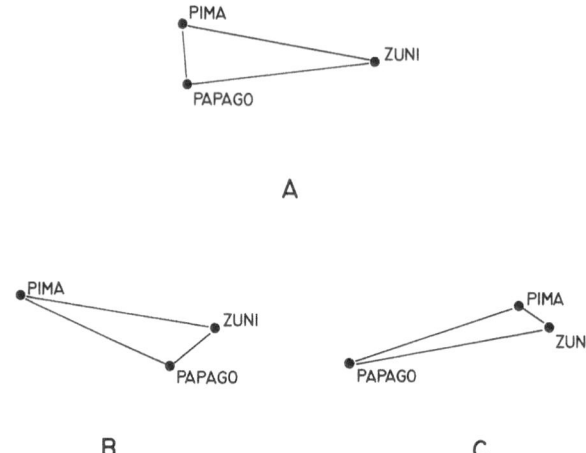

Figure 1. Diagrammatic representation of the patterns of relationship amongst the Pima, Papago, and Zuni Indian tribes of the American southwest. The comparative variables are blood group allelic frequencies (A), and hyperglycemia prevalence in males (B) and females (C). Distances between groups are relative approximations calculated from published data (1, 3).

indigenous southwestern Indians (Anasazi and Mogollon) and are genetically quite distinct from Pima and Papago (1, 3). Hence, the genetic pattern in a two-dimensional reduced space shows Pima and Papago in close association and Zuni as a remote outlier (Fig. 1).

The hyperglycemia pattern among these groups, also shown in Fig. 1, is very different form the genetic pattern. Among males, the proportion affected is most similar between Zuni and Papago. Among females, the proportion affected is most similar between Zuni and Pima. Most importantly, in neither sex are Papago and Pima at all close. The lack of coherence between the patterns has led Workman (1) to conclude that an explanatory model which accounts for tribal variation in hyperglycemia prevalence 'need not invoke genetic differentiation as an important causal factor'.

The historical background of gallbladder cancer

The earliest description of human carcinoma of the gallbladder has repeatedly been credited to Maximillian de Stoll, Professor of the Practice of Medicine in Vienna, who communicated his three cases, which had all come to autopsy, in 1777 in Pars Prima Rationis Medendi.

By the turn of the twentieth century a considerable amount of information about gallbladder cancer had been compiled. Illingworth (4) has summed up our indebtedness to early researchers, 'Indeed, it may be said that practically all of our present knowledge of carcinoma of the gall-bladder, except upon the detailed histology, is derived from these writers (of the last century), and more recent observations have served only to confirm and elaborate their findings.' It is not until the early 1950s that new aspects of gallbladder cancer began to become generally known. These new aspects revolve around the striking ethno-geographical patterning which is the focal point of the present paper.

Clinical features of gallbladder cancer: a review

Arminski (5) reviewed the contemporary knowledge about gallbladder cancer. During the intervening thirty years, several other reviews have been published (6, 7, 8). In this section an up-to-date summary of carcinoma of the gallbladder is presented which includes a description and analysis of 6,478 published cases of the disease as well as the most current information about an additional 521 cases from New Mexico. The present review should in no way be considered exhaustive. However, the cumulative data serve as a base-line for later discussion.

A chronological listing of sixty-nine published reports on the subject of gallbladder cancer is presented in Table 1. The quality and completeness of reporting has improved over time, particularly since 1950. Prior to that time few authors addressed the topic of average age at diagnosis. Nor had many authors reported median survival, preferring instead to describe this variable in qualitative terms. In addition, larger series (i.e., more than 100) have been reported most recently as researchers are now able to take advantage of Tumor Registry data and of large hospital and records office files which have needed years to accumulate.

Sex ratio

Soon after the initial description of gallbladder cancer by de Stoll, reports on the disease quickly established that women were at higher risk for this cancer than were men (9, 10). The sex ratio of the series in Table 1 (cols. 2 and 3) certainly supports this finding. Females outnumber males by 4,769 to 1,708, yielding a cumulative sex ratio of 2.8:1.

In my own experience at the New Mexico Tumor Registry (11) I have observed a sex ratio of 2.59:1 in a series of 521 cases (376 females to 145 males). Further, the ethnic origins, a variable which the New Mexico Tumor Registry is particularly well suited to assess, appear to have little influence on the sex ratio of the cases (Table 2). The sex ratio in the Anglo, or non-Hispanic Caucasian, sample is somewhat low at 1.55:1, while that in the Hispanic, persons having a Spanish surname or ancestry, sample is highest at 3.38:1, but both extremes do fall well within the expected range and should not be considered unusual.

Table 1. A chronological listing of sixty-nine published reports of gallbladder cancer encompassing 6,478 individual cases between 1889 and 1979.

	No. of cases	Sex ratio M	Sex ratio F	Mean age (years)	Prop. with stones	Median survival (months)
Musser, 1889[a] (6)	98	23	75		79.0	
Riechelmann, 1902[a]	39	11	28		66.6	
Krasting, 1906[a]	56	7	49			
Buday, 1908[a] (116)	9	1	8			
Fawcett and Rippman, 1913[a]	48	10	38		87.0	
Smithies, 1919 (137)	23	16	7	59.0	69.0	
von Berencsy and von Wolff, 1924[a]	161	28	133			
Lentze, 1926[a]	27	3	24		85.2	
Judd and Baumgartner, 1929 (24)	56	12	44		94.0	5.0
Finsterer, 1932[a]	46	9	37		93.5	
Judd and Grey, 1932 (17)	212	55	157	57.1	64.6	
Shelley and Ross, 1932 (5)	19	5	14[b]	60.7		0.75
Seide and Geller, 1933[a] (20)	35	11	24		48.5	
Illingworth, 1935 (7)	50	10	40	60.6	81.6[c]	
Cooper, 1937 (5)	48	13	35		79.0	
Rhodes and Greenblatt, 1937 (41)	24	8	16			
D'Aunoy, et al., 1938 (44)	11	8	3[b]	58.4	63.6	
Hochberg and Kogut, 1939 (122)	31	6	25		76.0[c]	
Liebowitz, 1939 (128)	28	5	23	64.1	71.4	4.47
Lam, 1940 (126)	34	11	23		90.0[c]	
Lichtenstein and Tannenbaum, 1940 (28)	75	31	44[b]		69.3	
Van Zandt, 1940 (140)	⌒	2	7	70.0	66.7	
Warren and Balch, 1940 (142)	84	21	63		80.0[c]	
Campbell, 1941 (117)	45	11	34[d]	57.7	83.0	
Gray and Sharpe, 1941 (29)	291	81	210		50.0	
Greenlee, et al., 1941 (22)	5	1	4	63.0	100.0	9.0
Kirshbaum and Kozell, 1941 (128)	55	6	25		76.0[c]	
Mattson, 1942 (132)	60	24	36	65.4	70.1	
Vadheim, et al., 1944 (39)	77	16	61		88.0	~6.0
Finney and Johnson, 1934 (119)	18	2	16	67.4		
Kelley and Speed, 1946 (21)	17	4	13	62.0	100.0[c]	
Benjamin, 1948 (30)	70	23	47		57.0	
Sainberg and Garlock, 1948 (135)	75	12	63		73.3	4.4
Arminski, 1949 (8)	25	2	23	58.7	100.0[c]	
Jones, 1950 (126)	50	14	36	61.3	82.0	
Russell and Brown, 1950 (145)	29	6	23[b]			
Ulin, et al., 1950 (140)	14	1	13	61.0	72.7[c]	
Tragerman, 1953 (94)	153	55	118[b]		79.8	
Rivkin, 1955 (9)	52	5	47	59.3	78.8	4.9
Strohl and Diffenbaugh, 1955 (40)	50	16	34	65.0		
Burdette, 1957 (31)	74	23	51[b]	67.0	55.0	1.6
Arner and von Schreeb, 1958 (115)	49	10	39	65.0	63.0	2.0
Thorbjarnarson and Glenn, 1959 (139)	90	25	65[b]		83.1[c]	
Strauch, 1960 (10)	70	16	54	67.9	90.6[c]	2.0
Gerst, 1961 (120)	132	28	104[b]	61.0	89.0[c]	~6.0
Bossart, et al., 1962 (25)	76	24	52[b]		90.0	~6.0
Chandler and Fletcher, 1963 (118)	66	30	36		79.0[c]	

Table 1. (continued).

	No. of cases	Sex ratio		Mean age (years)	Prop. with stones	Median survival (months)
		M	F			
Litwin, 1967 (26)	78	12	64		90.0[c]	
Robertson and Carlisle, 1967 (45)	52	15	37	65.0	93.9[c]	~6.0
Warren, et al., 1968 (27)	105	27	78	61.0	90.5[c]	
Andrews, et al., 1969 (99)	45	12	33	65.2	82.0	2.0
Gradisar and Kelly, 1970 (121)	41	10	31	70.0	68.3	4.0
Hardy and Volk, 1970 (122)	59	14	45[b]		84.2	
Neel, et al., 1970 (35)	14	4	10[b]	69.4	85.7	10.2
Tanga and Ewing, 1970 (138)	43	14	29	63.2	90.6[c]	2.0
Vaittinen, 1970 (141)	390	42	348[b]		83.3	2.0
Holmes and Mark, 1971 (125)	72	24	48	70.0	80.0	
Solan and Thompson, 1971 (32)	57	16	41	68.0	54.0	6.0
Klein and Finck, 1972 (95)	28	5	23[b]	68.3	89.3	~5.0
Krain, 1972 (18, 19)	1629	566	1063[d]	70.3		
Keill and DeWeese, 1973 (127)	33	3	30	67.8	75.8	2.95
Beltz and Condon, 1973 (33)	117	28	89	67.0	69.0	~6.0
Ohlsson and Aronsen, 1974 (133)	181	33	148[b]		88.4	9.3
Richard and Cantin, 1976 (134)	108	22	86[b]		83.0	2.5
Shani, et al., 1974 (136) Hart, et al., 1972 (123)	345	59	286		81.3	1.0
Treadwell and Hardin, 1976 (23)	43	12	31	64.0	95.3	
Weiskopf and Esselstyn, 1976 (144)	45	17	28	62.0	82.0	
Perpetuo, et al., 1978 (98)	75	12	63	62.0	98.0[c]	5.2
Maram, et al., 1979 (131)	32	4	28			
Total	6478	1709	4769			

[a] Data and reference from Arminski, 1949 (8).

[b] Data used to compile Fig. 1.

[c] Percentage of cases in which presence or absence of gallstones could be determined.

[d] Algebraically determined from the reported sex ratio and sample size.

Table 2. Sex ratio of 521 cases of gallbladder cancer in New Mexico by ethnic origins.

Ethnic group	Number of cases		Sex ratio
	Female	Male	
Anglo	87	56	1.55 : 1
Hispano	186	55	3.38 : 1
American Indian	101	33	3.06 : 1
Other[a]	2	1	2.00 : 1
Total	376	145	2.59 : 1

[a] 'Other' in New Mexico includes blacks and other non-whites, which comprise less than three percent of the total population.

202

Age at diagnosis

Gallbladder cancer is a 'disease of age' with the vast majority of cases diagnosed in the seventh decade of life or later (8). Naturally, there are some extremes to be found. Some half-dozen persons have been diagnosed for gallbladder cancer in the third decade of life, and I have reported on a 26 year old woman (11). A reliable case in a 13 year old Scandinavian girl and one in an 11 year old Navajo Indian girl have been reported (12, 13).

Among the 69 reports in Table 1, 36 report mean age at diagnosis (col. 4). The vast majority of these reported mean ages falls in the seventh decade as expected. The grand mean is 64.0 ± 3.93 years. The youngest mean age at diagnosis among these reports is 57.1 years (14) while the oldest is 70.3 years (15, 16).

I have obtained 17 reports from the survey in which age at diagnosis is provided by sex and decade. The cumulative age/sex distribution of the 1,506 individual cases recounted in these studies is presented in Fig. 2. While the absolute number of cases is higher in females (sex ratio 3.4:1), it can be seen that the shapes of the male and female distributions are quite similar. Further, the slightly higher mean age at diagnosis in females mentioned by several authors can also be seen in this figure.

New Mexico data show a mixed result when mean age at diagnosis is partitioned by sex and ethnicity (Table 3). The youngest mean age is 64.9 years in American Indian females while the oldest is 70.3 years in Hispanic males. The mean age of 72.0 years among females in the 'Other' category is based on two cases. Overall, the mean age at diagnosis for the New Mexico population is late in the seventh decade. None of the differences in mean age are significant regardless of sex or ethnicity.

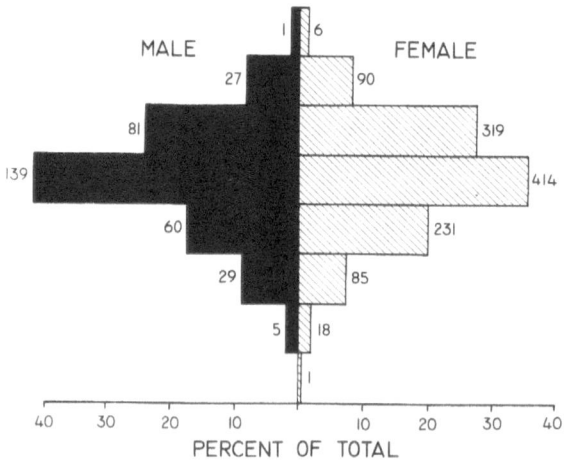

Figure 2. Age and sex distribution of 1506 cases of gallbladder cancer from the published literature. Sources used are indicated in Table 1.

Table 3. Mean age at diagnosis for 521 cases of gallbladder cancer in New Mexico by sex and ethnic origins.

Ethnic group	Mean age at diagnosis (years)		
	Female	Male	Total
Anglo	68.5	69.5	68.8
Hispano	67.6	70.3	68.2
American Indian	64.9	68.3	65.7
Other	72.0	58.0	67.3
Total	67.1	69.5	67.7

The role of gallstones

Between 1854 and 1904 Cowell collected figures regarding gallstones at the Middlesex Hospital in England. He observed that the occurrence of gallstones in patients with all types of cancers was roughly equal to the overall risk for cancers regardless of sex (17). A great deal of interest has been expressed concerning the occurrence of gallstones in gallbladder cancer. The earliest such association of cholelithiasis and gallbladder cancer is credited to Heschel in 1852 (18). Shelley and Ross (17) observed, as have countless authors since, that 'the occurrence of gallstones in carcinomatous gallbladders is unquestionable greater than that in non-carcinomatous gallbladders'. Naturally, the pivotal question has always concerned the exact nature of the association. The data which has been compiled is shown in Table 1, col. 5.

Among the reports summarized in Table 1, all but ten authors have reported on the proportionate occurrence of gallstones in the gallbladders they have examined. These reports discussed a grand total of 4,184 individual carcinomatous gallbladders of which 3,240 have been found to contain stones. This is an overall concordance of 77.4%. The lowest association is 48.5% in a series of 35 gallbladders (19). The maximum association (100%) is reported by several authors (5, 20, 21) on a series of 5, 17, and 20 gallbladders respectively. On the other hand, among those studies in which the concordance is greater than 90%, most are based on substantial numbers of cases (7, 22, 23, 24, 25, 26). However, reports in which the association is lower than 70% are equally numerous and are also based on substantial samples (27, 14, 28, 29, 30, 31, 32, 33). The lack of association in some patients may reflect the fact that cholelithiasis may be the result of diverse pathogenetic mechanisms, only some of which may be associated with carcinogenesis. It should not be expected, for instance, that cholelithiasis secondary to hemolytic anemia would lead to gallbladder cancer. In view of these results any formulation of a causal model which links gallbladder cancer and cholelithiasis should invoke a remote cause through which these two phenomena are correlated.

204

Survival

Gallbladder cancer has an extremely poor prognosis. It is this aspect which prompted Moertel (34) to characterize a gallbladder cancer as 'this dismal disease'. Dismal is certainly an apt description as evidenced by the survival figures reported (Table 1, col. 6). The range of median times of survival from diagnosis is from a low of only three weeks (17) to a 'high' of 10.2 months (35). Adson (8) reported in his review that only 3.2% of patients available to analysis survived five years or longer. Of these five year survivors, Adson points out that 92% had simple colecystectomy. A study of long term survivors by Appleman and colleagues (36) concluded that such occurrences are rare.

The unfavourable picture of survival painted by other authors is mirrored in the data from the New Mexico Tumor Registry (NMTR). A compilation of survival figures from NMTR is presented in Table 4. As can be seen, the survival of females is somewhat better than that of males with the exception of American Indian females.

Summary

The overall impression gained from this review of the clinical features of gallbladder cancer is that, regardless which sex or ethnic group has been examined, a number of basic generalizations may be made: the sex ratio will average about three to one in favor of females, the mean age of diagnosis will be somewhere in the seventh decade of life, gallstones will be present in approximately three of every four cases on the average, and the prognosis will run from extremely poor to miserable. In the two centuries over which these generalizations have been accumulated, the one area in which significant variation has appeared is with regard to ethnicity. Simply stated, whereas the clinical features of the disease do not vary from ethnic group to ethnic group, no two ethnic groups share a similar risk for the disease.

Table 4. Median survival from diagnosis for 521 cases of gallbladder cancer in New Mexico by sex and ethnic origins.

Ethnic group	Median survival (months)		
	Female	Male	Total
Anglo	4.50	2.31	3.44
Hispano	3.28	2.83	3.24
American Indian	2.20	2.96	2.49
Other	2.50	0.50	1.00
Total	3.21	2.61	3.01

Ethno-geographic variation

In the previous section nearly seven thousand cases of gallbladder cancer were presented. It is interesting to note that the vast majority of these cases, well above ninety percent, were reported from Caucasian patient populations in Europe or the United States. This compilation contributes a substantial body of knowledge about the characteristics of this cancer. However, such knowledge has been derived almost exclusively from a Caucasian perspective. In the present section what may be called the 'Caucasian base-line' will be addressed, and comparisons will be made with the world's two other major 'racial' groups, Negroid and Mongoloid.

The Caucasian base-line

The impression one gains from reading the numerous reports of gallbladder cancer among Caucasians is that it is a relatively rare cancer. According to the 'Third National Cancer Survey, (TNCS)', gallbladder cancer accounts for only 0.76% of the cancers among male cancer patients and 1.20% among female cancer patients. Even at these low figures gallbladder cancer does comprise the majority of all biliary tract malignancies (8), and ranks fifth or sixth in frequency among all gastrointestinal cancers (37, 38). Older reports of relative frequency range from 2.80% (4) to 4.50% (39). However, these figures are often based upon autopsy series and are, thus, misleading. It is best, therefore, to keep the newer TNCS estimates as base-line comparative data.

The negroid ethnic/racial group

Among the earliest references to the occurrence of gallbladder cancer in persons of African ancestry was the report by Rhodes and Greenblatt (40) who noted that four of the twenty-four cases in their survey were black. Though no incidence figures were cited, it was observed that gallbladder cancer appeared to be rarer in blacks than in whites. The authors noted that, in a 'Negro Hospital' in Savannah, Georgia, only '4 or 5 cases (of gallbladder cancer) had been operated on in the past 25 years'.

In a series of reports on the 'Pathology of Central African Natives', published during the 1940s, it was concluded that the cancer was indeed rarer among US blacks than among US whites (41). This report further showed that the incidence of gallbladder cancer among persons of African ancestry living in the West Indies was even lower than among US blacks, and that among African blacks themselves the disease was vanishingly rare. These conclusions were soon substantiated by Steiner (42) using data from the US, West Indies, Uganda, and South Africa.

Due to the rarity of the disease in the world's black population, little in the way of clinical information about gallbladder cancer is available for this group. However, even when a fair sample size has been obtained, any similarities or differences in the disease among blacks has often gone unnoted. For example, in one report from New Orleans, six of the eleven cases in the sample were black, but there was no mention that this was at all unusual (43). Indeed, there was no attempt to disaggregate blacks from whites with regard to any of the clinical features presented except to point out the racial composition of the sample. A similar situation obtained in a later report from Nashville, Tennessee, in which there were five blacks among the 52 cases reported (44).

More extensive information is available about cholelithiasis in blacks. In a report from Alabama, Cunningham (45) noted that the incidence of stones in blacks was far lower than in whites, being about one-fourth the white rate in both males and females. A similar finding was reported among blacks in the Philadelphia area (46). In the Alabama sample, the incidence of gallstones was 11.1% in white females compared to 4.8% in black females. The Philadelphia group showed a similar comparison of 21.7% among white females to 8.7% in black females. The same was true for males, being 6.9% in white males to 1.7% in black males in Philadelphia. Assuming that the general pattern of gallbladder cancer follows that of gallstones, then the average incidence of gallbladder cancer among black populations should be uniformly lower than the average incidence among white populations on a world-wide basis. Data from 'Cancer incidence in five continents', Vol. III, while having the problem of not disaggregating gallbladder per se from other biliary tract neoplasms, shows that black samples from the San Francisco Bay Area, Ibadan, Nigeria, and Bulawayo do exhibit some of the lowest rates in the world.

Insofar as disaggregated gallbladder cancer is concerned, the Philadelphia report (46) was one of the few papers in which gallbladder cancer in blacks was discussed with supporting data, and it was the only one for which data could be used for comparative purposes. The concurrence of gallstones in the cancerous gallbladders reported was only 25.0% in females (3 of 12) and 37.5% in males (3 of 8). The overall concordance of 30.0% for this black sample is far below that from any sample in the Caucasian base-line. While one should not make too much out of results from a sample of only 20 cases, it does suggest that blacks may be relatively less prone to developing gallstones than they are to developing gallbladder cancer when compared to whites.

Reports of biliary tract diseases from Africa shed more light on this problem even though the sample sizes observed are small. Trowell (47) noted the general rarity of all gallbladder disorders among sub-Saharan indigenous peoples. This assertion has repeatedly been confirmed by other authors. A retrospective study of biliary diseases in Uganda, for example, revealed only 22 cases during the seven year period from 1955 to 1961 (48). In addition, there were six cases of carcinoma of the gallbladder during the same time period. These six cases were somewhat unusual in that only one individual was female and two were under the age of 40 years. Also, in keeping with the low frequency of concomitant stones in the Philadelphia group, none of the Ugandan cases showed associated chole-lithiasis (48). Some black populations are known to be frequent carriers of some abnormal hemoglobins, such as S-hemoglobin, which may be associated with hemolisis and, therefore, predispose to lithiasis. It would appear that hemolisis-related cholelithiasis may not be etiologically related to gallbladder cancer and that the factors associated with other kinds of cholelithiasis and with gallbladder cancer are less frequent in blacks than in other races.

Whatever the reasons, some aspects of gallbladder cancer in the world's negroid 'racial' group appear to be clear. One is that black populations are a low risk group compared to white populations. However, when gallbladder cancer is found among blacks, the incidence of concomitant cholelithiasis is much lower than expected. More comparative data on these points are needed.

The Mongoloid ethnic/racial group

The Mongoloid 'racial' group presents a frustrating paradox in regard to gall-bladder cancer. This is the largest racial group in the world and, at the same time, they are the peoples about whom the least is known. For example, the 'Cancer incidence in five continents', Vol. III reports data only for Israel, Bombay, and Singapore from Asia. The Peoples Republic of China is virtually a blank as is Taiwan and the rest of southeast Asia. With the only truly solid gallbladder cancer information available from Japan, the world's largest racial group re-mains, for the most part, unaccounted for. Fortunately, some additional infor-mation is available from individual case studies, though much of it is anecdotal.

A survey of cancers among non-whites in the United States in the late 1960s showed that Japanese migrants experienced higher gallbladder cancer rates than whites (49). The survey further indicated that the disease was elevated among native Japanese women as well. This impression was later confirmed by a study of gallbladder cancer in California during the years 1955 to 1969 (15). A similar study in multi-racial Hawaii, however, failed to confirm those results, but it did show Chinese to be at high risk for the disease (50). While definitive statements about the nature of gallbladder cancer among Mongoloid peoples are not pos-sible, it may be reasonable to expect a somewhat higher incidence among Mon-goloid groups relative to the Caucasian base-line. Verification of such an asser-tion must await the accumulation of supporting data.

Part of the suspicion that Mongoloid peoples in Asia will be found to be at higher risk for gallbladder cancer is derived from the well documented and strikingly high rates of the disease among members of the only non-Asian indigenous Mongoloid group – the American Indians. Throughout much of this century there was an oft-repeated axiom that American Indians were not at high risk to cancer (51, 52). This characterization has been, for the most part, substantiated in subsequent reports (53, 54, 55). The lower incidence and low mortality among American Indians with regard to most cancers does not apply to gallbladder cancer, however. A study of cancer mortality among American Indians conclusively demonstrated that carcinoma of the gallbladder was a disease for which American Indians had significantly enhanced risks (56). Standardized Mortality Ratios (SMRs) of 296.8 for American Indian males and 377.7 for American Indian females compared to whites and of 469.3 for American Indian males and 681.1 for American Indian females compared to blacks, made it clear that carcinoma of the gallbladder was a condition to be reckoned with in this racial/ethnic group.

Subsequent compilations of gallbladder cancer data on American Indians revealed two inportant facts. The first was that the cancer was even more common in these groups than previously thought. In New Mexico, gallbladder cancer is the third most common malignancy in American Indian females, accounting for 8.5% of specific cancer diagnosis by site (57). A similar situation has been observed among the Pima Indians of Arizona (58). Such similarities in risk between two distinct American Indian groups illustrate the second important point about gallbladder cancer among these groups. A number of studies have reported consistently high rates of gallbladder cancer among American Indian groups living in a wide range of environments and practicing a wide range of cultural and dietary traditions (57, 59, 60, 61, 62).

Cultural, dietary, and environmental similarities among the American Indian groups so far studied have proved too sparse to permit a satisfactory environmental explanation for their high rates of gallbladder cancer. Populations as diverse as the Pima of southern Arizona, the Navajo of New Mexico, The Chippewa, Sioux, and Shoshone of the northern tier states and Canada, the native groups of Alaska, including Eskimo, the Aztec of Mexico and the Quechua-Aymara of South America have all been found to be high, not only for gallbladder cancer, but for cholecystitis as well (63). The overall coherence of the biliary abnormality pattern in the American Indian ethnic/racial group with the cultural/environment pattern of the same group is low on the basis of known information. On the other hand, the coherence of the biliary abnormality pattern with a biological/genetic pattern which takes as its first principle the documented fact that American Indians are biologically more similar to one another than they are to any non-Indian group, is much higher. The coherence of the biological/genetic pattern with the disease pattern is further enhanced by the fact that the root stock of all American Indians is Asian in origin (64, 65), and that indigenous Asian groups also appear to have elevated rates of these disease. It is, therefore, likely that a satisfactory explanation of gallbladder cancer will necessarily incorporate a substantial biological/genetic component, and that the cultural/environmental component will be of proportionately lesser importance. This is to say that the cultural/environmental component of gallbladder cancer will serve as a modifier of the basic pattern controlled by the biological/genetic component.

World-wide geographic patterning

The preceding discussion of racial/ethnic variation in the incidence of gallbladder cancer leads to a sense of what the world-wide patterning of the disease may look like. A hypothetical world-wide ethno-geographic pattern of gallbladder cancer, based on known ethnic/racial differences in the disease is presented in Fig. 3.

The 'Caucasian base-line' areas of the world include the United States and a large portion of Canada as well as England, Scandinavia, and most of Europe.

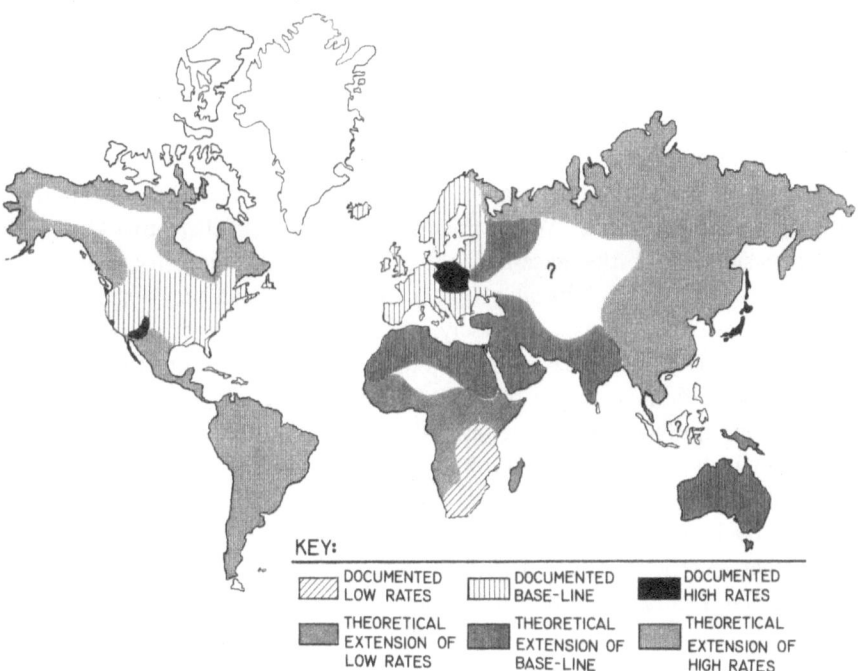

Figure 3. Theoretical world-wide distribution of gallbladder cancer rates based upon known racial/ethnic risks. See text for explanation.

Assuming all Caucasian populations to be at relatively equal risk under the model the theoretical extension of the base-line is shown to include the central and southern Soviet Union, the Indian sub-continent, all of the Middle East, and the African continent above the Sahara. One major exception to the overall Caucasian pattern is the anomalous high rate region in central Europe, which includes Poland, the German Democratic Republic, and the Federal Republic of Germany. Some rates among Hungarians are also known to be high. The known low regions of the world primarily include the West Indies and central and southern Africa. Some isolated areas of the United States are low due to the large black population of those regions. On this basis the theoretical extension of the low-rate region is limited only to sub-Saharan Africa and Madagascar. Finally, apart from the anomalous high region of central Europe, reliably documented high regions are difficult to find. Japan, of course, stands out as does the American southwest. Israel reports extremely high rates, but these must be considered extensions of the central European rates as this region is the historical home of the Ashkenazim Jews, upon whom these Israeli rates are based. Excluding the central European phenomenon, the extension of the high gallbladder cancer rates becomes a general inclusion of all Mongoloid peoples of the world. This covers the Peoples Republic of China, Korea, southeast Asia, and all American Indians and Eskimos. Mexico is included for reasons to be discussed below. Central and South America are also included as there is a growing body of data which suggests that they are in fact high rate areas and are so for the very same reasons which lead to the inclusion of Mexico (66, 67). A large region of western Asia is left blank because the historical mixing of Mongoloid and Caucasian populations is too confusing to even offer a reasonable guess.

Overall, the world-wide geographic patterning of gallbladder cancer falls quite distinctly along racial lines. Where the majority ethnic-racial group is Caucasian or Caucasian-based, the base-line obtains. Where the majority group is of African origin (i.e., sub-Saharan peoples), the average incidence is expected to be below the base-line figures. Conversely, when the predominant group is of Asian origin, the average incidence is expected to be above the base-line figures. In the United States, data provided by Mason and McKay (68) indicate that these expectations apply on a micro-geographical level as well. Regions of the United States in which the predominant non-white ethnic group is black, such as in the south and the industrial north central and northeast, gallbladder cancer rates are comparatively low. Where the predominant non-white ethnic group is Mongoloid, either American Indian or Asian, such as in the southwest and in the Los Angeles, San Francisco, and Seattle regions, rates are comparatively high.

Gallbladder cancer in hispanic-Americans

For this discussion, we will adopt Nostrand's (69, 70) definition of 'Hispanic' as those persons of mixed Spanish-Indian or Mexican descent. The geographical region in which the majority of such persons live includes southern and central California, southern Colorado, south and west Texas, and all of New Mexico and Arizona.

The distinctive ethno-geographic patterning of gallbladder cancer points to a conclusion that the disease has a strong Mongoloid focus. The lack of inter-population differences in gallbladder cancer among American Indians them-selves suggests that cultural and environmental factors are of reduced impor-tance in the overall ethno-geography of the disease (11, 63) and for the presence of a strong genetic component in gallbladder cancer and in gallbladder disease (63). This 'genetic hypothesis' has been extended to suggest that populations genetically admixed with American Indians would display rates of gallbladder cancer in proportion to the amount of such admixture (11, 71). Among groups whose history indicates American Indian admixture in significant amounts, the one with the largest membership and the one with the most complete and reliably documented history is the Hispanic-American ethnic group residing in the Ame-rican southwest.

Biosocial history of Hispanic Americans

In order to adequately assess the findings for the Hispanic ethnic group of the American southwest, one must first understand their unique biosocial history. The continued accumulation of knowledge regarding this indigenous Hispanic population suggests that the Hispanic-Americans of the southwest are a separate and distinct ethnic entity.

The unique biosocial history of the Hispano begins with the Spanish conquest of the Aztec Empire in 1529. Under Spanish rule, the combination of the King's interests and Catholic missionary zeal brought the Spaniards and the Indians into intimate contact (72). In 1607, the Viceroy of New Spain wrote that the miscegenation which had occurred as a result of the official policies designed to assimilate the Mexican Indians spiritually, culturally, and racially had produced an uncountable large population of *mestizos*, or persons of mixed Spanish and Indian ancestry (72, 73). The Spanish response to the success of their policies regarding assimilation was the establishment of a rigid class system based on racial distinctions. Within this system it was the *mestizo* who suffered most from a lack of status and privilege (73).

As Spanish colonization spread northward into the American southwest near the close of the sixteenth century, the rigid class system which was flourishing in central Mexico made life on the frontier appealing to the *mestizo*. The rigors of frontier life made class distinctions meaningless. If a *mestizo* proved to be the 'equal' of a Spaniard, the paramount yardstick of which was mere survival, he was treated equally (74). Evidence of this attitude of equality is found in the fact that the elaborate racial classifications used by the census takers in the rest of New Spain (73) never appeared on the frontier. Hence, by the middle of the seventeenth century, the inhabitants of New Spain's northern frontier were a complete amalgam of Spaniard, Indian, and *mestizo*.

The first permanent settlement of the northernmost frontier began in the area known then as *Nuevo Méjico* (New Mexico) with the founding of San Juan de los Caballeros by Oñate in 1598 (Fig. 4). The present capitol, Santa Fe, was established soon after, and the colonization of the upper Rio Grande Valley spread out from this location. As their predecessors to the south had done, the colonists of *Nuevo Méjico* proceeded to subdue and acculturate the local indigenous Indian groups. This process focused on the nearby sedentary Pueblo Indians. Unlike the acculturation of the Indians in central Mexico, the process was, after 1700, born out of mutual need more than out of missionary zeal or any thought of the King's interests. Both the Spanish colonists and the sedentary Pueblo Indians were subject to the constant harassment of marauding bands of horse-mounted, roving Indians. These nomadic Indian tribes, among whom were Navajo, Ute, Apache, and Comanche, had come to the southwest barely five centuries before the arrival of the Spanish. The Navajo, Ute, and Comanche were an impediment to colonization outside the upper Rio Grande and lower Chama River Valleys. The Apache presence was a constant threat to travel between the northern colony and the next closest *presidio* at El Paso del Norte (Fig 4). Separated from the south by the inhospitable Jornada del muerto, the colony was, in essence, an island surrounded by hostile Indians (75, 76).

The geographic and military situation in which the settlers found themselves forced an almost complete self-reliance and the formation of a defensive pact with the local Puebloan Indians. From this defensive alliance was born the group known historically as the *genízaros* (77). A military unit formed by the Spanish which was comprised of *genízaros*, the *Torzo de Genízaro* (Genizaro Column), became a mainstay of the frontier militia (78). The special status attained by the Torzo attracted many 'recruits' who were either American Indian captives and their descendants or out-and-out defectors. Many tribal groups contributed to the ranks including Ute, Navajo, Apache, Comanche, Wichita, Kiowa, Pawnee, and most of the local Puebloan tribes (76, 79).

The *genízaro*, who was genetically an Indian, became acculturated as a result of the *reducción*, the institutionalized method by which the Indian became a Christianized citizen of the Spanish Empire (77). Many later acquired high status (*vecino*) in the frontier society, and intermarriage between *genízaro* and Spanish families was commonplace. Chavez (80) writes that the *genízaros* had Spanish

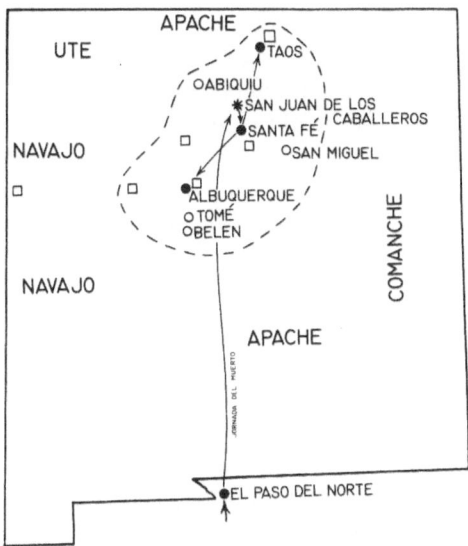

Figure 4. Map of New Mexico showing the area of original Spanish colonization. The closed circles (●) indicate the three major Spanish settlements, open circles (○) are *Genízaro* villages, and open squares (□) are the major local Pueblo Indian villages. As a point of reference, the distance from Albuquerque to El Paso del Norte is 300 miles.

names, many had Spanish blood, and all knew only the Spanish language. The unique position held by the *genízaro* on the northern frontier served to almost totally obscure any distinction between being Indian and being Spanish.

Whereas the *genízaro* was a uniquely New Mexican phenomenon, the practices of acculturation and miscegenation were ubiquitous on the northern frontier, the Hispanic-American borderland (69, 70, 81, 82). Unfortunately, while the biosocial history of the Hispanos has been carefully documented, the biological consequences of this history have been neglected. Among the few bio-medical and genetic studies which have been carried out on the Hispanic population, the results are fully coherent with historical prediction. That is, where either specific genetic traits or disease entities have been examined, the Hispanos appear to be more 'Indian-like' than do any other groups of Caucasians. These genetic traits and disease entities include: β-aminoisobutyric acid excretion (83, 84), isonicotinic acid (isoniazid) acetylation (85), diallelic red cell markers (86), HLA haplotypes (87), ischemic heart disease (88), and gallbladder disease (89). As will be seen, the same is true of gallbladder cancer.

Gallbladder cancer in Hispanics

An early observation of increased incidence of gallbladder cancer among persons of Hispanic descent was made by Steiner and co-workers in 1950 (90) who showed in a series of autopsies on California residents that Hispanic females displayed a relative frequency of primary carcinoma of the gallbladder that was three times higher than their Anglo counterparts. This observation was later confirmed by Tragerman (91) who reported on a similar California series. Combining males and females, Tragerman showed that the number of cases recorded under the age of fifty was 16 of 44 (36.7%) among Hispanics compared to 7 of 121 (5.8%) among Anglos. More recent data on the California Hispanic population have served to confirm these early impressions, particularly the significant excess incidence among Hispanic women (15, 92). The site by site distribution of cancers in the California Hispanic population shows striking similarities to the site by site distribution of cancers in American Indians described by Creagan and Fraumeni (93, 94). Reports on gallbladder cancer in the Texas Hispanic population reveal a similar pattern of increased incidence among Hispanics (95, 96). In one of these reports (95) it was noted that the Hispanic cancer experience in Texas showed marked affinities to that of the American Indian, particularly in the southwest.

Like gallbladder cancer, a number of reports note that cholecystitis occurs at high frequencies among American Indians (55, 60, 97, 98, 99, 100, 101). In a recent examination of the prevalence of cholecystitis in ambulatory patients in the Texas population, Diehl and co-workers (89) noted an excess of both cholecystitis and cholelithiasis in Hispanic women compared to Anglo and black women.

A report from the New Mexico tumor Registry (63) showed that this phenomenon applies to the New Mexico Hispanic population as well with regard to both gallbladder disease and gallbladder cancer. Age-adjusted mortality rates for gallbladder disease in New Mexico's tri-ethnic population presented in Table 5 show American Indians to have by far the highest rates while the Hispanic subpopulation lies intermediate between the rates for Indians and Anglos.

Gallbladder cancer in the New Mexico population has recently been reported in detail (11). A survey, based on the files of the New Mexico Tumor Registry and the New Mexico Department of Vital Statistics, revealed a total of 521 cases of gallbladder cancer which occurred during a span of 21 years from 1957 to 1977, inclusive. Using rates from the 'Third National Cancer Survey' the expected numbers of cases were computed and compared with observed numbers by sex

Table 5. Age-adjusted mortality rates for gallbladder disease in New Mexico by ethnic origins.

Ethnic group	Female	Male
Anglo	2.7	2.8
Hispano	7.3	4.1
American Indian	16.6	15.3

Table 6. Observed and expected gallbladder cancer cases for New Mexico from 1957 to 1977 by ethnic origins. *Source:* Devor and Buechley, 1980, reproduced by permission of the publisher.

Ethnic group	Male patients			Female patients		
	Observed	Expected[a]	Chi-square	Observed	Expected[a]	Chi-square
Anglo	56	71.52	3.38	87	125.00	11.55[b]
Hispano	55	26.75	29.83[c]	186	40.24	520.76[c]
American Indian	33	6.78	108.54[c]	101	10.88	746.30[c]
Total	144	100.28	19.06[c]	374	171.89	235.30[c]

[a] Expected results according to TNCS, age-adjusted to 1970 US population standard.
[b] $P < 0.01$.
[c] $P < 0.001$.

and ethnicity. Table 6 shows the American Indian males and females and Hispanic males and females to display significantly high excesses of the disease. The age/sex distribution of 241 recorded cases of gallbladder cancer among the New Mexico Hispanics in the survey is consonant with the conclusions offered above (see Table 2 and Table 3).

Historical genetics and gallbladder cancer in a Hispanic village

A striking feature of gallbladder cancer in New Mexico's Hispanic population is the non-uniform micro-geographic distribution of the disease. The geographic focus of gallbladder cancer among Hispanics is the region originally settled during the seventeenth century. Using age-adjusted Hispanic rates for New Mexico, a predicted county by county distribution of cases was computed and compared with the observed distribution with the result that a prime cluster was found in the lower Chama Valley in present-day Rio Arriba County (11). This is consonant with the seat of original colonization of New Mexico (Fig. 4). Historical documents further indicate that it was the southern region of Rio Arriba County or, more precisely, the lower Chama Valley, where the most pronounced intermixture of Spanish settlers and American Indians occurred (76, 81, 102).

The historical prominence of the lower Chama River region dictated that it should be studied in detail. Hence, I began a genetic and historical study of the village of Abiquiu in 1978. Abiquiu was chosen as it is the oldest settlement in the prime focus region, and there are complete and reliable records available for the area over a two-hundred year period (103). The major historical source utilized in the study of the village was the Church Marriage Book (Liber Matrimoniorum). An analysis of this source showed that the village has been genetically isolated for much of its history (104). Marital structure analysis revealed a high degree of assortative mating. Marriages were subdivided according to the birth places of the marriage partners and straight-line map distances between them were calculated. The resulting figures indicated that the median distances between the birth places of marriage partners increased from 11.5 miles during the period 1908 to 1910, to 20.0 miles during the period 1947 to 1977, revealing a strong local preference in mate choice in the village. The role of ethnicity was also considered using the family names registered in the Book. Of a total of 412 marriages recorded between 1947 and 1977, only 24 involved a person whose surname was not Hispanic, but more than half of these persons (14 of 24) had Hispanic ancestry confirmed by maternal maiden names. The ethnicity component in mate choice and its genetic effect are exemplified by the marital distances recorded for these 24 marriages. Among those persons for whom no Hispanic ancestry could be determined, the mean marital distance was 976.5 miles. For the remainder with proved Hispanic ancestry, the mean was 37.5 miles. These data suggest that outside genetic contribution to the Abiquiu gene pool has been quite small even in the most recent past.

Surname analysis further allows for the inference that there have been significant departures from random mating, in the direction of inbreeding. One may conclude on this basis that the original mixed racial origins of the Abiquiu gene pool have been retained to the present. In addition, the population structure is consonant with the struct..re of other isolated groups in which the enrichment of certain deleterious genes ha" come to be an expected consequence.

In the Abiquiu area, the disease which appears to fit the expectation of high incidence is gallbladder cancer. However, this is not due to inbreeding alone but to the simultaneous operation of two distinct genetic processes. On the one hand, the trait is present in the Abiquiu population as a result of admixture. On the other hand, the trait has persisted as a result of the genetic consequences of the groups isolation. Thus, the number of cases of gallbladder cancer found in the Abiquiu area does not necessarily indicate an increase over time but recognition of a condition that has been there all along. Further, this number of deaths is likely to be an underestimate as I have had extensive contact with the residents and have noted a decided reluctance on their part to seek medical assistance even in times of emergency. This reluctance is particularly true for the older persons in the community.

In addition to the microgeographic clustering of cases, more substantial evidence has been found in the form of two familial aggregations of gallbladder cancer in Abiquiu (71). Each was confirmed by the records of the Española Valley (Rio Arriba) Hospital, and by interviews with relatives. The two families involved, labeled Kindred 100 and Kindred 104, are shown in Fig. 5 and Fig. 6, respectively. Kindred 100 is particularly informative due to the presence of a direct Indian ancestor (confirmed by historical documentation and interview). Kindred 104 is also interesting in that the only other positively known sibling of the gallbladder cancer victims also succumbed to cancer. Given the characteristic

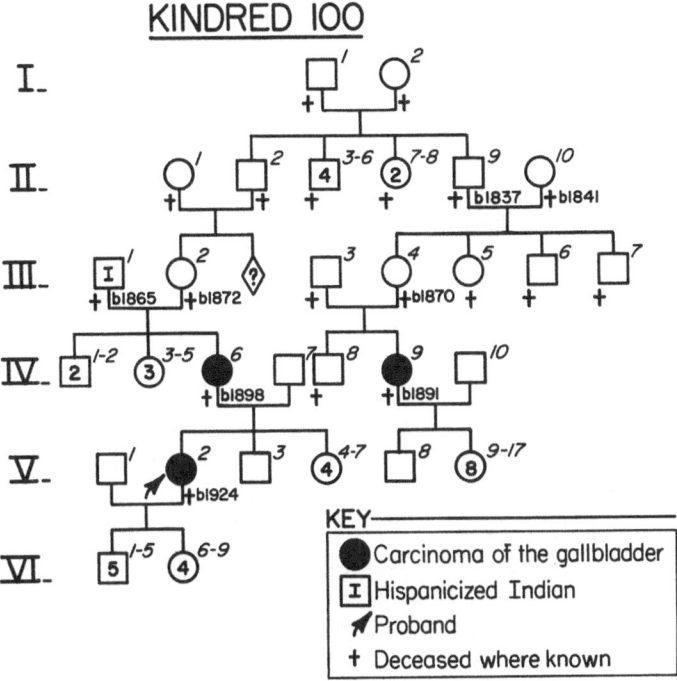

Figure 5. Pedigree of Kindred 100 from the Abiquiu area showing the mother–daughter–cousin association of gallbladder cancer. Selected, known birth dates are entered as an indication of time scale. *Source:* Devor and Buechley, 1979 (71), reproduced by permission of the publisher.

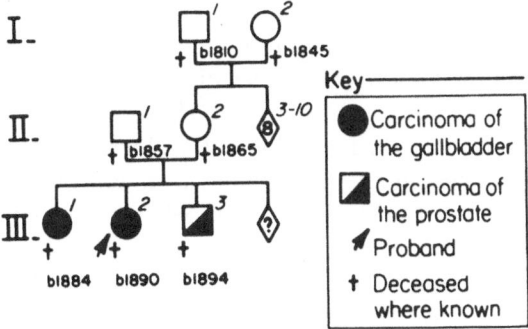

figure 6. Pedigree of Kindred 104 from the Abiquiu area showing the sister–sister association of gallbladder cancer. Selected, known birth dates are entered as an indication of time scale. *Source:* Devor and Buechley, 1979 (71), reproduced by permission of the publisher.

deficit of cancers of most types and sites among Hispanics, a familial grouping of this type is highly unusual.

Conclusions

Epidemiological observations concerning carcinoma of the gallbladder form an interesting and suggestive pattern when couched in the framework of ethno-geographic variation. First of all, the sex ratio of persons affected runs approximately three females to every male regardless of racial/ethnic group affiliation with the exception of US Chinese and Japanese. Secondly, the average age of onset of the cancer is consistently within the seventh decade of life regardless of racial/ethnic group affiliation. Further, no racial/ethnic group has yet been shown to be spared the low survival which characterizes gallbladder cancer. On the other hand, no two Ethnic groups have the same risk. Taking the Caucasian base-line set out in this paper as the benchmark, blacks are always at lower risk for the cancer, Asian peoples are apparently at higher risk as are Hispanic-Americans, and American Indians have the highest risk. This conclusion is supported by the observations made in New Mexico wherein a tri-ethnic population shows clear-cut differences in gallbladder cancer incidence without regard to residence, culture, or diet (11, 63). Therefore, it seems that the prominent host factor in gallbladder cancer is ethnicity.

With regard to environmental factors, studies of American Indians (wherein the complex of environmental milieu, cultural practices, and dietary traditions appear to have little or no influence on the distribution of gallbladder cancer incidence) lead to a conclusion that they are less important than ethnicity. The high coherence of the patterns of gallbladder disease and gallstones with those of gallbladder cancer and ethnicity adds additional power to the role of ethnicity in the incidence of both diseases.

Another highly coherent pattern has been found by the investigation of the Hispanic-American sub-population in the southwest. The genetic mixture between Anglos (who have low gallbladder disease, gallstone, and gallbladder cancer incidences) and American Indians (who have high incidences of the same conditions) has resulted in the formation of a biologically unique ethnic group whose rates for all three biliary abnormalities are intermediate between the two parental racial groups (11, 63). The fact that only this population displays this phenomenon among Latin ethnic groups in the United States and the fact that it is consistent without regard to residence further supports the primary role of ethnicity in the occurrence of gallbladder cancer as well as the other two biliary abnormalities.

A causal model for gallbladder cancer

The ethno-geographic patterning of gallbladder cancer and its high coherence with the two other biliary abnormalities renders the search for a cause for any one condition alone difficult since it appears that all three are linked together. Hence, a causal model which explains one should explain the other two to warrant serious consideration. In this section a causal model is presented which has as two of its features a mechanism for all three biliary abnormalities and an internally contained method for testing it. In addition, the model contains the quality of being predictive.

Early attempts to explain the origin of gallbladder cancer invariably invoked an etiologic role for gallstones. The range of association between the two is seen to vary from 48.5% to 100.0%. If the overall 77.4% concordance is due to the etiology of each operating through a common remote cause, both the lack of complete coherence and the variation are explainable. The basic form of the model is shown in Fig. 7. Both gallbladder cancer (Y_1) and gallstones (Y_2) are being caused by the same mechanism (X). The causal mechanism suggested is the development of lithogenic bile. Several studies have forged strong links between the size of the bile acid pool, lithogenic bile, and the development of gallstones (105, 106, 107). These reports present credible evidence that sex differences in bile-acids after puberty account for the sex-related differences in the frequency of gallstones. It is significant that similar sex-related differences apply for both gallbladder disease and gallbladder cancer. The obvious question remains as to the exact role of lithogenic bile in carcinogenesis. There is so far only anecdotal evidence to suggest that lithogenic bile may be both mutagenic and carcinogenic (108). Whatever the precise mechanism of carcinogenesis may be, it is clear that racial/ethnic variation in saturated bile, causing the development of gallstones and later nonvisualization of the gallbladder, fits well with all other racial/ethnic variations in biliary abnormalities (105).

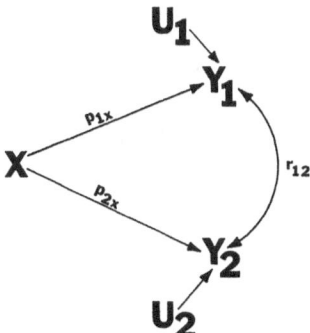

Fig. 7. Diagrammatic representation of the basic form of a model involving a common remote cause through which two dependent variables are related.

220

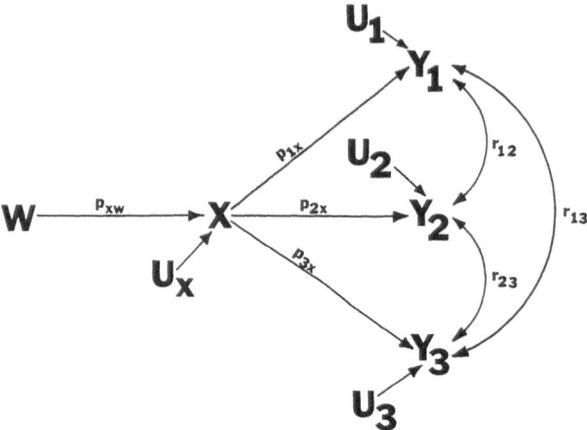

Figure 8. Diagrammatic representation of the causal model of biliary abnormalities. See text for explanation.

Taking these considerations in concert, it is possible to construct a testable causal model for all three major biliary conditions. The model, presented in Fig. 8, is simply an extension of the basic model shown in Fig. 7. It can be seen immediately from the model that the control of bile characteristics (X) is the common cause of observed variation in the occurrence of gallbladder cancer (Y_1), gallstones (Y_2) and chronic cholecystitis (Y_3). On the basis of the model, the remote cause, which is racial/ethnic, and sex-specific variation in the frequency of alleles controlling biliary response to pubertal changes (W), conditions the proximate cause (X) which in turn sets in motion a process that results in the development of biliary abnormalities. This model is appealing for a number of reasons. First of all, the universe of potential causality is parsimoniously reduced to a set of simple linear relationships. Secondly, these relationships are all confined to a small number of metrical biological variables. Hence, the model is subject to precise quantitative verification. Further, the model allows for the inclusion of environmental modification of causal pathways should they be required. Finally, the model, in its present form, will satisfactorily account for the following epidemiologic observations:

1. Sex related differences in the incidence of gallstones, gallbladder disease (cholecystitis), and gallbladder cancer are constant within all racial/ethnic groups.

Since the biliary responses to pubertal changes are primarily sex-mediated phenomena, the role of ethnicity should be limited to differences *within* sexes and not to differences *between* sexes.

2. Racial/ethnic differences in the incidence of gallstones, gallbladder disease, and gallbladder cancer are constant without regard to sex.

Sex-mediated response to pubertal changes maintains the relationship *between* sexes *within* racial/ethnic groups. Ethnic group specific differences in the frequencies of alleles responsible for sex-mediated response will, thus, be limited to differences *between* ethnic groups *within* sexes. Hence, the phenomenon that females are always at higher risk than males is accounted for regardless of the ethnic group's overall liability.

3. Ethnic sub-populations resulting from genetic admixture display intermediate incidences of gallstones, gallbladder disease, and gallbladder cancer in proportion to that admixture.
4. Racial/ethnic differences in the incidence of gallstones, gallbladder disease, and gallbladder cancer are consistent without regard to geographic location or environmental milieu.

Since pubertal changes are under canalized genetic control both within and between sexes and within and between ethnic groups, environmental interactions should be minimal.

5. Sex ratio, age of onset, clinical symptoms, histologic characteristics, and survival are consistent without regard to ethnic origin, geographic location, or environmental milieu.

As the true source of variation in biliary abnormalities lies in variation in the frequency characteristics of the remote cause, the clinical features of the diseases it produces should not be expected to vary.

Implications for future research

The nature of the causal model presented has an added advantage of immediately producing a method for testing it: examination of each causal pathway individually and, finally, collectively. Among the more obvious approaches for testing the model are: (1) population-based studies of bile characteristics, both before and after puberty in several ethnic groups. This will provide the necessary base line data and will establish the quantitative character of racial/ethnic differences; (2) case-control studies of the bile characteristics of persons diagnosed for any or all of the major biliary abnormalities. These results could then be compared to the base-line data by sex and ethnicity; (3) laboratory investigations of the potential deleterious effects of lithogenic bile.

The end result of this testing program will, hopefully, be the development of the long sought after early warning criteria for gallbladder cancer. In the long run, of course, the knowledge gained from such a systematic model evaluation may serve to better orient efforts to prevent the cancer.

222

Acknowledgments

The initial stages of the research in New Mexico were supported, in part, by Grant CA-19710 and Contract N01-CP-33344 from the National Cancer Institute. I gratefully acknowledge the New Mexico Tumor Registry, and in particular Dr Charles R. Key, M.D., for providing me with a place to conduct this research. I also thank Mr Charles Wiggins of NMTR for updating all of the clinical data reported in Tables 2, 3, and 4. Special thanks to the Laboratory of Biological Anthropology of the University of Kansas and to its Director, Dr Michael H. Crawford, for assistance in completing this project. Special thanks, too, to Dr Crawford and to Dr James H. Mielke and Dr Tibor Koertvelyessy for their valuable editorial assistance. Finally, I wish to dedicate this paper to Dr Robert W. Buechley, my friend and colleague, on the occasion of his retirement.

References

1. Workman PL: Genetic epidemiology and population structure. In: Morton NE, Chung CS (eds): Genetic Epidemiology. New York: Academic Press, 1978, pp 354–359.
2. Niswander JD, Brown KS, Iba BY, Leyshon WC, Workman PL: Population studies on southwestern Indian tribes: I. History, culture, and genetics of the Papago. Am J Hum Genet 22:7–23, 1970.
3. Workman PL, Niswander JD, Brown KS, Leyshon WC: Population studies on southwestern Indian tribes. IV. The Zuni. Am J Phys Anthrop 41:119–132, 1974.
4. Illingworth CFW: Carcinoma of the gallbladder. Brit J Surg 23:4–18, 1935.
5. Arminski TC: Primary carcinoma of the gallbladder: a collective review with the addition of twenty-five cases from the Grace Hospital, Detroit, Michigan. Cancer 2:379–398, 1949.
6. Rivkin LM: Carcinoma of the gallbladder: report of fifty-two operative cases and resume of the literature. Arch Surg 70:128–135, 1955.
7. Strauch GO: Primary carcinoma of the gallbladder: presentation of seventy cases from the Rhode Island Hospital and a cumulative review of the last ten years of the American literature. Surgery 47:368–383, 1960.
8. Adson MA: Carcinoma of the gallbladder. Surg Clin N Amer 53:1203–1215, 1973.
9. Villiard F: Étude sur le cancer primitif des voies biliares. Bul Soc Anat Paris 44, 1870 (cited in Cooper, 1937 (4)).
10. Ames D: Primary carcinoma of the gallbladder. Bull Johns Hopkins Hosp 5:74–80, 1894.
11. Devor EJ, Buechley RW: Gallbladder cancer in Hispanic New Mexicans. I. General population, 1957–1977. Cancer 45:1705–1712, 1980.
12. Beiring A: Galdeblaederecancer hos 13 aars pige. Nord Med 29:64–66, 1946.
13. Rudolf R, Cohen J: Carcinoma of the gallbladder in an 11 year old Navajo girl. J Pediatr Surg 7:66, 1972.
14. Judd ES, Grey HK: Carcinoma of the gallbladder and bile ducts. Surg Gynec Obstet 55: 308–315, 1932.
15. Krain LS: Carcinoma of the gallbladder in California: 1955–1969. J Chron Dis 25:65–71, 1972.
16. Krain LS: Gallbladder and extrahepatic duct carcinoma: analysis of 1808 cases. Geriatrics 27(11):111–117, 1972.
17. Shelley HJ, Ross LI: Primary carcinoma of the gallbladder: report of nineteen cases. Arch Surg 25:65–83, 1932.
18. Cooper WA: Carcinoma of the gallbladder. Arch Surg 35:431–448, 1937.

19. Seide J, Geller W: Beitrage zur Frage nach dem Zusammenhang von Gallensteinleiden und Krebs der Gallenblase. Arch f Verdawingskr 54:71–78, 1933.
20. Kelly FJ, Speed T: Primary carcinoma of the gallbladder. Texas State Med J 42:327–329, 1946.
21. Greenlee DP, Hamilton RC, Ferraro FP: Primary carcinoma of the gallbladder. Arch Surg 42:598–610, 1941.
22. Treadwell TA, Hardin WJ: Primary carcinoma of the gallbladder: the role of adjunctive therapy in its treatment. Am J Surg 132:703–706, 1976.
23. Judd ES, Baumgartner CJ: Malignant lesions of the gallbladder. Arch Intern Med 44:735–745, 1929.
24. Bossart PA, Patterson AH, Zintel HA: Carcinoma of the gallbladder: a report of seventy-six cases. Am J Surg 103:366–369, 1962.
25. Litwin MS: Primary carcinoma of the gallbladder: a review of 78 patients. Arch Surg 95: 236–240, 1967.
26. Warren KW, Hardy KJ, O'Rourke MGE: Primary neoplasia of the gallbladder. Surg Gynec Obstet 126:1036–1040, 1968.
27. Musser JH: Primary carcinoma of the gallbladder and bile ducts. Bost Med Surg J 121: 525–529, 1889.
28. Lichtenstein GM, Tannenbaum W: Carcinoma of the gallbladder: a study of seventy-five cases. Ann Surg 111:411–415, 1940.
29. Gray HK, Sharpe WS: Carcinoma of the gallbladder, extrahepatic bile ducts, and the major duodenal papilla. Surg Clin N Amer 21:1117–1124, 1941.
30. Benjamin EG: Carcinoma of the gallbladder: an analysis of 70 cases. Minn Med 31:537–540, 1948.
31. Burdette WJ: Carcinoma of the gallbladder. Ann Surg 145:832–844, 1957.
32. Solan MJ, Thompson BT: Carcinoma of the gallbladder: a clinical appraisal and review of 57 cases. Brit J Surg 58:593–597, 1971.
33. Beltz WR, Condon RE: Primary carcinoma of the gallbladder. Ann Surg 180:180–184, 1974.
34. Moertel CG: The Gallbladder. In: Holland JF, Frei E III (eds): Cancer Medicine. Philadelphia: Lea and Febiger, 1973, pp 1547–1551.
35. Neel HB III, Neel HB, Hammond WG: A reappraisal of primary gallbladder carcinoma. J Surg Oncol 2:131–143, 1970.
36. Appleman RM, Morlock CG, Dahlin DC, Adson M: Longterm survival in carcinoma of the gallbladder. Surg Gynec Obstet 117:459–464, 1963.
37. Fahim RB, McDonald JR, Richards JC, Ferric DO: Carcinoma of the gallbladder: a study of its modes of spread. Ann Surg 156:114–124, 1962.
38. Vadheim JL, Gray HK, Dockerty MM: Carcinoma of the gallbladder: a clinical and pathological study. Am J Surg 63:173–180, 1944.
39. Strohl EL, Diffenbaugh WG: Carcinoma of the gallbladder. Arch Surg 70:772–781, 1955.
40. Rhodes RL, Greenblatt RB: Carcinoma of the gallbladder: studies of 24 cases in Georgia. South Med J 30:315–318, 1937.
41. Davies JNP: Pathology of central African natives, Mulago Hospital post-mortem studies. 6: Cancer in Africans. East Afr Med J 25:117, 1948.
42. Steiner PE: Cancer: Race and Geography. Baltimore: Williams and Wilkins, 1954.
43. D'Aunoy R, Ogden MA, Halpert B: Primary carcinoma of the biliary system: a clinicopathological analysis of forty cases. Surgery 3:670–678, 1938.
44. Robertson WA, Carlisle BB: Primary carcinoma of the gallbladder: Review of 52 cases. Am J Surg 113:738–742, 1967.
45. Cunningham JA, Hardenberg FE: Comparative incidence of cholelithiasis in the Negro and white race. Arch Intern Med 97:68–72, 1956.
46. Lieber MM: The incidence of gallstones and their correlation with other disease. Ann Surg 135:394–405, 1952.
47. Trowell HC: Non-infective Diseases in Africa. London: Edward Arnold, 1960.
48. Shaper AG, Patel KM: Diseases of the Biliary tract in Africans in Uganda. East Afr Med J 41:251–253, 1964.
49. Haenszel W, Kurihara M: Studies of Japanese migrants; mortality from cancer. J Natl Cancer Inst 40:43–68, 1968.

50. Yamase H, McNamara JJ: Geographical differences in the incidences of gallbladder disease: influence of environment and ethnic background. Am J Surg 123:667–670, 1972.
51. Hrdlicka A: Physiological and medical observations among the Indians of southwestern United States and northern Mexico. Bureau of American Ethnology, Bulletin 34, 1908.
52. Salsbury CG: Incidence of certain diseases among the Navajos. Arizona Med 4:29–31, 1947.
53. Smith RL, Salsbury CG, Gilliam AG: Recorded and expected mortality among the Navajo, with special reference to cancer. J Natl Cancer Inst 17:77–89, 1956.
54. Palmer EP: The incidence of cancer among the Indians of the United States and Canada with specific reference to Arizona. Acat Un Int Cancer 9:373–391, 1953.
55. Kravetz RE: Etiology of biliary tract disease in southwestern American Indians. Analysis of 105 consecutive cholecystectomies. Gastroenterol 46:392–398, 1964.
56. Creagan ET, Fraumeni JF: Cancer mortality among American Indians, 1950–67. J Natl Cancer Inst 49:959–967, 1972.
57. Black WC, Key CR, Carmany TB, Herman D: Carcinoma of the gallbladder in a population of southwest American Indians. Cancer 39:1267–1279, 1977.
58. Justice, personal communication.
59. Lanier A: Survey of cancer incidence in Alaskan natives. In: Epidemiology and Cancer Registries in the Pacific Basin. National Cancer Institute Monograph, No 47, 1977, pp 87–88.
60. Nelson BD, Porvanik J, Benfield JR: Gallbladder disease in southwestern American Indians. Arch Surg 103:41–43, 1971.
61. Sampliner RE, Bennett PH, Comess LJ, Rose FA, Burch TA: Gallbladder disease in Pima Indians. N Engl J Med 283:1358–1364, 1970.
62. Thistle JL, Eckhart KL, Neusel RE, Norbrega FT, Pochline GG, Reimer M, Schoenfield LJ: Prevalence of gallbladder disease among Chippewa Indians. Mayo Clin Proc 46:603–608, 1971.
63. Morris DL, Buechley RW, Key CR, Morgan MV: Gallbladder disease and gallbladder cancer among American Indians in tricultural New Mexico. Cancer 42:2472–2477, 1978.
64. Smith, FH: The skeletal remains of the earliest American: a survey. Tenn Anth 1:116–148, 1976.
65. MSS Information Corporation (ed): Anthropological Studies Related to Health Problems of North American Indians. New York: ..SS Information Corporation, 1974.
66. Puffer RR, Griffith GW: Caracteristicas de la mortalidad urbana. Panamerican Health Organization Scientific Publication No 151. Washington, 1968.
67. Albores J, Alcantara A, Cruz H, Herrera R: The precursor lesions of invasive gallbladder carcinoma. Cancer 45:919–927, 1980.
68. Mason TJ, McKay, FW, Hoover R, Blot WJ, Fraumeni JF Jr: Atlas of Cancer Mortality Among U.S. Nonwhites: 1950–1969. Washington DC: US Government Printing Office, DHEW Publication No (NIH) 76–1204, 1976.
69. Nostrand RL: The Hispanic-American borderland: delimitation of an American culture region. Ann Assoc Am Geog 60:638–661, 1970.
70. Nostrand RL: Mexican Americans circa 1850. Ann Assoc Am Geog 65:378–390, 1975.
71. Devor EJ, Buechley RW: Gallbladder cancer in Hispanic New Mexicans. II. Familial occurrence in two northern New Mexico kindreds. Cancer Gen Cytogen 1:139–145, 1979.
72. Marshall CE: The birth of the mestigo in New Spain. Hispanic-Am Hist Rev 19:161–184, 1939.
73. Mörner M: Race Mixture in the History of Latin America. Boston: Little, Brown and Co, 1967.
74. Scholes FV: Church and State in New Mexico, 1610–1650. 1937 (cited in Jenkins and Schroeder (75)).
75. Jenkins ME, Schroeder AM: A Brief History of New Mexico. Albuquerque: University of New Mexico Press, 1974.
76. Swadesh FL: Los Primeros Pobladores: Hispanic Americans of the Ute Frontier. South Bend: University of Notre Dame Press, 1974.
77. Cordova GB: Missionization and Hispanicization of Santo Thomas Apostol de Abiquiu. Unpublished Ph.D. Dissertation, University of New Mexico.
78. Simmons M: Spanish Government in New Mexico. Albuquerque: University of New Mexico Press, 1968.
79. Gonzales NL: The Spanish-Americans of New Mexico. Albuquerque: University of New Mexico Press, 1969.

80. Chavez FA: Origin of New Mexico Families in the Spanish Colonial Period. Santa Fe, New Mexico: William Gannon, 1973.
81. Weber DJ: Foreigners in their Native Land: Historical Roots of the Mexican Americans. Albuquerque: University of New Mexico Press, 1973.
82. Bannon JF: The Spanish Borderlands Frontier, 1513–1821. New York: Holt, Rinehart and Winston, 1970.
83. Blumberg BS, Gartler SM: The urinary excretion of β-aminoisobutyric acid in Pacific populations. Hum Biol 33:355–362, 1961.
84. Lasker GW, Mast J, Tashian R: β-aminoisobutyric acid (BAIB) excretion in urine of residents of eight communities in the states of Michoacan and Oxaca, Mexico. Am J Phys Anthrop 30:133–136, 1969.
85. Harris H: The Principles of Human Biochemical Genetics. Amsterdam: North-Holland, 1961.
86. Gottlieb K, Kimberling WJ: Admixture estimates for the gene pool of Mexican-Americans in Colorado. Paper presented at the 48th Annual Meeting of the American Association of Physical Anthropologists, San Francisco, 1979.
87. Troup GM, Capper J, Devor EJ: Disparity between HLA-DRw typing and MLC responsiveness in a Hispanic isolate of northern New Mexico. Histocompatibility Testing (in press).
88. Buechley RW, Key CR, Morris DL, Morton WE, Morgan MV: Altitude and ischemic heart disease in tricultural New Mexico: an example of confounding. Am J Epidemiol 109:663–666, 1979.
89. Diehl AK, Stern MP, Ostrower VS, Friedman PC: Prevalence of clinical gallbladder disease in Mexican-American, Anglo, and Black women. South Med J 73: 438–443, 1980.
90. Steiner PE, Butt EM, Edmondson HA: Pulmonary carcinoma revealed at necropsy, with reference to increasing incidence in the Los Angeles County Hospital. J Natl Cancer Inst 2:497–510, 1950.
91. Tragerman LJ: Primary carcinoma of the gallbladder. Review of 173 cases. California Med 78:431–437, 1953.
92. Klein JB, Finck FM: Primary carcinoma of the gallbladder. Arch Surg 104:769–772, 1972.
93. Menck HR: Cancer incidence in the Mexican-Americans. In: Epidemiology and Cancer Registries in the Pacific Basin. National Cancer Institute Monograph, No 47, 1977, pp 103–105.
94. Menck HR, Henderson BE, Pike MC, Mack T, Martin SP, Soo Hoo J: Cancer incidence in the Mexican-American. J Natl Cancer Inst 55:531–536, 1975.
95. Perpetuo MDCMO, Valdivieso M, Heilbrun LK, Nelson RS, Connor T, Bodey GP: Natural History study of gallbladder cancer: a review of 36 years' experience at M.D. Anderson Hospital and Tumor Institute. Cancer 42:330–335, 1978.
96. Andrews EC, Bennett DE, Arbelger RB: Carcinoma of the gallbladder: Report of 45 cases. South Med J 62:573–578, 1969.
97. Brown JE, Christensen C: Biliary tract disease among the Navajos. JAMA 202:1050–1052, 1967.
98. Hesse FG: Incidence of cholecystitis and other diseases among Pima Indians of southern Arizona. JAMA 170:1789–1790, 1959.
99. Hesse FG: Incidence of diseases in the Navajo Indian: A necropsy study of coronary and aorticatherosclerosis, cholelthiasis, and neoplastic disease. Arch Pathol 77:553–557, 1964.
100. Lam RC: Gallbladder disease among American Indians. Lancet 74:305–309, 1954.
101. Sievers ML, Marquis JR: The southwestern American Indian's burden: Biliary disease. JAMA 182:172–174, 1962.
102. Walter PA: Race and Cultural Relations. New York: McGraw-Hill, 1952.
103. Devor EJ, Buechley RW: Population history and cancer incidence in Hispanic New Mexicans. Paper presented at the 49th Annual Meeting of the American Association of Physical Anthropologists, San Francisco, 1979.
104. Devor EJ: Marital structure and genetic isolation of a rural Hispanic population in northern New Mexico. Am J Phys Anthrop 53:257–265, 1980.
105. Bennion LJ, Knowles WC, Mott DM, Spagnola AM, Bennett PH: Development of lithogenic bile during puberty in Pima Indians. N Engl J Med 300:873–876, 1979.

106. Friedman GD, Kannel WB, Dawber TR: The epidemiology of gallbladder disease: observations in the Framingham study. J Chron Dis 19:273–292, 1966.
107. Heaton KW: The epidemiology of gallstones and suggested aetiology. Clin Gastroenterol 2:67–83, 1973.
108. Apisdorf, personal communication.

9. Epidemiology of Cancer of the Gallbladder and Extra-Hepatic Biliary Passages

THOMAS M. MACK and HERMAN R. MENCK

Introduction

It is customary to discuss cancers of the specialized tissues of the biliary tract as a unit even though each subsite has a particular function and a particular vulnerability. The following discussion pertains to adenocarcinomas of the gallbladder, right and left hepatic ducts, cystic duct, common bile duct, and ampulla of Vater.

The combined incidence of these malignancies is small, of the order of $2-3/10^5$/year in the United States during the 1970s (1). For several reasons, their importance is greater than their incidence would suggest. They tend to be aggressive tumors, and prognosis is poor if, as usual, they are not detected early (2). The most recent estimates from population-based registries suggest that fewer than 10% of patients are alive five years after diagnosis (3).

A second reason for special epidemiological interest can be given for cancer of the gallbladder, the site which accounts for approximately half of the total set of neoplasms. If it were possible to define a subset of the healthy population such that risk from subsequent cancer of the gallbladder were higher than the risk to be incurred from prophylactic cholecystectomy, surgical prevention might be warranted (4, 5, 6, 7). While physiologic considerations preclude this possibility for the other subsites, identification of those at extremely high risk, as for any disease, might still permit groups to be singled out for special diagnostic procedures in the expectation of earlier detection and longer survival.

Moreover, features of the descriptive epidemiology are sufficiently dramatic to suggest large variation in the distribution of important causes. An explanation for such patterns is the first step towards prevention.

Finally, the geographical occurrence of this group of diseases is different from that of other malignancies. In certain areas of Latin America and Asia, cancer of the biliary tract is a major gastrointestinal neoplasm and deserves an appropriate share of attention and resources.

Classification

The quality of epidemiologic interpretation depends on the meaningfulness and

Correa, P. and Haenszel, W. (eds.), Epidemiology of Cancer of the Digestive Tract.
© *1982 Martinus Nijhoff Publishers. The Hague/Boston/London. ISBN-13:978-94-009-7504-0*

consistency of the biologic classification. For gallbladder and biliary passages the classification of tumors is based on anatomic site, rather than tissue of origin. Lymphomas and sarcomas have been included along with adenocarcinomas in many tabulations, but they are fortunately too infrequent to have been responsible for serious error. In most pathologic series a small proportion of tumors is noted to exhibit squamous elements, and very occasionally a few homogeneously squamous carcinomas are distinguished from the adenocarcinomas which constitute the bulk of biliary tract malignancies (8).

With respect to grade of neoplasm, the full range of degree of differentiation has been noted, with sizeable numbers of tumors being described as both relatively differentiated and undifferentiated (8). Mucinous and papillary subcategories have been described among the more differentiated tumors (9). In few epidemiologic studies has there been serious consideration given to the subdivision of biliary tract malignancies, and in none has there been any indication that the presence of squamous, mucinous, or papillary elements, or that extremes of differentiation are related to demographic or putatively causal factors. Such subclassifications will therefore not be given further consideration.

Before leaving the subject of pathology and classification it should be said that benign papillary adenomas of the gallbladder and biliary tract do occur, but are not common (10). The most common variety are the unmistakable gallbladder masses which are composed of cells packed with cholesterol (8). One can therefore reasonably presume that the presence of benign neoplasms in biliary sites has not distorted the epidemiologic pattern of malignant neoplasms.

There is, however, major epidemiologic and therefore presumably etiologic heterogeneity within this group of anatomically diverse neoplasms. The descriptive epidemiology of gallbladder cancer is distinct from that of other biliary tract cancers in several aspects and must therefore be described separately insofar as possible. The distinctions can not always be made from published information because until recently the two sites were usually subsumed under the same anatomic rubric. In fact, prior to the 7th edition of the International Classification of Diseases in 1958, the two were counted conjointly with cancers of the liver.

A classificational problem that pertains only to gallbladder cancer is the error in estimates of biologic incidence that derives from the prevalence of past cholecystectomy. At present rates nearly 10% of Americans will have their gallbladders removed between the ages of 44 and 65 and will therefore not be at risk of disease (12). Because this practice has not been randomly distributed in populations over time, trends and patterns in incidence of gallbladder cancer must be interpreted with the phenomenon in mind. Similarly, routine pathologic examination of gallbladders removed at cholecystectomy done for indications other than cancer can be expected to distort the epidemiologic pattern to the extent that prevalent occult, slow-growing and in-situ lesions are included among the enumerated incident cases (13).

There are also special classificational problems pertaining to the other biliary sites. Although both intra-hepatic and extra-hepatic biliary duct cancers are rare and errors in classification are probably not important, the criteria for assignment to one group or the other are rarely made clear and assignment is probably based in most cases on gross pathology. Carcinomas of the ampulla are commonly misclassified as exocrine carcinomas of the pancreas, because of their anatomic position (14).

In general, although clinical distinctions have been made between cancers of the various biliary tract subsites, no epidemiologic distinctions have been proposed. For our present purposes they must be lumped together even though finer etiologic distinctions probably exist. In the one series large enough to permit quantitative evaluation of subsites, 40% of the carcinomas of the biliary ducts were thought to originate in the common bile duct (including the ampulla), about 25–30% in the hepatic ducts, a similar proportion at the confluence of the hepatic, common and cystic duct, and about 6% in the cystic duct itself (15).

Reported population-based incidence and mortality figures are derived from the count of microscopically verified diagnoses supplemented by clinical diagnoses which have not been verified. For these occult sites, the sensitivity and specificity of clinical diagnoses, which may account for more than a fifth of the total (16) must be presumed extremely low, since the more common malignancies of the pancreas and the vastly more common benign conditions of the biliary tract produce similar symptoms and may obscure the presence of the less common cancers (17, 18, 19). Because biliary malignancies are progressive and in the end usually produce obstructive jaundice, and because most such cases ultimately go to surgery, error derives mostly from those who refuse surgery or are spared it because of the obvious extent of disease. While errors of enumeration are not likely to be substantial within a population homogeneous with respect to referral patterns and the quality of medical care, it is possible that estimates of incidence from some countries represent serious underestimates, both on an absolute basis and in proportion to other cancers. Comparisons between countries and/or time periods should be interpreted with caution.

Descriptive epidemiology

Age. As with most cancers of the gastrointestinal epithelium, the strongest risk indicator for both gallbladder and other biliary cancers is age. Between age 40 and 60, there is an approximately 10-fold increase in risk within each sex group (Table 1).

Table 1. Average annual age-specific incidence rates (ASIR) for gallbladder and other biliary cancer, by age group, Los Angeles County, 1972–1979.

| | Gallbladder cancer | | | |
| | Spanish surnamed | | Other whites | |
Age group	Males ASIR (N)[b]	Females ASIR (N)	Males ASIR (N)	Females ASIR (N)
35–44	0.2 (1)	0.6 (3)	0.2 (5)	0.1 (3)
45–54	0.8 (3)	4.9 (19)	0.4 (11)	0.3 (9)
55–64	3.6 (8)	14.4 (37)	2.0 (38)	2.4 (51)
65–74	8.2 (10)	44.9 (65)	4.5 (47)	7.5 (116)
75 +	46.9 (18)	66.4 (45)	10.3 (60)	17.4 (203)
All[a]	2.7 (40)	7.2 (171)	0.9 (162)	1.4 (383)
	Other biliary cancer			
35–44	0.6 (4)	0.2 (1)	0.3 (6)	0.1 (3)
45–54	0.3 (1)	1.8 (7)	0.9 (22)	0.8 (22)
55–64	4.1 (9)	6.2 (16)	3.7 (72)	2.0 (43)
65–74	5.7 (7)	10.4 (15)	5.5 (57)	3.9 (60)
75 +	2.6 (1)	16.0 (11)	11.7 (68)	8.4 (98)
All[a]	0.9 (22)	2.0 (50)	1.2 (226)	0.8 (227)

[a] Age-adjusted to 1970 US population.
[b] (N) = Number of cases.

Race. The second dramatic component in the pattern of occurrence is that of race (Table 2). High rates of gallbladder cancer have been observed in Amerindians generally (20) and in particular among Pimas (21), Navajos (22), Pueblos (23), Alaskan natives (24), and, anecdotally, Choctaws (25). They are also high in natives of Peru (26), Bolivia (27), and Mexico (28), among other Latin American countries. Rates of other biliary tract cancers are less dramatically increased in Amerindians, but have been observed to be especially high in persons of Japanese origin, whose rates for gallbladder cancer is less dramatically increased (29, 30). Chinese, other Asians, and Polynesian groups experience rates which are unexceptional (31, 32). For both anatomic rubrics, rates in African and US blacks are even lower than rates in US whites (1, 16).

Geography. Within racial groups there are also differences by place of origin. Especially for gallbladder cancer, rates are high in white residents of central and eastern Europe (16). High rates of biliary cancer appear to prevail in Chile (33) and Costa Rica (34), with populations of predominately European origin, but not in the similarly Hispanic and European residents of Cuba (16) and Puerto Rico (35). In North America, high risk from gallbladder cancer is present in

Table 2. Average annual age-adjusted incidence rates for cancers of the gallbladder, bile ducts and ampulla Vater by registry.[a]

Ethnic group	Registry	Gallbladder		Bile ducts		Ampulla Vater	
		Male	Fe-male	Male	Fe-male	Male	Fe-male
Latin America	Recife	0.8	2.1	0.7	1.7	0.6	0.5
	Cali	1.3	3.5	1.4	1.9	0.5	0.2
	New Mexico	1.1	6.6	1.1	1.8	0.4	0.4
	Puerto Rico	0.7	2.4	0.6	0.6	0.3	0.2
Amerindian	New Mexico	5.8	12.4	0.7	1.1	0.0	0.0
European white	Germ Dem Repub	2.1	6.1	1.2	1.5	0.5	0.3
	Szabolcs	1.5	2.9	0.1	0.5	0.3	0.2
	Norway	0.3	1.0	0.5	0.5	0.2	0.2
	Katowice	1.3	3.9	0.3	0.6	0.4	0.4
	Sweden	1.9	3.7	0.2	0.4	0.1	0.1
	Birmingham	0.5	1.1	0.7	0.5	0.4	0.2
	Slovenia	0.9	3.3	0.9	0.9	0.5	0.3
	Geneva	0.7	2.4	0.8	1.0	0.2	0.0
North American white	British Columbia	1.1	2.2	0.9	0.6	0.5	0.3
	Alameda County	1.0	0.9	0.8	0.4	0.4	0.2
	New Mexico	0.6	0.8	0.7	0.1	1.1	0.2
	Connecticut	0.7	1.5	1.1	0.6	0.4	0.4
Japanese	Miyagi	1.6	2.0	3.8	2.4	0.0	0.2
	Osaka	0.9	1.2	1.4	1.1	0.1	0.1
Black	Detroit	0.2	2.1	0.8	0.5	0.2	0.4
South Asian	Bombay	0.4	0.6	0.2	0.1	0.1	0.0
Polynesian	New Zealand	1.5	2.1	1.3	0.0	0.0	0.0

[a] From Reference (16), 'Cancer in 5 continents' (rates adjusted to world population).

residents of Appalachia (36) as well as in American Indians and Hispanics. In Los Angeles, immigrant Hispanics, Jews and other Europeans seem to experience a higher risk than do US-born Hispanics, Jews and other Europeans (Table 3).

Sex. The third important and consistent indicator of risk is gender, with females experiencing a rate of gallbladder cancer as high as several times that of males in the same population. This high sex ratio is somewhat variable from race to race and population to population, and the extreme values of the ratio do not coincide with the extremes of risk. In general, the sex ratio seems to correlate with the mean parity of women in the population (Table 4). Consistent with the above, gallbladder cancer risk is higher in married than in unmarried women (Table 5).

In contrast with gallbladder cancer, cancer of the other biliary subsites occurs with approximately equal frequency in the two sexes within each racial and geographic population (Table 2).

Table 3. Proportional incidence ratios (PIR)[a] for gallbladder and other biliary cancer by birthplace, Los Angeles, 1972–1979.

Birthplace	Gallbladder		Other Biliary	
	Male PIR (N)	Female PIR (N)	Male PIR (N)	Female PIR (N)
Spanish surnamed				
North America	121 (19)	52 (37)	64 (7)	68 (15)
Central/South America	96 (16)	155 (115)	164 (12)	146 (30)
Jews				
North America	98 (10)	48 (9)	105 (15)	87 (10)
Europe	106 (8)	158 (27)	97 (12)	124 (9)
Other whites				
North America	92 (99)	87 (215)	98 (142)	97 (143)
Europe	134 (24)	153 (55)	121 (24)	130 (25)

[a] PIR = 100 for referent standard: all cases of known class.

Socio-economic class and religion. Risk for gallbladder cancer has been found to be higher in lower socio-economic persons, especially in women (Table 5). In Los Angeles it is more common in Catholics (Table 5), and it has been reported to be less common in Mormons (37) and Seventh-Day Adventists (38). These factors have not been adequately studied by eliminating the confounding effects of race and origin. Rates in Protestants and American Jews are similar (Table 5).

Clusters. Anecdotal reports of conjugal (39) and sibship (25, 40) clusters have appeared as has a description of an apparently high risk locale (40). Certain occupational groups, such as rubber workers (41), have been observed to be at high risk. That observed excess was not large, was not based on a substantial number of observations, and it has not been confirmed by others (42, 43, 44).

Table 4. Female to male (F/M) risk ratio for gallbladder and other biliary cancer in relation to average parity in four ethnic groups of Los Angeles county, 1972–1979.

Ethnic group	Gallbladder F/M	Other biliary F/M	Average parity[a]
Spanish surnamed	2.7	2.2	3.5
Black	3.2	1.0	3.2
Other white	1.6	0.7	2.6
Japanese-American	1.8	0.8	2.3

[a] Average number of children born per married woman, age 35–44, 1970 (96, 97).

Table 5. Proportional incidence ratios (PIR^a) for gallbladder and other biliary cancer by selected demographic variables, other whites, Los Angeles county, 1972–1979.

Variable	Gallbladder		Other biliary	
	Male PIR (N)	Female PIR (N)	Male PIR (N)	Female PIR (N)
Marital status				
single	99 (11)	65 (17)	128 (20)	88 (14)
ever married	103 (150)	104 (362)	99 (203)	101 (209)
Social class				
1 (high)	111 (14)	67 (17)	119 (22)	77 (13)
2	97 (38)	81 (72)	109 (61)	91 (50)
3	86 (35)	101 (106)	109 (62)	102 (63)
4	98 (54)	115 (151)	83 (63)	113 (86)
5 (low)	161 (20)	125 (36)	109 (18)	95 (15)
Religion				
Catholic	113 (33)	144 (95)	122 (51)	126 (51)
Protestant	103 (73)	91 (168)	95 (95)	92 (100)
Jewish	107 (19)	93 (41)	130 (31)	81 (21)

^{a} PIR = 100 for referent standard: all cases of known class.

Trends. The final demographic factor of interest is secular trend. Because of trends in the methods used to classify tumors, the increasing frequency of cholecystectomy, and changes in algorithms of diagnosis, nothing useful can be said about the trends in incidence of these diseases over time.

Biliary lithiasis

The single most important foundation upon which to base conjecture about the etiology of gallbladder cancer is the strong relationship between that disease and cholelithiasis. Gallstones have been found prior to or at the time of diagnosis of gallbladder cancer in the majority of affected men and especially women (45), a proportion several times that to be expected on the basis of chance. Like gallbladder cancer, gallstones themselves occur more commonly in women (46), in Amerindians (47, 48, 49), Latin Americans (50), residents of Appalachia (51), and northern Europeans (52), and in persons of advanced age (53). The idea that gallstones might play a role in the etiology of the associated cancer is biologically appealing and interest is therefore generated in those factors which are, in turn, known or suspected antecedents of cholelithiasis (54).

Among the former, in addition to age, sex and ethnicity, are obesity and relatively high caloric intake, drugs which lower blood cholesterol, drugs and conditions which decrease the reaborption of bile acids from the gut, and relative cumulative excess of endogenous end exogenous estrogens (55).

As suspected determinants of cholelithiasis, one group which must be listed includes those conditions likely to result in cholesterol supersaturation, whether by increasing cholesterol secretion, by reducing the pool of bile acids, by decreasing the secretion of phospholipids, or by altering the water and electrolytic content of bile. Over-secretion or under-secretion of one of these crucial elements might result from the inherited capacity or incapacity to produce a given liver enzyme, from a quantitative alteration in a feedback system normally regulating one of these constituents (i.e., from a defect in gallbladder or small bowel function), or from a simple anomaly of diet (calories, cholesterol, polyunsaturated fat, fiber).

A second group of suspected factors would include conditions which produce precipitation in saturated bile, or which provide the necessary nidus for stone formation. Among these factors would be all determinants of pigment stone production (see below) in addition to those conditions which might result in the presence of other nucleating agents, such as salt crystals, parasite eggs or fragments, or foreign bodies of other kinds.

Finally, the list must also include conditions which affect the ability of the gallbladder to efficiently mix and discharge stagnant bile, and to discharge microscopic stones. In addition to various pathologic conditions, such a list would include the cumulative effects of successive pregnancies and exposure to estrogens (58, 59).

Despite this large number of inherited, physiological and environmental factors that can be putatively linked indirectly to gallbladder cancer through a common relationship with cholelithiasis, direct links have not been conclusively demonstrated.

Biliary lithiasis is also of interest in relation to cancer of the extra-hepatic bile ducts, and not only because of simple analogy (60). While the link between the presence of stones and the appearance of cancer in individuals in this case has not yet been conclusively shown, the patterns of the two conditions in the population are more similar to each other than either resembles the pattern of gallbladder stones or that of gallbladder cancer. Stones in the ducts tend to the composed of more pigment, mostly bilirubin, than of cholesterol, and among patients with such stones the sex ratio is closer to unity, as it is for cancer of the biliary passages (53). Moreover, pigment stones have been observed to be relatively common among ethnic Japanese, a group historically at higher risk from extra-hepatic biliary cancer (61).

The genesis of pigment stones must be considered in the context of different physiologic dynamics than of those operating in the gallbladder. Unconjugated bilirubin is relatively insoluble in bile and is present in increased concentration in the bile of patients with pigmented stones (62). While the bilirubin itself could be secreted in excess by the liver in certain individuals, there is less interaction with other secreted bile components. Pigmented stones do occur more commonly in the presence of hemolytic anemia, which greatly increases blood levels (63, 64). However, bile from patients with pigmented stones appears to hydrolyse conjugated bilirubin and thereby to produce unconjugated bilirubin in the bile, presumably because biliary levels of beta-glucuronidase are increased (62). The predominate source of the excess enzyme in such individuals is not known; while it could in theory be produced by resident bacteria, it has been observed often in the presence of sterile bile.

One presumes that no matter what the composition of the stones formed, the factors leading to their initial nucleation and those which have inhibited the efficient clearance of stagnant bile and incipient stone nuclei are also important. It is notable that in Asia, pigmented stones have commonly been found in the past to contain fragments of Ascaris roundworms (65), and Clonorchis sinensis infestation in Hong Kong is thought to be more commonly present in patients with intra-hepatic cholangiocarcinomas than chance would predict (66, 67). In one follow-up study of chronic typhoid carriers, who can be presumed to have had biliary infection, an apparent excess of both gallbladder and biliary tract cancers was observed to occur, although the numbers were very small (68, 69).

Other coexisting conditions

Carcinoma of the biliary passages has been observed to occur in patients with congenital anomalies of the biliary tract (70), and familial polyposis coli (71). It appears to occur in excess with ulcerative colitis (72); in particular in the presence of a related and often coincident condition of unknown etiology, sclerosing cholangitis (73). In this condition the biliary lumen is encroached by fibrotic thickening, although the relationship between antecedent disease and subsequent biliary cancer appears to be independent of lithiasis (74).

Pigmented stones are also found in excess in patients with alcoholic cirrhosis (75, 76) although the mechanism for the excess is not known and there are no reports of an excess of biliary carcinoma.

Animal studies

Biliary anatomy and physiology and the composition of bile varies greatly from species to species, and no single species appears to offer a convenient model for human disease; indeed that most generally useful model, the rat, has no gallbladder at all (77). Biliary cancers are not common in clinical veterinary practice, although one unexplained cluster of biliary carcinomas in bears successively residing in a single grotto at the San Diego Zoo has been reported (78). Neither has a satisfactory animal model for biliary cancer been accepted. Biliary malignancies were produced in a large number in the majority of dogs fed a toxic dose of a mixture of organic sulfites (79). This experiment has never been repeated, and others have not been successful in producing consistent biliary cancers in dogs using other means (80). In guinea pigs, metastatic carcinomas have been produced by the insertion of inert glass bodies into the lumen (81), although similar results have been obtained by others (82), and even more drastic physical action has failed to produce tumors in mice (83).

Placement of methylcholanthrene in the gallbladder has produced cancers in hamsters (84) and in cats but not dogs (85), although direct placement of at least two *azo* compounds has produced biliary cancers, along with tumors at other sites, in dogs (86).

One animal model demonstrates a synergistic effect that may be especially pertinent to the disease in man. Several different nitrosamines, when fed to hamsters, not only produced liver cancers but also resulted in anatomically widespread dysplastic foci in the bile duct epithelium (87). No frank cancers of the biliary tree were produced, however, until cholesterol pellets, made to stimulate cholesterol stones, were also placed in the lumen of the biliary system; then the majority of animals developed adenocarcinomas of the gallbladder or bile duct.

Hypothesis generation

To be plausible, hypotheses offered in explanation of the existence of cancers of the biliary tract must provide for a selective effect upon the distribution of lesions to the target cell, and within the biliary tree, and the means of access to the organ, if environmental agents are invoked. Chronological relationships must be consistent with known facts. Because of the descriptive pattern of disease, such a hypothesis must also provide an explanation for the ethnic predominance of disease, in particular with respect to Amerindians and Japanese, for the female excess, and for the strong association with gallstones. Beyond these few facts, so little information is available that few additional constraints need be imposed.

The most basic hypotheses are those which invoke the traditionally alternative influences of heredity and environment. In the case of biliary cancer, as in most cases, there are strong indications that both factors play an etiologic role. The high risk of both biliary stones and cancer in culturally diverse groups with Amerindian heritage, and the biologic plausibility of a role for a heritable enzyme in bile lithogenicity argue strongly for a hereditary component to etiology.

The differences in risk within the members of a single racial or ethnic group which are associated with birthplace, social class, and marital status, and the paucity of reported familial clusters and disease-concordant twins argue for a major environmental role. Chronologic trends, or the absence thereof, are not interpretable and cannot contribute to the discussion.

The apparent effects of long antecedent events, such as migration and marriage/parity, need not actually represent long distant etiologic events but may represent fundamental and long-lasting choices in lifestyle which have made recent environmental exposures inevitable. Otherwise, there is no evidence bearing on the length of the interval between any environmental event and the biologic onset of biliary cancer.

The fact of carcinogenic transformation of the lining of the biliary tract seems to imply that constituents in bile are responsible, at least in part, for that transformation. Before following that path, it must be said that even the association with gallstones could occur on the basis of common blood-borne determinants, or even because of some altered physiologic circumstance which appeared quite independently of bile production and excretion. Moreover, whatever the pertinent bile constituents, both physiologic and epidemiologic evidence suggests that they are not identical for gallbladder cancer on the one hand, and cancer of the biliary passages on the other. In fact, to the extent that factors which determine stone formation are initially responsible for the appearance of cancer, it must be presumed that the physical determinants which affect the availability of stone nuclei or the retention of stagnant bile or microscopic stones are qualitatively and/or quantitatively different for each of the biliary passages.

The evidence that determinants of bile lithogenicity are also causes of cancer is strong; especially for the gallbladder, because of the parallel trends in the epidemiology of tumors and stones, and because of the wealth of information linking the two phenomena in individuals. The major environmental components in the etiology of both conditions, or at least those which now comprise the frontier of knowledge, begin with diet, because of the many indications from epidemiology, physiology and biochemistry. The second component is estrogenic activity, indicated by animal work, epidemiology, and, to a lesser extent, biochemistry. It is tempting but premature to tie these two major factors together into an integrated hypothesis which also accounts for the possible role of heredity. Although the most probable interaction between the nutritional and endocrine factors is at the biochemical level, in the genesis of stones, there are other possibilities. Pregnancy affects the quantity and quality of the diet, results in a profound alteration in lipid metabolism (88) and affects the efficiency of gallbladder function. It also alters the clinical course of gastrointestinal infections (89), increases the prevalence of measurable infection with certain organisms (90) and may affect the composition of the population of functional lymphocytes (91). The long-term effects of any or all of these relationships might cumulate in impoverished women who spend a large proportion of their youth pregnant.

Diet must also be presumed an important determinant of stones of the biliary

238

passages, again on both epidemiological and biochemical grounds, although the particular nutritional factors are likely to be different, and both inherited enzyme availability and physiological considerations are sure to be additional determinants of bilirubin availability. Although some drugs and conditions may affect pertinent gastrointestinal physiology, there is no reason to postulate a role for endocrine factors, nor any need to presume that gallbladder function is pertinent at all.

It will be difficult to speculate about the role played by non-lithogenic environmental influences until there is greater understanding of the role of stones and the factors which determine them. It is intuitively appealing to presume that, as in the hamster model, stones act to increase the access of environmental carcinogens to otherwise protected sites. Although many carcinogens are known or presumed to be excreted in bile, such as the products of incomplete combustion from smoking, conjugation of large molecular weight carcinogens into polarized, bile soluble conjugates greatly reduces carcinogenicity (92). The presence of local glucuronidases, however, might partially restore such activity. Such compounds could present to the liver after ingestion as food contaminants, after occupational or non-occupational exposure to environmental carcinogens, or as a result of smoking or drinking. Because of the rarity of biliary cancers, there is little empiric evidence from available cohort studies to implicate such specific environmental factors (93).

A role for radiation as a cause of biliary cancer has not been detected. External radiation from the Hiroshima atomic bomb exposure has not thus far produced an increase in risk from cancers of the biliary tract (94). Patients having received thorium-232 dioxide are subject to an increased risk from liver cancer, including cholangiocarcinoma, but no extra-hepatic biliary cancer excess has been noted (95).

There having been no studies of individuals in which postulated factors such as those listed above could have been distinguished from each other, no more can be said about the etiology of biliary cancer, and the conduct of case-control studies in populations at various degrees of risk should be pursued.

Acknowledgment

This work was supported by Grants Nos. CA19171 and CA14089, awarded by the National Cancer Institute, DHEW.

References

1. Cutler S, Young J: Third National Cancer Survey: Incidence data. Natl Cancer Inst Monogr 41, 1975.
2. Gerst P: Primary carcinoma of the gallbladder. Ann Surg 153:369–372, 1961.
3. Axtell L, Asire A, Myers M: Cancer Patient Survival, Rpt No 5. Wash DC: US Govt Print Off, DHEW Pub No (NIH) 77–992, 1977.
4. Graham E: The prevention of carcinoma of the gallbladder. Ann Surg 93:317–322, 1931.
5. Lund J: Surgical inductions in cholelithiasis. Ann Surg 151:153–162, 1960.
6. Colcock B, Perey B: The treatment of cholelithiasis. Surg, Gynec & Obstet 117:529–534, 1963.
7. McLaughlin C: Carcinoma of the gallbladder, an added hazard in untreated calculous cholecystitis in older patients. Surgery 56:757–759, 1964.
8. Edmundson H: Tumors of the gallbladder and extrahepatic ducts. Atlas of Tumor Pathology Section VII, Fascicle 26, Armed Forces Inst of Pathology, 1964.
9. Strauch G: Primary carcinoma of the gallbladder. Surgery 47:368–383, 1960.
10. McGregor J, Cordiner J: Papilloma of the gallbladder. Brit J Surg 61:356–358, 1974.
11. Burhaus R, Myers R: Benign neoplasms of the extrahepatic biliary ducts. Amer Surgeon 37:161, 1971.
12. Ranofsky A: Surgical operations in short-day hospitals. DHEW NCHS Series 13, No 34, 1978.
13. Appleman R, Morlock C, Dahlin D, Adson M: Long term survival in carcinoma of the gallbladder. Surg, Gynec & Obstet 117:459–464, 1963.
14. Cubilla A, Fitzgerald P: Surgical pathology aspects of the ampulla-head-of-pancreas region. In: Fitzgerald PJ, Morrison AB (eds): The Pancreas, Baltimore: Williams and Wilkins, 1980, pp 67–81.
15. Sako K, Switzinger G, Garsede E: Carcinoma of the extrahepatic bile ducts. Surgery 41:416–437, 1957.
16. Waterhouse J, Muir C, Correa P, Powell J: Cancer incidence in five continents, Vol III. IARC Sci Pub No 15. Lyon: IARC, 1976.
17. Tragerman L: Primary carcinoma of the gallbladder. Review of 173 cases. Calif Med 78:431–437, 1953.
18. Donhauser J: Primary carcinoma of the gallbladder. Arch Surg 77:918–924, 1958.
19. Bauer F, Robbins S: An antopsy study of cancer patients. JAMA 221:1471–1474, 1972.
20. Creagan E, Fraumeni J: Cancer mortality among American Indians, 1950–1967, J Natl Cancer Inst 49:959–967, 1972.
21. Hesse F: Incidence of cholecystitis and other disease among Pima Indians of southern Arizona. JAMA 170:1789–1790, 1959.
22. Smith R, Salsbury C, Gilliam A: Recorded and expected mortality among the Navajos, with special reference to cancer. J Natl Cancer Inst 17:77–89, 1956.
23. Morris D, Buechley R, Key C, Morgan M: Gallbladder disease and gallbladder cancer among American Indians in tricultural New Mexico. Cancer 42:2472–2477, 1978.
24. Lanier A, Bender T, Blot W, Fraumeni J, Hurlburt W: Cancer incidence in Alaska natives. Int J Cancer 18:409–412, 1976.
25. Sperling M: Familial biliary tract carcinoma. JAMA 190:944–945, 1964.
26. Olivares L: Presentation at Third Symposium on Epidemiology and Cancer Registries, Maui, Hawaii, January, 1981.
27. Rios-Dalenz J, Correa P, Haenszel W: Morbidity from cancer in La Paz, Bolivia. Int J Cancer 28:000–000, 1981.
28. Menck H, Henderson B, Pike M, Mack T, Preston-Martin S, SooHoo J: Cancer incidence in the Mexican-American. J Natl Cancer Inst 55:531–536, 1975.
29. Haenszel W, Kurihara M: Studies of Japanese migrants I. Mortality from cancer and other diseases among Japanese in the United States. J Natl Cancer Inst 40:43–68, 1968.
30. Tominaga S, Kuroishi T, Ogawa H, Shimizu H: Epidemiologic aspects of biliary tract cancer in Japan. Natl Cancer Inst Monogr 53:25–34, 1979.
31. Fraumeni J, Mason T: Cancer mortality among Chinese Americans, 1950–69. J Natl Cancer Inst 52:659–665, 1974.

32. Menck H, Henderson B: Cancer incidence rates in the Pacific Basin. Natl Cancer Inst Monogr 53:119–124, 1979.

33. Armijo R: The epidemiology of cancer in Chile. Natl Cancer Inst Monogr 53:115–118, 1979.

34. De Madrigal L: Epidemiological Study of Cancer by Site in Costa Rica, Mortality and Hospital Discharges 1956–1969. Thesis presented to the University of Oklahoma Health Sciences Center, Oklahoma City, 1972.

35. Young J, Asire A, Pollack E: SEER Program: Cancer Incidence and Mortality in the United States, 1973–1976. Wash DC: US Govt Print Off, DHEW Pub No (NIH) 78–1837, 1978.

36. Mason T, McKay F: US Cancer Mortality by County: 1950–1969. Wash DC: US Govt Print Off, DHEW Pub No (NIH) 74–615, 1974.

37. Lyon J, Gardner J, West D: Cancer risk and life-style: Cancer among Mormons from 1967 to 1975. In: Cairns J, et al. (eds): Banbury Report 4. Cancer Incidence in Defined Populations, pp 3–30. Cold Spring Harbor, NY: Cold Spring Harbor Laboratory, 1980.

38. Phillips R, Garfinkel L, Kuzma J, Beeson L, Lotz T, Brin B: Mortality among Seventh-Day Adventists for selected cancer sites. J Natl Cancer Inst 65:1097–1107, 1981.

39. McCarthy C, Espiner H: Carcinoma of bile ducts in husband and wife. Gut 10:94–97, 1969.

40. Devor E, Buechley R: Gallbladder cancer in Hispanic New Mexicans, I. General population, 1957–1977. Cancer 45:1705–1712, 1980.

41. Mancuso T, Brennan M: Epidemiological considerations of cancer of the gallbladder, bile ducts and salivary glands in the rubber industry. Occup Med 12:333–341, 1970.

42. McMichael A, Spirtas R, Kupper L: An epidemiologic study of mortality within a cohort of rubber workers, 1964–72. Occup Med 16:458–464, 1974.

43. Williams R, Stegens N, Goldsmith J: Associations of cancer site and type with occupation and industry from the Third National Cancer Survey Interview. J Natl Cancer Inst 59:1147–1185, 1977.

44. Monson R, Fine L: Cancer mortality and morbidity among rubber workers. J Natl Cancer Inst 61:1047–1053, 1978.

45. Maram E, Ludwig J, Kurland L, Brian D: Carcinoma of the gallbladder and extrahepatic biliary ducts in Rochester, Minnesota, 1935–1971. Am J Epidem 109:152–157, 1979.

46. Friedman G, Kannel W, Rawber T: Th epidemiology of gallbladder disease: Observations in the Framingham study. J Chron Dis 19:273–292, 1966.

47. Comess L, Bennett P, Burch T: Clinical gallbladder disease in Pima Indians: Its high prevalence in contrast to Framingham, Massachusetts. New Engl J Med 277:894–898, 1967.

48. Brown J, Christensen C: Biliary tract disease among the Navajos. JAMA 202:1050–1052, 1967.

49. Thistle J, Echart K, Nensel R, Nobrega F, Poehling G, Reimer M, Schoenfield L: Prevalence of gallbladder disease among Chippewa Indians. Mayo Clin Proc 46:603–608, 1971.

50. Marinovic I, Guerra C, Larach G: Incidencia de litiasis biliar en material de autopsias y analisis de composición de los cálculos. Rev Med Chil 100:1320–1327, 1972.

51. Richardson J, Scutchfield F, Proudfoot W, Benenson A: Epidemiology of gallbladder disease in an Appalachian community. Health Serv Repts 88:241–246, 1973.

52. Heaton K: The epidemiology of gallstones and suggested aetiology. Clin Gastroenterol 2:67–83, 1973.

53. Trotman B, Soloway R: Pigment vs cholesterol cholelithiasis: Clinical and epidemiological aspects. Am J Dig Dis 20:735–740, 1975.

54. Bennion L, Grundy S: Risk factors for the development of cholelithiasis in man. New Engl J Med 299:1161–1167, 1221–1227, 1978.

55. Lynn J, Williams L, O'Brien J, Wittenberg J, Egdahl R: Effects of estrogen upon bile: Implications with respect to gallstone formation. Ann Surg 178:514–524, 1973.

56. Boston Collaborative Drug Surveillance Program: Surgically confirmed gallbladder disease, venous thromboembolism, and breast tumors in relation to postmenopausal estrogen therapy. New Engl J Med 290:15–19, 1974.

57. Bennion L, Ginsberg R, Garnick M, Bennett P: Effects of oral contraceptives on the gallbladder bile of normal women. New Engl J Med 294:189–192, 1976.

58. Wilcox L, Englert E Jr: Sex, biliary stasis and gallstones in American Indians and Caucasians. Clin Res 20:223, 1972.

59. Braverman D, Johnson M, Kern F: Effects of pregnancy and contraceptive steroids on gallbladder function. New Engl J Med 302:362–364, 1980.
60. Soloway R, Trotman B, Ostrow J: Pigment gallstones. Gastroenterol 72:167–182, 1977.
61. Miyake H, Johnston C: Gallstones: Ethnological studies. Digestion 1:219–228, 1968.
62. Boonyapisit S, Trotman B, Ostrow J; Unconjugated bilirubin, and the hydrolysis of conjugated bilirubin, in gallbladder bile of patients with cholelithiasis. Gastroenterol 74:70–74, 1978.
63. Cameron J, Maddrey W, Zuidema G: Biliary tract disease in sickle cell anemia: Surgical considerations. Ann Surg 174:702–710, 1971.
64. Merendino K, Manhas D: Man-made gallstones, a new entity following cardiac valve replacement. Ann Surg 177:694–704, 1973.
65. Maki T: Cholelithiasis in the Japanese. Arch Surg 82:599–612, 1961.
66. Belamaric J: Intrahepatic bile duct carcinoma and C sinensis infection in Hong Kong. Cancer 31:468–473, 1973.
67. Baker M, Baker B, Woo R: Biliary clonorchiasis. Arch Surg 114:748, 1979.
68. Welton J, Marr J, Friedman S: Association between hepatobiliary cancer and typhoid carrier state. Lancet i:791–794, 1979.
70. Richards S: Congenital absence of the gallbladder and cystic duct associated with primary carcinoma of the common bile duct. Can Med Assoc J 94:859–860, 1966.
71. Mir-Madjlessi S, Farmer R, Hawk W, Turnbull R: Adenocarcinoma of the ampulla vater associated with familial polyposis coli: Report of a case. Dis Colon & Rectum 16:542–546, 1973.
72. Ritchie J, Allan R, MacCartney J, Thompson H, Hawley P, Cooke W: Biliary tract carcinoma associated with ulcerative colitis. Quart J Med 43:263–279, 1974.
73. Smith M, Loe R: Sclerosing cholangitis. Am J Surg 110:239–246, 1965.
74. Akwari O, Van Heerden J, Foulk W, Boogenstoss A: Cancer of the bile ducts associated with ulcerative colitis. Ann Surg 181:303–309, 1975.
75. Bouchier I: Postmortem study of the frequency of gallstones in patients with cirrhosis of the liver. Gut 10:705–710, 1975.
76. Nicholas P, Rinaudo P, Conn H: Increased incidence of cholelithiasis in Laennec's cirrhosis: A post-mortem evaluation of pathogenesis. Gastroenterol 63:112–121, 1972.
77. Nakayama F: Composition of gallstone and bile: Species difference. J Lab Clin Med 73:623–630, 1969.
78. Dorn C: Biliary and hepatic carcinomata in bears of the San Diego Zoological Gardens. Nature XXX:513–514, 1964.
79. Sternberg S, Popper H, Oser B, Oser M: Gallbladder and bile duct adenocarcinomas in dogs after long term feeding of aramite. Cancer 13:780–789, 1960.
80. Fortner J, Leffal L: Carcinoma of the gallbladder in dogs. Cancer 14:1127–1130, 1961.
81. Petrov N, Krotkina N: Experimental carcinoma of the gallbladder. Ann Surg 125:241, 1947.
82. Desforges G, Desforges S, Robbins S: Carcinoma of the gallbladder: An attempt at experimental production. Cancer 3:1088–1096, 1950.
83. Zeppa R, Womack N: Carcinoma of the gallbladder: Attempt of experimental induction. South Med J 50:1267–1271, 1957.
84. Bain G, Allen P, Silberman O, Kowalewski K: Induction in hamsters of biliary carcinoma by intracholecystic methylcholanthrene pellets. Cancer Res 19:93–96, 1959.
85. Fortner J: Experimental induction of primary carcinomas of the gallbladder. Cancer 8:698, 1955.
86. Nelson A, Woodard G: Tumors of the urinary bladder, gallbladder, and liver in dogs fed 0-aminoazotoluene or P-dimithylaminoazobenzine. J Natl Cancer Inst 13:1497–1501, 1953.
87. Kowalewski K, Todd E: Carcinoma of the gallbladder induced in hamsters by insertion of cholesterol pellets and feeding dimethylnitrosamine. Proc Soc Exp Biol Med 136:482–486, 1971.
88. Turtle J: Carbohydrate and lipid metabolism during pregnancy. In: Shearman R (ed), Human Reproductive Physiology. Oxford: Blackwell, 1972.
89. Plotz E: Virus disease in pregnancy. NY State Med 65:1239–1251, 1965.
90. Stagno S, Reynolds D, Tsiantos A: Comparative serial neurological and serological studies of symptomatic and subclinical congenitally acquired cytomegalovirus infection. J Infect Dis 132:568–577, 1975.

242

91. Ong K, Grieco M, Goel Z: Increased subpopulations of thymus - derived lymphocytes bearing Fc receptors for IgG in pregnancy. J Allergy Clin Immunol 61:143, 1978.
92. Reddy B, Weisburger J, Wynder E: Colon cancer. Bile salts as tumor promoters. In: Slaga TJ, et al. (eds): Carcinogenesis, Vol 2. Mechanisms of Tumor Promotion and Carcinogenesis, New York: Raven Press, 1978, pp 453–464.
93. Surgeon General: Smoking and Health. Wash DC: US Govt Print Off, 1979.
94. Robertson J, Kato H, Schreiber W: Carcinoma of the gallbladder, bile ducts, and Vater's ampulla, Hiroshima and Nagasaki. ABCC Technical Report: 7–70, 1970.
95. Committee on the Biological Effects of Ionizing Radiation, NAS-NRC: The Effects on Populations of Exposures to Low Levels of Ionizing Radiation. Wash DC: National Academy Press, 1980.
96. US Bureau of the Census: Census of Population: 1970 General Social and Economic Characteristics, Final Report PC (1)-C6 California. Washington DC: US Govt Printing Off, 1972.
97. US Bureau of the Census: Census of Population: 1970 Subject Reports, Final Report PC (2)-16, Japanese, Chinese, and Filipinos in the United States. Washington DC: US Govt Printing Office, 1973.

10. Epidemiology of Cancer of the Pancreas

ELIZABETH T.H. FONTHAM

Introduction

Pancreatic cancer which ranks second in the United States as a cause of death attributed to neoplasms of the gastrointestinal tract (1) is easily ranked first in terms of challenge presented to the clinician and epidemiologist alike. Just as early diagnosis and improved prognosis for patients have eluded the clinician, so substantive etiologic associations have eluded the epidemiologist investigating cancer of the pancreas. Several excellent review articles on carcinoma of the pancreas have been published, including Fraumeni's comprehensive review in 1975 (2, 3, 11, 18).

There has been a steady increase in death rates for pancreatic carcinoma over the past four to five decades in the United States, and this increase has been paralleled in recent years in other western industrialized countries (3). Mortality rates reflect incidence rates so closely that they are essentially the same. Patients with pancreatic carcinoma have one of the poorest prognoses among all cancer cases with the number of deaths equal to 95 percent of the number of new cases (1). The five-year survival rate is only 1–2% (4). Occupational exposures, diet, tobacco usage, alcohol, predisposing medical conditions, genetic factors, and other variables have been examined as potential etiologically-associated factors. While some associations have been found between various factors and carcinoma of the pancreas, the etiology is at best poorly understood.

The reasons why this disease etiology has remained so elusive are complex. Difficulties associated with diagnostic accuracy have certainly contributed to the problem. Gudjonsson et al. (5) investigated the reliability of diagnosis of pancreatic cancer and found a 40 to 62.5% error in the histologic confirmation of diagnosis of pancreatic carcinoma. Engel et al. (6) compared original death certification with autopsy findings and pertinent clinical data among 257 autopsied cases in a general hospital in Atlanta, Georgia, in 1970. While all malignant neoplasms were found to be under-reported, pancreatic carcinoma was accurately recorded only 25% of the time. Only one of four cases was noted on the death certificate. Errors in classification of primary site. or histologic type were also noted in greater than 25% of the cancer cases, and the more inaccesible the tumor the greater the likelihood of discrepancies and inaccuracies. When statis-

Correa, P. and Haenszel, W. (eds.), Epidemiology of Cancer of the Digestive Tract.
© *1982 Martinus Nijhoff Publishers. The Hague/Boston/London. ISBN-13:978-94-009-7504-0*

tics are found to have this margin of error in a developed country, international comparisons between and among developed and developing nations may obscure true geographic differences or exaggerate differences between countries which are only minimal. Diagnostic uncertainties affect time trends as well as intercountry comparisons.

Pancreatic cancer falls into two broad types, endocrine and exocrine; however, endocrine tumors account for only a small fraction of all cases. Over 90% of all malignant exocrine tumors of the pancreas are adenocarcinoma (7); therefore, what is known about the epidemiology of pancreatic carcinoma is based primarily on a relatively histologically homogeneous entity when cases are diagnosed accurately. Although most tumors are adenocarcinomas, there are several morphological subtypes as described by Cubilla and Fitzgerald (8). At this time it is not known whether they have any epidemiologic meaning.

International comparisons

There is a ten-fold difference in both incidence and mortality rates when comparisons are made between the countries at highest risk for pancreatic carcinoma and the countries at lowest risk (3, 9, 10).

The highest incidence rates for males and females are found in western industrialized countries led by blacks in the United States, and the lowest incidence rates recorded are in Hungary, Nigeria and India (9). See Figs. 1 and 2. An exception to the low risk generally found in non-westernized societies is the high incidence reported for males in several Polynesian groups, including the Maoris of New Zealand and native Hawaiians. The female Maoris and native Hawaiians, however, have incidence rates in the intermediate range.

The ranking of countries in order of incidence rates is similar for males and females, but the magnitude is different. The range of rates for males is from 15.8 per 100,000 in native Hawaiians to 1.5 per 100,000 in Hungary. For females the range is lower and less broad with a rate of 9.4 per 100,000 for blacks in Alameda, California to a rate of 1.7 per 100,000 in Ibadan, Nigeria. Populations at higher risk have a higher male/female ratio.

While there is a ten-fold difference in the international range of incidence rates, the range is not nearly as broad as it is for many other cancers such as cancer of the stomach or lung. This finding may be an indication that non-environmental factors also play an important role in cancer of the pancreas.

Time trends

International mortality trends reviewed by Aoki and Ogawa (3) are similar to the

Rate per 100,000 population

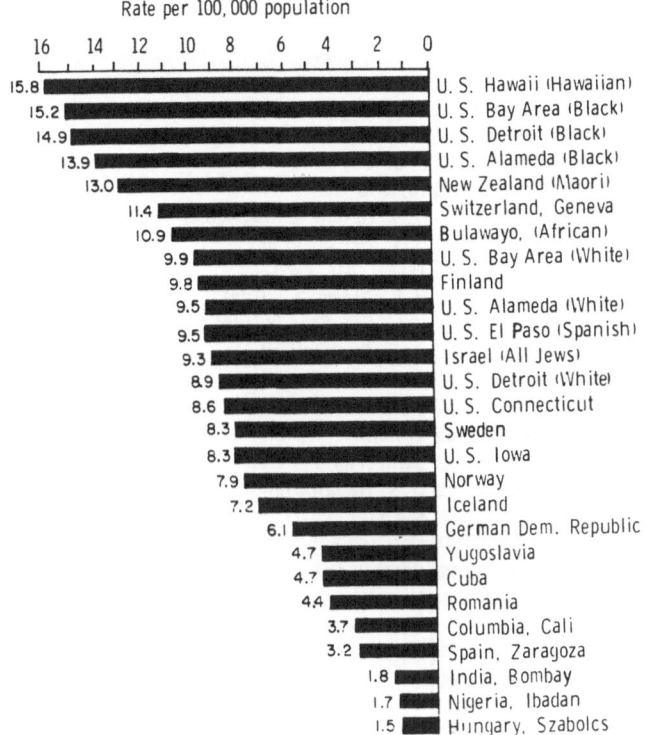

Source: Waterhouse J., Muir C., Correa P., Powell J.: Cancer incidence in
five continents, Vol III. IARC Scientific Publications No 15, Lyon, France, 1976.

Figure 1. Selected age-standardized incidence rates for malignant neoplasms of the pancreas for males by country of residence.

trends in incidence rates. As they point out, valid comparisons of mortality rates for pancreatic cancer between different countries are difficult because of differences in health care systems and diagnostic criteria resulting in both over-diagnosis and under-diagnosis. Differences in treatment and stage at diagnosis unfortunately at this time have only a minimal effect on prognosis.

The report by Aoki and Ogawa documents an increase in pancreatic cancer from 1950 to 1972 based on age-adjusted death rates. The increase in mortality rates over time has occurred for both sexes in all countries with available data in Africa, America, Asia, Europe, and Oceania; however, the rise in rates is more dramatic in countries with the lowest rates in 1950. Rates have begun to level off in North America where the rise in rates began several decades prior to 1950. The increase in death rates has occurred in all age groups forty-five years and above.

Mortality trends over time may be a function of changes other than real increases or decreases in mortality. Improvement in the quality of diagnosis can

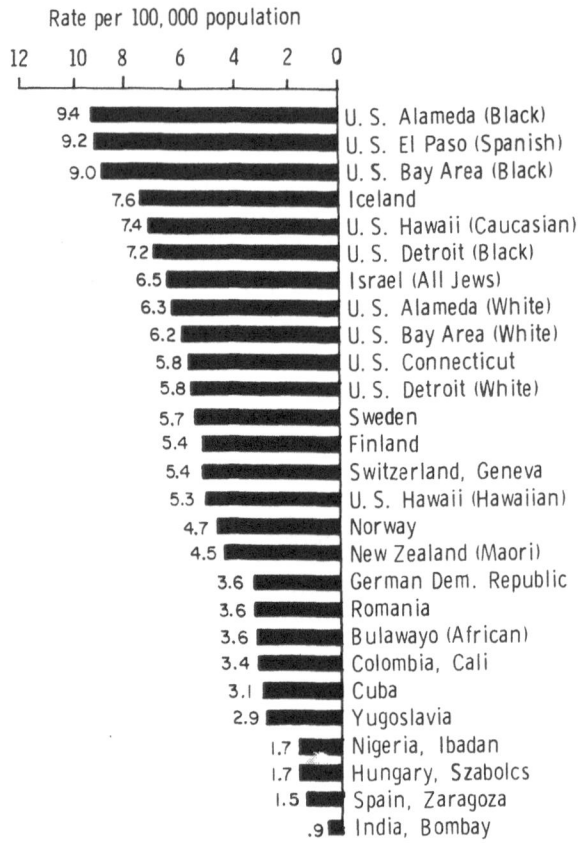

Rate per 100,000 population

9.4	U. S. Alameda (Black)
9.2	U. S. El Paso (Spanish)
9.0	U. S. Bay Area (Black)
7.6	Iceland
7.4	U. S. Hawaii (Caucasian)
7.2	U. S. Detroit (Black)
6.5	Israel (All Jews)
6.3	U. S. Alameda (White)
6.2	U. S. Bay Area (White)
5.8	U. S. Connecticut
5.8	U. S. Detroit (White)
5.7	Sweden
5.4	Finland
5.4	Switzerland, Geneva
5.3	U. S. Hawaii (Hawaiian)
4.7	Norway
4.5	New Zealand (Maori)
3.6	German Dem. Republic
3.6	Romania
3.6	Bulawayo (African)
3.4	Colombia, Cali
3.1	Cuba
2.9	Yugoslavia
1.7	Nigeria, Ibadan
1.7	Hungary, Szabolcs
1.5	Spain, Zaragoza
.9	India, Bombay

Source : Waterhouse J., Muir C., Correa P., Powell J, : Cancer
incidence in five continents, Vol III. IARC Scientific Publications
No 15, Lyon, France, 1976.

Figure 2. Selected age-standardized incidence rates for malignant neoplasms of the pancreas for females by country of residence.

yield an increase in the number of accurately diagnosed cases without a change in the true number. While Levin and Connelly (11) show that the increasing death rates for pancreatic carcinoma are in great part a reflection of improved accuracy in death certification, there appears to be a real rise in incidence which cannot be accounted for by improved diagnostic accuracy, an aging population, ICD changes or increasing histologic confirmation of cases. Krain (12) analyzed statistics from twenty-five countries and concluded that the rise could not be attributed to those factors.

Demographic factors

Age and sex

Silverberg (13) has estimated that 24,000 new cases of primary pancreatic cancer will occur in the United States in 1980. This number will account for 3% of all new cancer cases for males and females. He estimates that 5% of all male and female cancer deaths in the US in 1980 will be attributed to pancreatic cancer. Mortality data from other countries presented by Segi et al. (10) reflect a similar proportion of cancer deaths attributed to primary pancreatic cancer as a percentage of cancer of all sites with a range of 3–6%.

Age-specific death rates increase with age and this relationship is remarkably consistent for both sexes throughout the world (2). For most countries the mortality rate distribution reached the highest level in the oldest age group, 75 years and older. See Figs. 3 and 4. Cook et al. (14) analyzed the age distribution

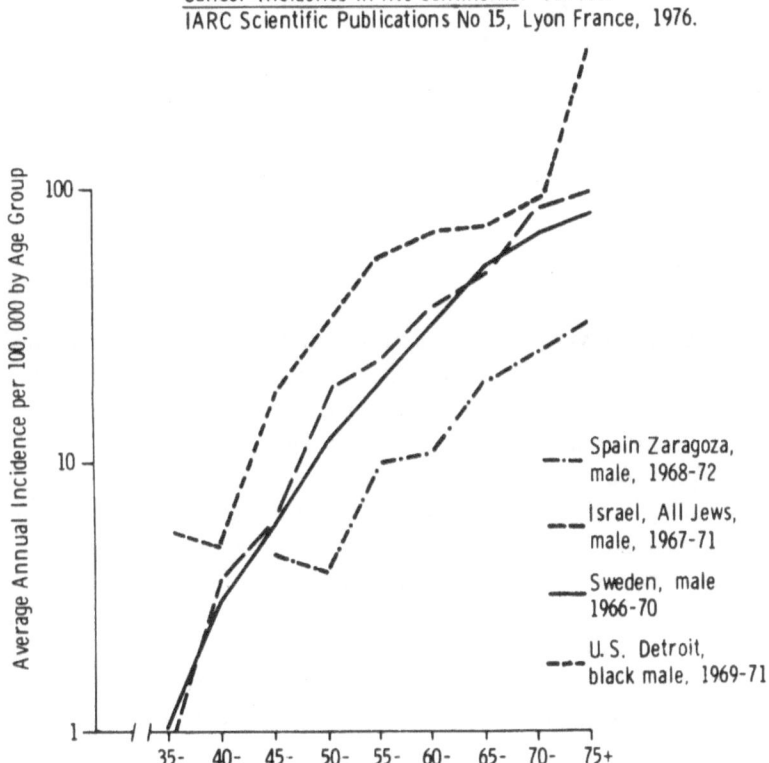

Source : Waterhouse J, Muir C, Correa P, Powell J :
Cancer incidence in five continents. Vol III.
IARC Scientific Publications No 15, Lyon France, 1976.

Figure 3. Selected age-specific incidence rates for malignant neoplasms of the pancreas for males by country of residence.

248

Source : Waterhouse J, Muir C, Correa P, Powell J :
Cancer incidence in five continents. Vol III.
IARC Scientific Publications No 15, Lyon, France, 1976.

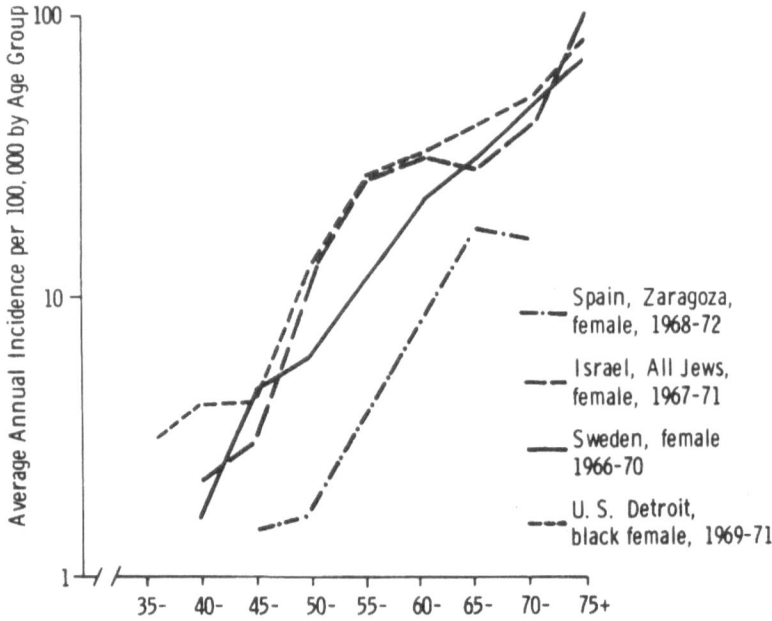

Figure 4. Selected age-specific incidence rates for malignant neoplasms of the pancreas for females by country of residence.

of cancer by site for various countries throughout the world plotting the logarithm of five-year age-specific incidence rates against age. The slopes of the lines were tested to determine whether they differed significantly from one population to another. For carcinoma of the pancreas the slopes were found to be invariant over all populations for both sexes.

The mean age at diagnosis for pancreatic cancer patients is greater for women than men, with an average age of approximately 67 years for females and 63 for males (15). Cases below 40 years of age are uncommon in both sexes.

The sex ratio has been variously reported to be between 1.5:1 and 2:1 in the United States (15, 16). In a recent report Berg and Connelly (17) found it to be 1.7:1, quite similar to the world-wide median ratio of 1.6:1. As Aoki and Ogawa (3) point out, although the male excess has been consistent over time and nations, the sex ratio is smaller than that found for most cancers. It has not yet been determined whether this male excess is a reflection of biological differences in susceptibility or differences in exposure to etiologic agents.

Race, religion and migration

Incidence data show the age-adjusted rates for blacks of both sexes in the United States to be among the highest in the world (9) (Figs. 1 and 2). One of the lowest reported incidence rates is in Ibadan, Nigeria, which calls into question any genetic/racial association for blacks and emphasizes environmental factors. Again comparability of the data between the two countries must be considered.

As mentioned previously, the high rates among Polynesian males of Hawaii and New Zealand are noteworthy and have been interpreted by some as an indication of a genetic factor.

In Israel, Jews have incidence rates three times higher than non-Jews (9). Israeli Jews born in Europe or America have incidence rates four-fold higher than Israeli Jews born in Asia or Africa. Similarly, within the United States Jews have a greater risk than non-Jews (18).

A recent study compared cancer incidence rates for the Mormon and non-Mormon populations of Utah. While Mormons had a lower incidence of all cancers associated with cigarette smoking ($p < .00001$), pancreatic cancer rates were low for both Mormons and non-Mormons compared to the Third National Cancer Survey (19).

Migrant studies have historically provided clues as to the relative importance of environmental and endogenous factors. Both Smith (20) and Haenszel and Kurihara (21) found that in contrast with patterns normally found, Japanese migrants to the United States (Issei) have mortality rates higher than the low rates found in Japan and higher than the rates of the native white population of the United States. The rates than subside in offspring (Nisei) to a level intermediate between rates in Japan and the US. Recently McMichael et al. (22) examined patterns of gastrointestinal cancer in migrants from Europe to Australia and found this unusual pattern of pancreatic cancer mortality among migrants to exist for this group of immigrants as well. They found that migrants from seven different European countries all experienced mortality rates higher than those in each respective country of origin and higher than the rate for native Australians. They postulate that major dietary changes in the years immediately following migration may alter the exocrine activity of the pancreas such that the probability of carcinogenesis is increased. This hypothesis of increased risk due to dietary changes rather than the diet itself is consistent with the finding that rates subside in offspring who presumably do not undergo major dietary changes.

Socio-economic status (SES)

Reports of studies which have examined socio-economic class and its relationship to cancer of the pancreas have produced conflicting results. The Second National Cancer Survey (23) found greater pancreatic cancer risk among persons in the lowest socio-economic class. A large study in Connecticut (15) found no apparent association between socio-economic status and pancreatic cancer incidence rates. An interview study from the Third National Cancer Survey (24) found college attendance as one indicator of socio-economic status to have a positive association with pancreatic cancer in males. Unlike some gastrointestinal cancers such as cancer of the stomach, any association of socio-economic status with pancreatic cancer is likely weak and may be confounded by differences in diagnosis and treatment according to social class.

Because social class reflects not only differences in life-style, but occupational differences as well, the investigation of specific factors which are associated with social class such as diet, alcohol consumption by both type and amount, and specific job categories and exposures should provide more enlightening results.

Intracountry variation for the United States

Geographic variation within the United States, as illustrated by maps depicting mortality rates for pancreatic cancer at a county level, is not striking (25). In general the maps reflect higher rates in urban areas. It should be noted, however, that they are based on mortality rates over a 20-year period, 1950–1969, urban–rural differences in certification cannot be discounted. The only unusual cluster can be seen in white male residents of 24 south Louisiana parishes (counties). Currently a case-control study is being conducted in this region to examine specific residential and occupational exposures which may contribute to the high rates in this area.

Recently Wellington et al (26) published a series of cancer mortality models analyzing state patterns of cancer mortality. Multiple regression models were derived by linear least squares methodology and the stability of the coefficient estimates tested by ridge regression techniques for each mortality pattern. The dependent variables were the death rates by site for white males and white females for each of the continental 48 states and the District of Columbia. The independent variables included population distribution variables, climate variables, air contamination variables, radiation variables, income variables, consumption variables, and ethnic variables. The models for both male and female mortality from cancer of the pancreas fail to explain as much as 50% of the variation in either sex; however, in all models for males the strongest positive effect is from the variable PRELEV a score based on precipitation and elevation. A wet climate at a low elevation, similar to that found in south Louisiana, was associated with high pancreatic mortality.

Predisposing conditions

No premalignant lesion of the pancreas has been clearly defined as yet; however, two possible precursor lesions have been described. Cubilla and Fitzpatrick (27) compared the pancreas duct epithelium of 195 patients with pancreas carcinoma to duct epithelium in a control group of 100 pancreata from autopsies of patients with nonpancreatic cancer. They found atypical duct hyperplasia in 14% of the pancreatic cancer cases and carcinoma in situ in 19% of the cases while no hyperplasia or carcinoma in situ was found in the control group Longnecker et al. (28) examined the pancreas of 108 autopsied persons for lesions of the ductal and acinar cells. Ductal epithelial abnormalities were more common than dysplastic acinar cell nodules which were present in 44% of the persons. The incidence of nodules was higher among patients with a history of heavy cigarette smoking and/or alcohol abuse than among nonsmokers and/or abstainers and may reflect exposure to potential pancreatic carcinogens.

Some attention has been given to two diseases which also affect the pancreas, diabetes mellitus and chronic pancreatitis, in order to determine whether either is associated with primary carcinoma of the pancreas.

Diabetes mellitus

Overall cancer mortality in diabetics is low. The incidence of all cancer in diabetic patients compared to nondiabetic patients is less than one half. Pancreatic carcinoma, however, as a proportion of all cancers in diabetics is three times greater than in nondiabetics indicating an association between cancer of the pancreas and diabetes (29, 30).

While the genetic mechanisms, if any, are not known, the association of diabetes and pancreatic cancer has been well established. The nature of the relationship is not understood; however, several studies (31, 32, 33) have reported diabetes mellitus in pancreatic cancer patients at a rate of 13 to 14%. These reported prevalence rates were based on case series alone without companion control groups. Bell (29) found that when cases of diabetes diagnosed after or concurrent with the onset of symptoms of the cancere were excluded, the incidence of diabetes in pancreatic cancer cases did not differ significantly from the age-specific rates in the general necropsy population. Bell's study illustrates the difficulties associated with time of onset of diabetes mellitus in relation to diagnosis of the carcinoma. Similarly, when diabetics diagnosed just prior to diagnosis of pancreatic cancer were excluded from a recent study, no increased risk was found for males; however, a markedly elevated risk remained for females (15).

At the population level, rates of pancreatic cancer are correlated with rates of

252

diabetes world-wide, most notably the high rates of each disease in Maoris and Hawaiians (9, 34) and in the United States at the county level positively corelated with diabetes in females, but not in males (35).

Pancreatitis

No association has been found for chronic pancreatitis as a predisposing condition for pancreatic carcinoma. Most reports in the literature are based on clinical observations of a single case, and it is felt that in cases of individuals with both conditions, the pancreatitis is the result of pathologic changes due to the carcinoma rather than predisposition toward the development of cancer (36, 37, 7, 15).

Tobacco

Cigarette smoking has been clearly established as one of the important risk factors for pancreatic cancers. The elevated risk for pancreatic cancer among smokers has been found in both retrospective and prospective studies and further a dose-response relationship has been demonstrated (18, 24, 12, 38). Hammond additionally found no sex differential among nonsmokers, while overall rates for pancreas cancer indicate a small, but consistent, sex differential (38). Use of tobacco products other than cigarettes such as pipe tobacco, snuff and chewing tobacco has not been associated with increased risk and so it is likely that one or more components of inhaled cigarette smoke act to increase risk (24). Several nitrosamines have been shown to be carcinogenic in animal models and, as a component of cigarette smoke, nitrosamines may be among those components which act on the pancreas carcinogenically (39). Wynder (40) suggests several possible mechanisms of pancreatic carcinogenesis by tobacco smoke: the absorbed carcinogens may reach the pancreas through the blood stream; inactive carcinogen precursors are activated by the liver, excreted into bile, and are refluxed from the bile duct to the pancreatic duct; and finally, smoking may elevate blood lipids which in turn increase risk of pancreatic cancer. Wynder bases this last potential mechanism on the positive interpopulation correlation found between high fat diets and pancreatic cancer. At this time the mechanism of action has not been proven, but the fact of increased risk among cigarette smokers is not questioned.

Alcohol

An association has been reported based on a retrospective study of chronic alcoholism and pancreatic carcinoma (41). In the analysis of state patterns of cancer mortality by Wellington et al. (26) using multiple regression models, wine consumption per capita had a strong positive correlation in both the male and female adults. Hakulinen et al. (42) studying Finnish alcoholics found a moderate excess of pancreas cancer, 2.2 cases expected versus 4 observed. While this finding was not statistically significant because of the small numbers, it was in a positive direction. Most recent studies, however, call into question any alcohol consumption association which persists after controlling for tobacco use. Monson and Lyon (43) found no association in their study of proportional mortality among alcoholics and this finding is consistent with the results of Wynder et al. (18) and Williams and Horm (24). The conflicting results of these studies may be due in part to failure to control for tobacco usage since this known risk factor for pancreas cancer is so highly correlated with alcohol consumption.

Occupation

Carcinoma of the pancreas has been linked to several occupational groups, but more studies are needed to identify specific high risk exposures.

While Blot et al. (35) found no correlation between county mortality rates and chemical or primary metal manufacturing plants, other mortality studies reviewed by Wynder et al. (18) have reported an association between both the chemical industry and the metal industry and pancreatic carcinoma. Mancuso and El-Attar (44) found a greatly increased mortality rate for a cohort of white males ages 25–64 who were employed in a chemical plant manufacturing β-naphthylamine and benzidine in 1938 and 1939 and were followed for over 25 years. They found a mortality rate of 39 per 100,000 for the cohort in contrast to a rate of 7.5 for white male residents of Ohio, ages 25–64. In a study of occupational mortality in England and Wales, there was a higher than expected rate of mortality due to cancer of the pancreas observed among employees of coke and gas plants (45).

Li et al. (46) found a significantly greater than expected number of deaths attributed to pancreatic cancer among members of the American Chemical Society who died between 1948 and 1967. The total number of deaths due to pancreatic cancer was 36 out of 3,637 deaths studied.

Lin and Kessler (47) found that males with pancreatic cancer were more often employed in the dry cleaning business or in occupations involving close exposure to gasoline than controls, increasing risk up to five-fold, and risk increased with increasing duration of exposure.

In a recent investigation of the high pancreatic cancer mortality rates among white males in south Louisiana, a two-fold increase in risk was found for workers in the oil refining and paper manufacturing industries (48). This case-control study was a preliminary one in which 876 pairs of death certificates were examined and all information was obtained from the certificate. These industries and others will be examined in greater detail using information obtained by interview in an on-going case-control study of lifestyle, diet, residence, occupation, and the association of each to pancreatic cancer.

In 1977 Mancuso, Stewart and Kneale (49) published an analysis of the mortality experience of 24,939 male workers at the Hanford Works, Richland, Washington, employed between 1943 and 1971 and followed through 1972. The Hanford Works is one of the largest atomic plants in the United States, and most of the individuals employed there are in some way concerned with the manufacture of radioactive substances. The analysis was based primarily on a case-control comparison of mean cumulative radiation in cancer vs non-cancer deaths and a proportionate mortality comparison of Hanford deaths with general US mortality patterns. Both methods of analysis were consistent in indicating excess deaths from cancer of the pancreas among workers exposed to radiation. In a subsequent review of this report, Hutchinson et al. (50) reanalyzed the data adjusting for age and calendar year of death. While the number of cancer sites for which a radiation dose relationship could be suggested was greatly reduced, the relationship persisted for cancer of the pancreas. As Anderson (51) suggests in his critique of the original report, a thorough investigation of the work histories of these cases is called for. The increased incidence of pancreatic cancer among these workers which has been attributed in some way to radiation exposure might be a result of other occupational exposures common to these men since radiation exposure in humans has not been shown to single out pancreas cancer (52, 53).

Diet

The study of the role of diet as a factor associated with mortality from pancreatic cancer has been limited primarily to correlation studies.

Lea (54) was one of the first to report a significant positive correlation between pancreatic cancer mortality and per capita consumption of fats and oils. This correlation has also been reported by Maruchi (55) and Zaldivar et al. (56) both of whom found a significant positive correlation between average amount of oils and fats consumed and pancreatic mortality in 19 countries. This correlation needs to be examined in greater detail using data on individual consumption by cases and controls.

Lin and Kessler (47) recently reported one such case-control study in which diet histories were analyzed. They found that habitual consumption of de-caffeinated coffee was significantly greater among pancreatic cases than controls.

MacMahon et al. (57) reported a strong association between coffee consumption and pancreatic cancer for both males and females. For the sexes combined, there was a significant dose-response relation ($p \sim 0.001$). However, in this case-control study, patients with gastroenterologic conditions were overrepresented in the control group in relation to the general hospital population, and this particular group of patients may have had decreased coffee consumption. This situation could have biased the results causing an overestimation of risk. Further studies are needed to confirm the association and to determine whether the association is causal.

While information on individual consumption is certainly a necessary step in establishing the link, if any, between diet and cancer of the pancreas, the present methodology for obtaining dietary histories needs to be refined to obtain more reliable data.

Animal models

Investigation of pancreatic carcinogenesis in the recent past has been limited by the paucity of animal models. Spontaneous carcinomas are rare in the exocrine pancreas of common experimental animals. During the decade of the 1970s, however, several animal models were reported which have contributed to our knowledge of chemical induction of pancreatic carcinogenesis and which may provide leads for future epidemiologic investigations.

Pour et al. (58) first demonstrated the selectivity of response by the Syrian hamster pancreas to the neoplastic effect of a simple dose of N-nitrosobis (2-onopropyl)amine.

Longnecker and co-workers (59, 60, 61) have developed a model of pancreatic cancer in the rat with the induction of atypical acinar cell nodules, adenomas and adenocarcinomas by azaserine (O-diazoacetyl-L-serine). Other animal models of pancreatic carcinogenesis include induction by N-methyl-N-nitrosourea in strain 13 guinea pigs (62, 63) by 4-(hydroxyamino)quinoline 1-oxide in rats (64, 65) and by 2,2'-dihydroxydi-N-propylnitrosamine in Syrian golden hamsters (66).

Shinozuka et al. (67) have further explored the azaserine model to investigate the effect of dietary modification. They found that a diet devoid of choline reduces the induction of precancerous lesions of the pancreas of rats and suggest that the role of nutrition and dietary factors should be investigated in greater detail.

256

Summary

Pancreatic cancer has had a steadily increasing impact on most populations throughout the world as incidence of this cancer has risen. Epidemiologic discoveries have not kept pace with the growing need to understand this disease. Recent developments, however, are encouraging and the coming years will hopefully prove more fruitful than the past.

The decade of the 1970s witnessed development of new and better techniques for diagnosis of cancer of the pancreas which should lead to more accurate diagnosis with a larger proportion of histologically confirmed cases. This accuracy should extend to distinctions between true primary lesions of the pancreas and lesions of adjoining sites, such as the ampulla of Vater, which in the past have been included in case series but which may have a distinct epidemiology.

The role of nutrition and the interaction of the various components of diet need to be examined in detail in light of correlations with fat and oil consumption at the population level and in view of the animal models developed. In several of these models pancreatic cancers are induced by various nitrosamines, a class of compounds known to be carcinogenic in many animal species and believed to be associated with other gastrointestinal cancers. Diet may play a greater role in the etiology of pancreatic cancer than has been uncovered to date.

The other area which warrants further exploration is occupational exposure to chemicals. While death certificate analyses serve as a useful source for preliminary investigations, accurate data on extent and duration of exposures is essential if meaningful associations are to be demonstrated.

References

1. Young JF Jr, Asire AJ, Pollack ES (eds): SEER Program. Cancer Incidence and Mortality in the United States 1973–1976. Bethesda: US Dept HEW, 1978.
2. Fraumeni JF Jr: Cancers of the pancreas and biliary tract: epidemiological considerations. Cancer Res 35:3437–3446, 1975.
3. Aoki K, Ogawa H: 1. Cancer of the pancreas, international mortality trends. World Health Stat Rep 31(1):2–27, 1978.
4. Hirayama T, Waterhouse JAH, Fraumeni JF Jr (eds): Cancer Risks by Site. UICC Technical Report Series Vol 41. Geneva, 1980, pp 78–83.
5. Gudjonsson B, Livstone EM, Spiro HM: Cancer of the pancreas: diagnostic accuracy and survival statistics. Cancer 42:2494–2506, 1978.
6. Engel LW, Strauchen JA, Chiazze L, Heid M: Accuracy of death certification in an autopsied population with specific attention to malignant neoplasms and vascular diseases. Am J Epidemiol 111:99–112, 1980.
7. Malagelada JR: Pancreatic cancer: an overview of epidemiology, clinical presentation, and diagnosis. Mayo Clin Proc 54:459–467, 1979.
8. Cubilla AL, Fitzgerald PJ: Cancer of the pancreas (nonendocrine): a suggested morphologic classification. Seminars in Oncol 6(3):285–297, 1979.

9. Waterhouse J, Muir C, Correa P, Powell J (eds): Cancer incidence in five continents, Vol III, IARC Scientific Publication No 15. Lyon, France, 1976.
10. Segi M, Kurihara M (eds): Cancer mortality for selected sites in 24 countries. No 6 (1966–1967). Japan Cancer Society, 1972.
11. Levin DL, Connelly RR: Cancer of the pancreas: available epidemiologic information and its implications. Cancer 31:1231–1236, 1973.
12. Krain LS: The rising incidence of carcinoma of the pancreas. J Surg Oncol 2:115–124, 1970.
13. Silverberg E: Cancer statistics, 1980. CA 27:23–38, 1980.
14. Cook PJ, Doll R, Fellingham SA: A mathematical model for the age distribution of cancer in man. Intl J Cancer 4:93–112, 1969.
15. Moldow RE, Connelly RR: Epidemiology of pancreatic cancer in Connecticut. Gastroenterol 55:677–686, 1968.
16. Go VL, Dimagno EP: The pancreas: pancreatic exocrine adenocarcinoma. Br J Hosp Med 18(6):567–576, 1977.
17. Berg JW, Connelly RR: Updating the epidemiologic data on pancreatic cancer. Semin Oncol 6(3):275–283, 1979.
18. Wynder EL, Mabuchi K, Maruchi N, Fortner JG: Epidemiology of cancer of the pancreas. J Natl Cancer Inst 50:645–667, 1973.
19. Lyon JL, Klauber MR, Gardner JM, Smart CR: Cancer incidence in Mormons and non-Mormons in Utah. N Engl J Med 294:129–133, 1976.
20. Smith RL: Recorded and expected mortality among Japanese of the United States and Hawaii with special reference to cancer. J Natl Cancer Inst 17:459–473, 1956.
21. Haenszel W, Kurihara M: Studies of Japanese migrants. I. Mortality from cancer and other diseases among Japanese in the United States. J Natl Cancer Inst 40:43–68, 1968.
22. McMichael AJ, McCall MJ, Hartshorne JM, Woodings TL: Patterns of gastrointestinal cancer in European migrants to Australia: the role of dietary change. Int J Cancer 25(4):431–437, 1980.
23. Dorn HG, Cutler SJ: Morbidity from cancer in the United States, Parts I and II. Public Health Monograph 56, US Dept HEW. Washington DC: US Govt Printing Office, 1959.
24. Williams RR, Horm JW: Association of cancer sites with tobacco and alcohol consumption and socioeconomic status of patients: interview study from the Third National Cancer Survey. J Natl Cancer Inst 58:525–547, 1977.
25. Mason TJ, McKay FW, Hoover R, et al.: Atlas of cancer mortality in U.S. counties: 1950–69. Department of Health, Education and Welfare, Publ No (NIH) 75–780. Washington DC: US Govt Printing Office, 1975.
26. Wellington DG, Macdonald EJ, Wolf PF: Cancer mortality: environmental and ethnic factors. New York, NY: Academic Press, 1979.
27. Cubilla AL, Fitzgerald AJ: Morphological patterns of primary nonendocrine human pancreas carcinoma. Cancer Res 35:2234–2248, 1975.
28. Longnecker DS, Shinozuka H, Dekkar A: Focal acinar cell dysplasia in human pancreas. Cancer 45(3):534–540, 1980.
29. Bell ET: Carcinoma of the pancreas. I. A clinical and pathological study of 609 necropsied cases. II. The relation of carcinoma of the pancreas to diabetes mellitus. Am J Path 33:499–523, 1957.
30. Kessler II: Cancer mortality among diabetics. J Natl Cancer Inst 44:673–685, 1970.
31. Lazar HP, Spellberg MA, Fox RE: The increasing incidence of carcinoma of the pancreas. A clinical and statistical study. Am J Gastroenterol 34:235–247, 1960.
32. Marble A: Diabetes and cancer. New Engl J Med 211:339–349, 1934.
33. Miller TR, Fuller LM: Radiation therapy of carcinoma of the pancreas. Am J Roentgenol 80:787–792, 1958.
34. Prior IAM, Davidson F: The epidemiology of diabetes in Polynesians and Europeans in New Zealand and the Pacific. New Zealand Med J 65:375–383, 1966.
35. Blot WJ, Fraumeni JF Jr, Stone PF: Geographic correlations of pancreas cancer in the United States. Cancer 42:373–380, 1978.
36. Robinson A, Scott J, Rosenfeld DD: The occurrence of carcinoma of the pancreas in chronic pancreatitis. Radiology 94:289–290, 1970.
37. Howard JM, Jordan GL Jr: Cancer of the pancreas. Curr Probl Cancer 2(3):15–52, 1977.

258

38. Hammond EC: Smoking in relation to the death rates of one million men and women. Natl Cancer Inst Monograph 19:167–204, 1966.
39. Hoffman D, Wynder E: Chemical composition and tumorgenicity of tobacco smoke. In: Schmeltz I (ed): The Chemistry of Tobacco and Tobacco Smoke, pp 123–147. New York: Plenum Press, 1972.
40. Wynder EL: An epidemiological evaluation of the causes of cancer of the pancreas. Cancer Res 35:2228–2233, 1975.
41. Burch GE, Ansari A: Chronic alcoholism and carcinoma of the pancreas: a correlative hypothesis. Arch Intern Med 122:273–275, 1968.
42. Hakulinen T, Lehtimäki L, Lehtonen M, Teppo L: Cancer morbidity among two male cohorts with increased alcohol consumption in Finland. J Natl Cancer Inst 52(6):1711–1714, 1974.
43. Monson RR, Lyon JL: Proportional mortality among alcoholics. Cancer 36:1077–1079, 1975.
44. Mancuso TF, El-Attar AA: Cohort study of workers exposed to betanaphthylamine and benzidine. JOM 9:277–285, 1967.
45. The Registrar General's Decennial Supplement, England and Wales, 1951: Occupational Mortality Part II, Vol I. Commentary. London: Her Majesty's Stationery Office, 1958.
46. Li FP, Fraumeni JF, Mantel N, Miller RW: Cancer mortality among chemists. J Natl Cancer Inst 43:1159–1164, 1969.
47. Lin RS, Kessler II: A multifactorial model for pancreatic cancer in man. JAMA 245(2):147–152, 1981.
48. Pickle LW, Gottlieb MS: Pancreatic cancer mortality in Louisiana. AJPH 70(3):256–259, 1980.
49. Mancuso TF, Stewart A, Kneale G: Radiation exposures of Hanford workers dying from cancer and other causes. Health Phys 33:369–385, 1977.
50. Hutchinson GB, MacMahon B, Jablon S, Land CE: Review of report by Mancuso, Stewart and Kneale of radiation exposure of Hanford workers. Health Phys 37(2):207–220, 1979.
51. Anderson TW: Radiation exposures of Hanford workers: a critique of the Mancuso, Stewart and Kneale report. Health Phys 35(6):743–750, 1978.
52. International Commission on Radiological Protection: Radiosensitivity and Spatial Distribution of Dose. Oxford: Pergamon Press, 1969.
53. Angevine DM, Jablon S: Late radiation effects of neoplasia and other diseases in Japan. Ann NY Acad Sci 114:873–831, 1964.
54. Lea AJ: Neoplasms and environmental factors. Ann Roy Coll Surg Engl 41:432–437, 1967.
55. Maruchi N: An epidemiologic study on pancreatic cancer with special reference to U.S.-Japanese comparison. Jap J Cancer Clin 19:73–81, 1973.
56. Zalvidar R, Wetterstrand WH, Ghai GL: Relative frequency of mammary, colonic, rectal and pancreatic cancer in a large autopsy series. Statistical associations between mortality rates from these cancers: dietary fat intake as a common aetiological variable. Zentralbl Bakterial B 169(5–6):474–481, 1979.
57. MacMahon B, Yen S, Trichopoulos D, Warren K, Nardi G: Coffee and cancer of the pancreas. New Engl J Med 304(11):630–633, 1981.
58. Pour PM, Salmasi SZ, Runge RG: Selective induction of pancreatic ductular tumors by single doses of N-nitrosobis(2-oxopropyl)amine in Syrian golden hamsters. Cancer Letters 4:317–323, 1978.
59. Longnecker DS, Curphey TJ: Adenocarcinoma of the pancreas in azaserine-treated rats. Cancer Res 35:2249–2258, 1975.
60. Longnecker DS, Crawford BG: Hyperplastic nodules and adenomas of exocrine pancreas in azaserine-treated rats. J Natl Cancer Inst 53:573–577, 1974.
61. Longnecker DS, French J, Hyde E, et al.: Effect of age on nodule induction by azaserine and DNA synthesis in rat pancreas. J Natl Cancer Inst 58:1769–1775, 1977.
62. Reddy JK, Svoboda DJ, Rao MS: Susceptibility of an inbred strain of guinea pigs to the induction of pancreatic adenocarcinoma by N-methyl-N-nitrosourea. J Natl Cancer Inst 52:991–993, 1974.
63. Reddy JK, Rao MS: Pancreatic adenocarcinoma in inbred guinea pigs induced by N-methyl-N-nitrosourea. Cancer Res 35:2769–2279, 1975.
64. Hayashi Y, Furukawa H, Hasegawa T: Pancreatic tumors in rats induced by 4-nitroquinolene-

1-oxide derivatives. In: Hakahara W, Takayama S, Sugimura T, et al. (eds): Topics in chemical carcinogenesis. Baltimore: Univ Park Press, 1972, pp 53–72.

65. Konishi Y, Denda A, Inui S, et al.: Pancreatic carcinoma induced by 4-hyroxyaminoquinoline-1-oxide after partial pancreatectomy and splenectomy in rats. Ganu 67:919–920, 1976.

66. Pour P, Krüger FW, Althoff J, et al.: A new approach for induction of pancreatic neoplasms. Cancer Res 35:2259–268, 1975.

67. Shinozuka H, Katyal S, Lombardi B: Azaserine carcinogenesis: organ susceptibility change in rats fed a diet devoid of choline. Int J Cancer 22(1):36–39, 1978.

Subject Index